D0897507

Community Based Participatory Research for Health

Community Based Participatory Research for Health

Edited by
Meredith Minkler
Nina Wallerstein

Foreword by
Budd Hall

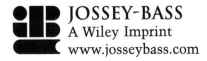

JOSSEY-BASS
A Wiley Imprint
www.josseybass.com

RA
440.85
.C65
2003

Copyright © 2003 by John Wiley & Sons, Inc. All rights reserved.

Published by Jossey-Bass
A Wiley Imprint
989 Market Street, San Francisco, CA 94103-1741   www.josseybass.com

No part of this publication may be reproduced, stored in a retrieval system, or
transmitted in any form or by any means, electronic, mechanical, photocopying,
recording, scanning, or otherwise, except as permitted under Section 107 or 108 of
the 1976 United States Copyright Act, without either the prior written permission
of the Publisher, or authorization through payment of the appropriate per-copy
fee to the Copyright Clearance Center, Inc., 222 Rosewood Drive, Danvers, MA
01923, 978-750-8400, fax 978-750-4470, or on the web at www.copyright.com.
Requests to the Publisher for permission should be addressed to the Permissions
Department, John Wiley & Sons, Inc., 111 River Street, Hoboken, NJ 07030
(201) 748-6011, fax (201) 748-6008, e-mail: permcoordinator@wiley.com.

Limit of Liability/Disclaimer of Warranty: While the publisher and author have
used their best efforts in preparing this book, they make no representations or
warranties with respect to the accuracy or completeness of the contents of this
book and specifically disclaim any implied warranties of merchantability or
fitness for a particular purpose. No warranty may be created or extended by sales
representatives or written sales materials. The advice and strategies contained
herein may not be suitable for your situation. You should consult with a
professional where appropriate. Neither the publisher nor author shall be liable
for any loss of profit or any other commercial damages, including but not limited
to special, incidental, consequential, or other damages.

Jossey-Bass books and products are available through most bookstores. To
contact Jossey-Bass directly call our Customer Care Department within the U.S.
at 800-956-7739, outside the U.S. at 317-572-3986 or fax 317-572-4002.

Jossey-Bass also publishes its books in a variety of electronic formats. Some
content that appears in print may not be available in electronic books.

Library of Congress Cataloging-in-Publication Data
Community based participatory research for health/edited by Meredith
Minkler and Nina Wallerstein.
      p. cm.
Includes bibliographical references and index.
  ISBN 0-7879-6457-3 (alk. paper)
  1. Public health—Research—Citizen participation. 2. Public
health—Research—Methodology. 3. Community health services.
  [DNLM: 1. Consumer Participation—United States. 2. Health Services
Research—methods—United States. 3. Community Health Planning—United
States. W 84.3 C734 2003] I. Minkler, Meredith. II. Wallerstein, Nina, 1953-
  RA440.85 .C65 2003
    362.1'07'2—dc21   2002008544

FIRST EDITION

PB Printing   10 9 8 7 6 5 4

CONTENTS

TABLES, FIGURES, AND EXHIBITS

TABLES

FIGURES

EXHIBITS

FOREWORD

Don't mourn—organize
—Joe Hill, 1915

How is it that the most intimate sphere of our knowledge—the knowledge of our own culture, families, lives, and bodies—can have been colonized so fully by the portrayal by others: researchers, epidemiologists, medical sociologists, and even health promotion experts?

How is it that the people living in the lands of some of the largest store of richness in the forms of natural resources—the peoples of rural Appalachia, urban black and Latino America, Indian nations, and internationally, of the Brazilian Amazon, Africa, subtroptical regions—are among the poorest people in the world?

Community Based Participatory Research for Health, edited by Meredith Minkler and Nina Wallerstein, is a wonderful resource for anyone who wonders as I do about such questions. Meredith and Nina wonder about these questions and about much more. They and the colleagues who have joined them in this extremely useful compilation believe in the capacity of all women and men to create knowledge about their own lives. They know that the limited advances that have been made in dealing with HIV/AIDS would never have been possible without the early interventions of the gay, lesbian, transgendered, and transsexual movements into the world of science and medicine. The writers featured in this collection are among the most experienced and thoughtful persons that I know working in the broad fields of health promotion, health education, popular epidemiology, and community health.

This book is a unique collection of writing, ranging from basic explanations of the history and origins of community based participatory research through working in complex layers of race, gender, sexuality, and ability differences to influencing public health policy. The chapters are informative, practical, challenging, and wonderfully documented and referenced. The authors come, like the ideas for the work itself, from a global diaspora. They "dance," to use a metaphor from the book, their stories, their knowledge seeking, their celebrations, and their commitment to social justice. Some of the scholar-activists are known around the world; others may be appearing here for the first time. The result is a work that is both local and global in concept, interdisciplinary in execution, and dramatically current in focus.

Community based participatory research tells us as scholars and researchers that the ideas of poor women, indigenous peoples, workers in hotels, and the homeless in Michigan count. These ideas remind us as scholars and researchers to be more modest and more humble in how we label the world. Such ideas carry with them responsibilities for those of us in universities, community based organizations, and government research organizations. We must listen in new ways, learn to follow in new ways, develop a capacity for long-term engagement. We must learn that sometimes the best way to be of service in a social movement is to stay away or remain respectfully in the background.

We live in a world out of balance—a world dominated by a solitary and militant political superpower, which works for hegemonic acceptance of its own views of what constitutes security and happiness. This book is about something else—it is about critique, survival, relationships, and hope. Read this book, take part in the alternative global movements of the majority world, and support the struggles for justice and democracy in your own communities. The choices you make about the work you do and the life you lead are important and powerful. If you work in health and community, as you engage in the combined activities of research, education, and action, this book will strengthen you on your journey.

Budd L. Hall
Dean, Faculty of Education,
University of Victoria, Canada

ACKNOWLEDGMENTS

It is often said that if you want something done, ask someone who is already overcommitted. This book owes its existence to many such people who believed enough in this volume to carve out time they didn't have so that it might come to fruition. Our deepest gratitude therefore goes to our community, academic and professional coauthors who gave so generously of their time, insights, and experiences in crafting this book, a truly collaborative undertaking.

We owe a great debt to many other friends and colleagues who have left a profound mark on our own thinking, research, and community engagement through their scholarship, their commitment to working "with" rather than "on" communities, and their dedication to social justice and the elimination of health disparities. High on this list are our current and former colleagues and mentors at the University of California, Berkeley, and the University of New Mexico. Key among them at UC Berkeley are Robin Baker, Henrik Blum, Paul Chown, Fred Collignon, Troy Duster, Len Duhl, Andy Furco, Denise Herd, John Hurst, Joyce Lashof, Jack London, Pat Morgan, S. Leonard Syme, and Lawrence Wallack. At New Mexico, we thank Edward Bernstein, Lily Dow Velarde, Bonnie Duran, Jo Fairbanks, Clark Hansbarger, Deborah Helitzer, Marianna Kennedy, Lorraine Halinka Malcoe, Frances Varela, Howard Waitzkin, and William Wiese.

Many other colleagues in community health education and related fields have had an important influence on our thinking that is reflected in this undertaking. We thank especially in this regard Marco Akermann, Ben Amick,

Elsa Auerbach, Beth Baker, Deborah Barndt, David Buchanan, Maria Teresa Cerqueira, Camy Condon, Galen El-Askari, Eugenia Eng, Esme Fuller-Thomson, John Gaventa, Robert Goodman, Eda Gordon, Budd Hall, Amparo Herrera, Marcia Hills, Michele Kelley, Marshall Kreuter, Ron Labonté, Kay Lovelace, Kristine Maltrud, Chuck McKetney, Rosilda Mendes, Michelle Minnis, Pia Moriarty, Michel O'Neill, Rena Pasick, Michele Polacsek, Ann Robertson, Kathleen M. Roe, Lisbeth Schorr, Sheryl Walton, Merri Weinger, and Irene Yen. As distant mentors and teachers, Paulo Freire and Myles Horton have been ever present.

We have both been fortunate to have worked over the years with many outstanding students, and their insights, too, are reflected in this volume. Ultimately, we have gained immense wisdom from the community, health department, and Indian Health Service partners with whom we've been privileged to work and who have often been our most important teachers. These include, for Meredith, the community residents, staff, and volunteers of the former Tenderloin Senior Organizing Project, the Gray Panthers, the communities of grandmothers raising grandchildren and of people with disabilities, the Oakland-based Community Health Academy, and the Contra Costa County Health Department's Healthy Neighborhoods Project. Colleagues at PolicyLink, and particularly Mildred Thompson and Angela Glover Blackwell, have also been wonderful sources of education and inspiration on connecting local community-building efforts with regional and national public policy.

For Nina, such teachers and collaborators have included the staff, middle school, and high school students and faculty of the Adolescent Social Action Program; the New Mexico Healthier Communities Department of Health and community partners, in particular Patricia Erickson, Anita Laran, and Louisa Rogers; the Youth-Link and Women to Women projects; the community advisory groups from Jemez and Sandia Pueblo's participatory research project on tribal community capacities; and the dedicated professionals and community members engaged with the Pan American Health Organization's Healthy Municipalities participatory evaluation efforts in Latin America.

Finally, a special debt of gratitude is extended to the W. K. Kellogg Foundation's Community Health Scholars Program, whose network of community, academic, and other partners has made major contributions to the inception and maturation of this project.

Edited books of necessity involve an inordinate amount of paperwork and organization, and we owe many thanks to Lisa Butler, Donna Odierna, Chris Roebuck, and Jennifer Sarché for their help in making the pieces come together. Particular thanks go to Laura Spautz, whose unfailing assistance, sense of humor, and commitment to the cause were invaluable in helping this project come to fruition.

We have had the great good fortune of working with Andy Pasternack, a superb senior editor who believed in this project from its inception and provided unparalleled support and assistance throughout. Amy Scott, Erin Jow, and other staff at Jossey-Bass, as well as production editor Susan Geraghty and copyeditor Bruce Emmer, deserve our deep thanks for their timely help and flexibility. Thanks as well go to the anonymous reviewers of our book proposal for their contributions to the final product.

The energy for a project like this one truly comes from within, and we are both blessed with families that provide much of that inner strength. We are deeply grateful to our parents and grandparents, who always believed in us and instilled in their children a desire to make a difference. Our husbands and children help keep even the most daunting of tasks in perspective. Although they may not always succeed in pulling us away from the computer, especially late at night and at the crack of dawn, their love and support have provided the backdrop to make this book possible.

THE EDITORS

MEREDITH MINKLER, DrPH, MPH, is a professor of health and social behavior at the School of Public Health, University of California, Berkeley, and assistant to the vice chancellor on national and community service. She has more than twenty-five years' experience working with underserved communities on community-identified issues through community building, community organizing, and community based participatory research. Her current research interests include local efforts to foster CBPR among diverse groups and national studies on the health and social circumstances of grandparents raising grandchildren and their implications for policy. Minkler is coauthor or editor of six books and more than one hundred articles and book chapters in community based participatory research, community health education, health promotion, community building, and gerontology, including *Forgotten Caregivers: Grandmothers Raising Children of the Crack Cocaine Epidemic* (with Kathleen M. Roe), *Critical Perspectives on Aging* (with Carroll L. Estes), and *Community Organizing and Community Building for Health.*

NINA WALLERSTEIN, DrPH, MPH, is a professor in the Department of Family and Community Medicine at the University of New Mexico and founder and director of the university's MPH program. She earned her master's and doctoral degrees in community health education at the School of Public Health, University of California, Berkeley. For more than twenty-five years, she has been involved in empowerment and popular education, participatory research, and community-building efforts with youth, women, and tribes. She is the coauthor of *Participatory Evaluation Workbook for Community Initiatives: New Mexico Healthier Communities*, three adult education books, and more than seventy-five articles and book chapters on participatory intervention research, adolescent health promotion, empowerment theory, and popular health education. She was senior editor of a two-volume special issue of *Health Education Quarterly* on community empowerment, participatory education, and health in 1994. Her current research interests focus on understanding and assessing the role of social capital and community capacity in tribal communities.

THE CONTRIBUTORS

ALEX J. ALLEN III, MSA, is director of the Butzel Family Center in Detroit, Michigan, a multipurpose service center housing over a dozen family-serving agencies and organizations. Allen leverages community resources and support in community health and related areas and partners on community well-being projects. He also frequently serves as a facilitator, bringing diverse groups together to promote collaborative partnerships that address community issues and maximize resources. He is a member of the National Advisory Committee of the W. K. Kellogg Foundation's Community Health Scholars Program (CHSP) headquartered at the University of Michigan, Ann Arbor.

CAROL A. ALLEN is the project coordinator for Healthy Homes, an asthma-related intervention project in Seattle, Washington. Formerly, she spent eleven years as director of the Central Area Senior Center. A native of California, Allen has been a Seattle resident for fifteen years and has represented community interests on a number of community based participatory research projects. Because of her strong ties to the community, she has been a valuable resource as a board member of Seattle Partners for Healthy Communities (SPHC) and as an employee of the Public Health Department of Seattle & King County.

MAGDALENA M. AVILA, DrPH, MPH, MSW, is an assistant professor of health education in the College of Education, University of New Mexico. She works with communities to identify and address public health problems and develop culturally relevant community-driven research in areas such as environmental health and social justice, substance abuse, migrant health, and children with special needs. Avila also has studied alcohol-related problems and their impact on Chicano and Mexican American families, as well as issues of environmental racism. She was the West Coast representative to the First People of Color Environmental Leadership Summit in Washington, D.C., and continues to be actively involved in public health education issues on the local, state, and national levels. She received her graduate training at the University of California, Berkeley, School of Public Health.

ARI BACHRACH, BA, is a research associate on the HOPE (Homebased Outcomes Program Evaluation) study at Continuum-Homebase, an HIV services agency in San Francisco. He was referral coordinator and a member of the Community Advisory Board for the Transgender Community Health Project. Bachrach received his bachelor's degree in community studies from the University of California, Santa Cruz.

QUINTON E. BAKER is a consultant in community health, leadership, and development residing in Hillsborough, North Carolina. He formerly served as executive director of the Center for the Advancement of Community Based Public Health in Durham and as a member of the National Advisory Board of the Community Health Scholars Program. His professional activities include working with communities, coalitions, community leaders, and community based organizations in their efforts to improve community health and well-being.

GEORG F. BAUER, MD, DrPH, MPH, is chair of the Department of Health and Intervention Research at the Institute of Social and Preventive Medicine of the University of Zurich, Switzerland. He holds an MD from the University of Tübingen, Germany. He obtained an MPH in community health education and a DrPH in community health sciences at the University of California, Berkeley, School of Public Health. Prior to his current position, Bauer worked with the Oakland Community Based Public Health Initiative and the Center for Family and Community Health at Berkeley.

ADAM B. BECKER, PHD, is an assistant professor in the Department of Community Health Sciences at Tulane University. His current projects include a participatory investigation with high school students to explore and address root causes of violence, a participatory evaluation emphasizing youth leadership development as an HIV prevention strategy among young African American men who have sex with men, and a grounded theory study of internal and external factors in the development of community based organizational capacity.

KLAUS BLUM, BA, is a retired computer programmer and formerly served as a consultant to organizations including the World Institute on Disability and an instructor with the Computer Training Center. He earned his bachelor's degree in business administration at San Francisco State University. He is a former member of the Albany (California) Water Commission and of the Albany–El Cerrito Access Disabled Society and served as a member of the Community Advisory Group of the Death with Dignity study.

WILLIAM R. BOWIE, MD, FRCPC, is a professor of medicine in the Division of Infectious Diseases at the University of British Columbia. He obtained his MD from the University of Manitoba in 1970, was a Medical Research Council of Canada Fellow in infectious diseases at the University of Washington with King K. Holmes, MD, PhD, from 1974 to 1977, and has been at UBC since 1977. He has been president of the Canadian Infectious Diseases Society and a member of numerous local, national, and international committees.

HILARY BRADBURY is an assistant professor in the Department of Organizational Behavior at the Weatherhead School of Management, Case Western Reserve University, in Cleveland, Ohio. Her research and teaching focus on sustainable organizational change and action research. Born in Ireland, Bradbury received her bachelor of arts degree from Trinity College in Dublin, her master's degree in religion and literature from the University of Chicago, and her doctorate in organization studies from Boston College. She has published in Academy of Management journals and is coeditor (with Peter Reason) of the *Handbook of Action Research.*

LELAND BROWN, MPH, is founder and director of the Global Bridges Group, a minority-owned business whose mission is to enhance collaboration, promote dialogue, and increase understanding between diverse communities, cultures, and institutions. He currently works with the California Center for Public Dispute Resolution on issues including land use, air quality, and environmental concerns. Brown teaches a graduate course on conflict resolution at John F. Kennedy University. He received his degree in health policy and planning from the School of Public Health, University of California, Berkeley.

MARIANNE P. BROWN, MPH, is director of the University of California at Los Angeles (UCLA) Labor Occupational Safety and Health program and has twenty-five years of experience in workplace health and safety training. Brown is principal investigator on grants from the National Institute of Environmental Health Sciences, the National Institute of Occupational Safety and Health, and the California Endowment to provide training for workers and has published articles in occupational health and safety journals on a variety of topics. She is also a lecturer in the UCLA School of Public Health and a member of the advisory boards of various state, county, and local occupational health programs.

VALORIE LYNN CARSON, M.S., is a doctoral student in developmental and child psychology in the Human Development and Family Life Department at the University of Kansas and a graduate research associate of the KU Work Group on Health Promotion and Community Development. Her work involves evaluating and providing technical assistance to community health initiatives. Carson's research interests are focused primarily on how to reduce risk factors for chronic disease through community based efforts, especially among racial and ethnic minority populations.

STELLA S. CHAO, MSW, is executive director for the International District Housing Alliance, a community based nonprofit in Seattle focusing on services for Asian and Pacific Islander communities. She left twelve years in medical research at the University of Washington to work for three years in community development at a health project in Kenya. Afterward she was a community fellow at the Massachusetts Institute of Technology's Department of Urban Studies and Planning and completed her master's in social work at the University of Washington. These experiences are the foundation for her interest in community and cultural competency in health and research.

VIVIAN CHÁVEZ, DrPH, MPH, is an assistant professor in the Department of Health Education at San Francisco State University. She is author of numerous multimedia presentations that integrate health, community, and culture, including *A Bridge Between Communities*, a thirty-two-minute documentary video on Detroit's Urban Research Center community-academic partnership. Her interests range from teaching and research on nonviolent social action to developing youth leadership among college students and "digital storytelling," the process of using video as a tool for evaluation.

ANN CHEATHAM is a PhD candidate in epidemiology and received her master's degree in community health education at the University of California, Berkeley. She is research coordinator at Asians and Pacific Islanders for Reproductive Health (APIRH). Cheatham has worked on social change issues using popular education, participatory action research, epidemiology, and organizing with Southeast Asian girls in California, with farmworkers and day laborers in Ohio and California, and with other communities in California.

KRISTEN CLEMENTS-NOLLE, PhD, MPH, is assistant research professor at the University of Nevada, Reno Department of Health Ecology. She received her master's of public health degree in behavioral sciences and her doctorate in epidemiology from the University of California, Berkeley. She formerly worked as an epidemiologist for the San Francisco Department of Public Health, conducting HIV research with hard-to-reach populations. Clements-Nolle emphasizes participatory research approaches when conducting epidemiologic and evaluation studies.

MARK DANIEL, PhD, is an assistant professor in the School of Public Health, University of North Carolina at Chapel Hill, jointly appointed in the Department of Health Behavior and Health Education and the Department of Epidemiology. He specializes in health promotion and disease prevention, chronic disease epidemiology, and participatory research and is currently studying the impact of social context on health.

BONNIE DURAN, DrPH, is an assistant professor in the School of Family and Community Medicine at University of New Mexico. She has worked in the field of public health education practice and research with Native Americans and other communities of color for twenty-seven years. Duran has planned, directed, and evaluated mental health, HIV/AIDS, substance abuse, and maternal child health prevention, intervention, and treatment projects in urban Indian and reservation communities. Currently she is principal investigator on an NIMH grant investigating mental health among Native American women, co-PI on projects investigating social capital measures, and evaluator of a Health Resources and Services Administration AIDS treatment demonstration project.

PAMELA FADEM, MPH, a longtime community organizer and social justice activist, received her master's degree in health and social behavior from the University of California, Berkeley, School of Public Health in 2002, where she also served as project director for the Death with Dignity study and managing editor for the *Wellness Guide.* She works as an educator, trainer, and advocate in the disability and prisoners' rights communities.

STEPHANIE ANN FARQUHAR, PhD, is an assistant professor in the School of Community Health at Portland State University in Oregon and was formerly a postdoctoral fellow in the Community Health Scholars Program at the University of North Carolina, Chapel Hill. Her work addresses the structural and social determinants of health, and she is currently working with community organizations and local agencies to examine environmental justice issues in Oregon.

STEPHEN B. FAWCETT, PhD, is Kansas Health Foundation Professor of Community Leadership and University Distinguished Professor of Human Development at the University of Kansas. He is also director of the KU Work Group on Health Promotion and Community Development. A former VISTA volunteer, he worked as a community organizer in public housing and low-income neighborhoods. In his work, he uses behavioral science and community development methods to help understand and improve health and social concerns of importance to communities.

VINCENT T. FRANCISCO, PhD, is associate director of the KU Work Group on Health Promotion and Community Development; assistant research professor with the Schieffelbusch Institute for Life Span Studies; courtesy assistant professor with the Department of Human Development and Family Life, all at the University of Kansas; and adjunct assistant professor with the Department of Preventive Medicine at the University of Kansas Medical School. Francisco is primarily interested in research in community development and work toward the empowerment of marginalized groups. He is also concerned with the provision of technical support for the development of coalitions and the evaluation of community based intervention programs focusing on adolescent development for reducing the risks of teen substance abuse, assaultive violence, teen parenthood, and cardiovascular and other chronic diseases.

C. JAMES FRANKISH, PhD, is associate director of the Institute of Health Promotion Research and associate professor in graduate studies and the Department of Health Care and Epidemiology at the University of British Columbia. A registered clinical psychologist, he has held a BCHRF Research Scholar Award and awards from the Healthway Foundation in Western Australia and the Association of Pacific Rim Universities. He has published papers on community participation, mental health and population health, health impact assessment, and participatory research and is developing a research training program on community based health promotion.

NICHOLAS FREUDENBERG, DrPH, is Distinguished Professor and director of the Program in Urban Public Health at Hunter College, City University of New York. For twenty-five years he has worked with communities in New York City on a variety of public health and policy issues including asthma, environmental hazards, HIV, and substance abuse.

SANDRO GALEA, MD, MPH, is a medical epidemiologist at the Center for Urban Epidemiologic Studies at the New York Academy of Medicine. He is interested in the social determinants of health and in particular in the role social determinants play in the health of marginalized populations. Galea is also the epidemiologist for the Harlem Urban Research Center in New York City.

M. ANNE GEORGE, PhD, is assistant professor in the Department of Pediatrics at the University of British Columbia (UBC) and works at the Centre for Community Child Health Research at the Children's and Women's Health Centre in Vancouver. She completed graduate studies at UBC's Institute of Health Promotion Research after many years as an independent research consultant. Her research focuses on population based studies, particularly in the areas of prevention and health promotion, and prenatal alcohol and tobacco exposure.

CHARLES GOETCHIUS is staff director at the Hotel and Restaurant Employees Union (HERE) Local 2 in San Francisco. He has worked for four different international unions over the past two decades and has organized with room cleaners for most of that period. Goetchius has worked with a number of community groups, involving them in organizing and often using health as an organizing issue.

LAWRENCE W. GREEN directs the Office of Extramural Prevention Research at the Centers for Disease Control and Prevention (CDC) in Atlanta, guiding federal research toward more participatory approaches. He has served as director of the federal Office of Health Information and Health Promotion, in the CDC's World Health Organization Collaborating Center on Global Tobacco Control, and as acting director of the Office on Smoking and Health. In his previous professorships at the University of British Columbia, the University of Texas, and Johns Hopkins University, he helped develop participatory approaches in health education, prevention, and community interventions for health promotion and risk reduction.

J. RICARDO GUZMAN, MSW, MPH, is the executive director of Community Health and Social Services Center, Inc. (CHASS). CHASS is a Section 330 Federally Qualified Health Center (FQHC) with two locations in the city of Detroit. Guzman is a long-standing community leader and activist in southwest Detroit. He has played a leadership role in increasing access to culturally appropriate, high-quality, affordable, comprehensive health services to community members who historically have not had access to such services. Guzman also is an influential member of the National Association of Community Health Centers and in 1994 received the National Hispanic Health Leadership Award.

TREVOR HANCOCK is an independent public health physician and health promotion consultant and one of the creators of the Healthy Cities/Communities concept. He has worked as an adviser to the World Health Organization and was founding chair of the Ontario Healthy Communities Coalition. As an associate medical officer of health for the city of Toronto, he helped develop community health worker programs and has long been an advocate of community development and participatory research in public health.

CAROL P. HERBERT is professor of family medicine and dean of the Faculty of Medicine and Dentistry at the University of Western Ontario. She was chair of the Department of Family Practice from 1988 to 1998 and was a founder and executive member of the Institute for Health Promotion Research at the University of British Columbia. She has conducted participatory research in aboriginal communities in British Columbia. Her current research interests are clinical health promotion, patient-physician communication, and physician behavior change.

YOLANDA R. HILL, MSW, received her bachelor's degree in social sciences from Tuskegee University in 1992 and her master of social work degree from Wayne

State University in 1998. She is community health coordinator at the Detroit Health Department and in that capacity directs the citywide Village Health Worker program. Hill is a member of the National Association of Social Workers, the National Association of Black Social Workers, and the American Public Health Association.

BARBARA A. ISRAEL, DrPH, MPH, is a professor in the Department of Health Behavior and Health Education at the University of Michigan School of Public Health and is the deputy editor of the journal *Health Education and Behavior.* She received her doctorate in public health from the University of North Carolina at Chapel Hill. Israel has published widely in the areas of community based participatory research, community empowerment, evaluation, stress and health, and social networks. She has extensive experience conducting community based participatory research in collaboration with partners in diverse ethnic communities.

AHOUA KONÉ, MPH, is a native of the Ivory Coast, an alumna of the University of Washington School of Public Health, and a second-year law student at Seattle University School of Law. She worked for several years as an epidemiologist with the Public Health Department of Seattle & King County and several community health organizations where she was involved in numerous local community health projects. In addition, she has worked as a public health consultant in the Ivory Coast, Mozambique, Burkina Faso, and Ghana.

NIKLAS KRAUSE, MD, PhD MPH, received his medical degree and a doctoral degree in orthopedic medicine from the University of Hamburg, Germany. He earned a master's degree in public health and a doctoral degree in epidemiology at the University of California at Berkeley. His research focus has been the epidemiology and prevention of work-related musculoskeletal diseases and disability. He is currently an assistant professor of medicine in the University of California at San Francisco's Division of Occupational and Environmental Medicine.

JAMES KRIEGER, MD, MPH, is chief of the Epidemiology, Planning, and Evaluation Unit at the Public Health Department of Seattle & King County and a clinical associate professor of medicine and health services at the University of Washington. He oversees public health community assessment activities, develops and evaluates community based asthma control activities, and directs Seattle Partners for Healthy Communities, a collaboration among community members, public health authorities, and the university that develops and evaluates interventions to promote health among low-income, diverse communities by addressing social determinants of health.

PAM TAU LEE is a labor and community services coordinator with the Labor Occupational Health Program (LOHP) at the University of California, Berkeley, School of Public Health. Her work focuses on labor-management training and facilitation, policy and environmental justice, and the coordination of participatory research projects. She is the author of two LOHP publications, and her articles have appeared in the *Journal of Public Health Policy* and elsewhere. Lee was the recipient of the APHA Lorin Kerr Award and a Bannerman Fellowship. She was formerly a union organizer and union staff director.

MURLISA LOCKETT, MA, received her bachelor's degree in family life education from Spring Arbor College in 1998 and her master's in adult education from Central Michigan University in 2000. She is assistant community health coordinator at the Detroit Health Department and project coordinator for the East Side Village Health Worker Partnership. Lockett is a member of the American Public Health Association.

LEROY MOORE is founder and director of Disability Advocates of Minorities (DAMO), the only organization for and by people of color with disabilities. In addition to his leadership in the disability movement, Moore is a poet and artist who conducts frequent tours and presentations of his work around the United States.

MICHEL O'NEILL is a professor of community health and health promotion in the Faculty of Nursing of Laval University in Quebec City, Quebec, Canada. He has been involved in community and public health for three decades as a community health worker, professor, researcher, consultant, and activist. He is coeditor of three books, has published extensively in the scientific and professional literature, and has presented papers at scientific and professional meetings all over the world.

ANN-GEL S. PALERMO, MPH, is a research associate for the Institute for Medicare Practice of Mount Sinai School of Medicine. She is responsible for research and analysis on issues related to benefit and coverage issues for low-income Medicare beneficiaries and on health financing issues affecting the Medicare program and the health care system in general. Palermo is chairperson of the Community Action Board of the Harlem Urban Research Center.

EDITH A. PARKER, DrPH, MPH, is an associate professor in the Department of Health Behavior and Health Education at the University of Michigan School of Public Health. She received her master's and doctoral degrees at the University of North Carolina School of Public Health. Her work focuses on the development, implementation, and evaluation of community based participatory public health interventions. She is currently involved with the Community Action Against Asthma project, the Eastside Village Health Worker Project, and the Detroit Community–Academic Urban Research Center, all located in Detroit, Michigan.

MARTHA PERRY, RN, is a private duty nurse in Washington State. She received her bachelor's degree in psychology from the University of California, Berkeley, and has a special interest in gerontology and work with older populations.

MARTINE PIERRE-LOUIS, MPH, manages interpreter and translator services for the University of Washington Medical Center in Seattle. She holds a master's in public health with a focus on international health. A Haitian Creole and French interpreter for more than a decade, she is a founding member and past board member for both the Society of Medical Interpreters and the National Council on Interpreting in Health Care. Pierre-Louis has been involved for years in community based public health efforts with a focus on access to health care and equity for refugees and immigrants.

PETER REASON is a professor of action research and practice at the University of Bath, England, and director of the Centre for Action Research in Professional Practice in the university's School of Management. His many publications include the edited volumes *Human Inquiry: A Sourcebook of New Paradigm Research* (with John Rowan), *Human Inquiry in Action,* and *Participation in Human Inquiry.* He and Hilary Bradbury recently coedited the *Handbook of Action Research* and will shortly be launching the new *Action Research Journal* with Sage Publications.

VALERIE A. RENAULT is a writer and coordinator for the Community Tool Box, a project of the KU Work Group on Health Promotion and Community Development at the University of Kansas. She previously taught English at the University of Kansas and has also been a professional editor, writer, and coordinator of public relations. She has a master of arts degree in English from the University of Southern California and a bachelor's degree in secondary education from the University of Kansas.

CASSANDRA RITAS, MPP, is a policy analyst with the Center on AIDS, Drugs, and Community Health at Hunter College, City University of New York. For the past decade she has worked with diverse New York City communities on issues ranging from HIV prevention to police oversight. She is personally committed to creating effective public policy through community involvement. Ritas is the chairperson of the Policy Work Group of the Harlem Urban Research Center's Community Action Board.

JUDITH ROGERS, OT, is an occupational therapist specializing in disabled women's issues and a parenting specialist with Through the Looking Glass in Berkeley, California. She is the author of *Mother-to-Be: A Guide to Pregnancy and Birth for Women with Disabilities* and was a key architect of the Breast Health Access for Women with Disabilities (BHAWD) project.

JERRY A. SCHULTZ, PhD, is associate director of the KU Work Group for Health Promotion and Community Development at the University of Kansas. He teaches courses on building healthy communities, directs research on urban community development, and develops content for the Community Tool Box. His research interests are participatory action research, building community capacity for change, evaluation, and the empowerment of at-risk community groups. He has written numerous articles and reports and consults with a variety of foundations, state agencies, and local community organizations on these topics.

AMY J. SCHULZ, PhD, MPH, is an assistant research scientist in the Department of Health Behavior and Health Education at the University of Michigan School of Public Health. Her current research focuses on social factors that contribute to health, with a particular focus on health disparities and urban communities. Her work emphasizes a community based participatory approach, linking research with community-level interventions to address social conditions linked to health. She received her doctorate in sociology in 1994 and her MPH in 1981, both from the University of Michigan.

SARENA D. SEIFER, MD, is executive director of Community-Campus Partnerships for Health and a research assistant professor in the Department of Health Services at the University of Washington School of Public Health and Community Medicine. She serves on the national advisory committees for the Community Health Scholars program and the CDC Bridges to Healthy Communities program. Her teaching and research interests include health-promoting partnerships between communities and higher educational institutions. Seifer has written numerous publications on service learning, the principles of partnership, the scholarship of engagement, and the civic role of higher education and was recognized for her work as a "Young Leader of the Academy" by the American Association of Higher Education.

EVELINE SHEN received her MPH in community health education at the University of California, Berkeley. She is currently the executive director of Asians and Pacific Islanders for Reproductive Health (APIRH), where she worked with staff and members to develop an innovative social change model integrating community organizing, popular education, participatory action research, and community building. Before coming to APIRH, she organized with communities to address issues related to housing and economic justice.

JANE SPRINGETT, PhD, is a professor of health promotion and public health at Liverpool John Moores University, England, where she is also director of the Institute for Health. She has a doctorate in urban geography and a long-standing research interest in healthy cities and communities. Her main research interests are joint work and organizational change, participatory evaluation, and action research in a variety of settings. She has considerable experience in curriculum development in health promotion, grounded in a theoretical understanding of the way people learn.

RANDY STOECKER is a professor of sociology at the University of Toledo. He has been doing community based research since the mid-1980s when a community activist made him agree to contribute something to the community in exchange for granting an interview. He works mostly with community organizing and development groups and with community Internet efforts, including managing the COMM-ORG Web site and listserv (http://comm-org.utoledo.edu). He also publishes regularly on community based research, community organizing and development, and community Internet.

MARIANNE SULLIVAN, MPH, is a researcher with the Public Health Department of Seattle & King County and Seattle Partners for Healthy Communities. Her research interests are in community based participatory approaches and intervening to address social determinants of health. Most recently she has been working on a social support intervention with refugee and immigrant survivors of domestic violence.

MAKANI N. THEMBA is executive director of the Praxis Project, a not-for-profit organization providing capacity-building assistance for media and policy advocacy for health justice. Themba has published numerous articles and case studies on media, public policy, and race. She is coauthor of *Media Advocacy and Public Health: Power for Prevention.* Her latest book is *Making Policy, Making Change.*

JULIANA VAN OLPHEN, PhD, MPH, is an assistant professor in the department of health education at San Francisco State University. She has extensive experience developing, implementing, and evaluating community-level interventions and formerly worked with the Harlem Urban Research Center on a policy-level intervention to reduce the harm caused by drug use. Her research interests include social inequalities in health, community capacity and social capital, and the impact of policy on health.

WILLIAM A. VEGA, DCrim, is a professor of psychiatry at the Robert Wood Johnson Medical School–University of Medicine and Dentistry of New Jersey, and the director of the Behavioral Research and Training Institute, University Behavioral Health Care. His research projects on health, mental health, and substance abuse in the United States and Mexico have resulted in several books, as well as articles in journals including the *New England Journal of Medicine* and *Archives of General Psychiatry*. Vega's specialties are comparative health research and immigrant social adaptation and mental health adjustment. He is the president of the National Latino Council on Tobacco and Alcohol Prevention, a founding member of the International Consortium of Psychiatric Epidemiology, and a member of the Institute of Medicine advisory group on the future of public health education.

CAROLINE C. WANG, DrPH, MPH, is an assistant professor in the Department of Health Behavior and Health Education at the University of Michigan's School of Public Health. She has directed and consulted on photovoice projects in rural China; Ann Arbor and Flint, Michigan; and the San Francisco Bay Area. She is coeditor of the book *Visual Voices: 100 Photographs of Village China by the Women of Yunnan Province* and editor of *Strength to Be: Community Visions and Voices*. Additional information can be found at http://www.photovoice.com.

ROCHELLE WILLS is an East Side Village Health Worker, massage therapist, doula, community organizer, and advocate for women and children. In addition, she is a certified phlebotomist and medical assistant. Wills works as a mentor specialist for women in community service and as a community liaison for the Butzel Family Center in Detroit.

STEVE WING, PhD, received his doctorate in epidemiology from the University of North Carolina, Chapel Hill, where he has been on the faculty since 1985. He teaches and conducts research in the area of occupational and environmental health. His research areas include health effects of ionizing radiation, environmental justice in North Carolina, health impacts of industrial animal agriculture, health of women slaughterhouse workers, and environmental health research ethics. He is a founding member of the North Carolina Environmental Justice Network.

Community Based Participatory Research for Health

PART ONE

INTRODUCTION TO COMMUNITY BASED PARTICIPATORY RESEARCH

CHAPTER ONE

Introduction to Community Based Participatory Research

Meredith Minkler
Nina Wallerstein

Many of the complex health and social problems that have accompanied us into the twenty-first century—problems such as HIV/AIDS, homelessness, environmental injustice, and violence—have proved ill suited to traditional "outside expert" approaches to research and the often disappointing community interventions they have helped spawn. Growing disillusionment with the pitfalls and drawbacks of such approaches have been accompanied by increasing community demands for truly collaborative research that addresses locally identified issues. Funders too have stepped up the call for research that is collaborative and community *based,* rather than merely community *placed,* dramatically increasing funding for such research over the past five years (Blackwell, Tamir, Thompson, & Minkler, in press; Chopyak & Levesque, 2001). Finally, the past decade has seen a rapid escalation in the demand for research aimed at eliminating health disparities and promoting community and broader social change (Bruce & Uranga McKane, 2000; George, Daniel, & Green, 1998–1999; Israel, Schulz, Parker, & Becker, 1998; U.S. Department of Health and Human Services, 2000). Together, these forces have helped focus increasing attention on alternative orientations to inquiry that stress community partnership and action for social change and reductions in health inequities as integral parts of the research enterprise.

In public health, social work, and related fields, *community based participatory research* (CBPR) is increasingly acknowledged as the term that may best capture this paradigm. Building on the work of Barbara Israel and her colleagues

(1998) and Lawrence W. Green and his colleagues (1995), the W. K. Kellogg Foundation's Community Health Scholars Program (2001) suggests that "community based participatory research in health is a collaborative approach to research that equitably involves all partners in the research process and recognizes the unique strengths that each brings. CBPR begins with a research topic of importance to the community with the aim of combining knowledge and action for social change to improve community health and eliminate health disparities."

This book is designed to excite students, practitioners, and scholars in public health, social work, community psychology, and related disciplines about the potentials of CBPR as a potent alternative to "outside expert"–driven research approaches to eliminating health disparities. We hope that both "old hands" at CBPR and newcomers to this paradigm will find themselves challenged by the theoretical frameworks offered, the ethical and methodological dilemmas explored, and the theory-driven case studies used throughout to illuminate this approach.

Together with many related action research and participatory research traditions, CBPR "turns on its head" the more traditional applied research paradigm in which the outside researcher largely determines the questions asked, the tools employed, the interventions developed, and the kinds of results and outcomes documented and valued (Gaventa, 1993). For in the words of Budd Hall (1992, p. 22), "participatory research fundamentally is about who has the right to speak, to analyze and to act."

Although often and erroneously referred to as a research method, CBPR and other participatory approaches are not methods at all but *orientations to research.* As Andrea Cornwall and Rachel Jewkes (1995, p. 1667) have pointed out, what is distinctive about such approaches "is not the methods but methodological contexts of their application"; what is new is "the attitudes of researchers, which in turn determine how, by and for whom research is conceptualized and conducted" and "the corresponding location of power at every stage of the research process."

Central to CBPR and related approaches, for example, are their shared commitments to consciously blurring the lines between the "researcher" and the "researched" (Gaventa, 1981, p. 19) and "the strengthening of people's awareness of their own capabilities" as researchers and agents of change (Hagey, 1997, p.1). As Lawrence W. Green and Shawna Mercer (2001, pp. 1926–1927) suggest, CBPR thus effected a change in the balance of power such that "research subjects became more than research objects. They gave more than informed consent; they gave their knowledge and experience to the formulation of research questions" and to many other aspects of the research process. In epidemiology, often described as the "basic science" of public health, movement toward a more participatory and action-oriented approach has also increasingly been advocated (Schwab & Syme, 1997; Wing, 1998). Michael Schwab and

S. Leonard Syme (1997, p. 2050) are among those pointing up the potential of such an approach, which embraces "the experience and partnership of those we are normally content simply to measure." Environmental epidemiologist Steve Wing (1998, p. 250) similarly notes that if we are to transform society to eliminate health disparities and promote social justice, "a more democratic and ecological approach to scientific study is necessary," one in which "education between scientists and the public must take place in both directions." It is with this *orientation to research,* with its heavy accent on issues of trust, power, dialogue, community capacity building, and collaborative inquiry toward the goal of social change to improve community health and well-being and eliminate health disparities, that this book is concerned.

WHAT'S IN A NAME?

Our choice to use the term *community based participatory research* in the title of this volume was not made lightly. Numerous variations of the term exist, key among them *participatory action research, participatory research, action research, mutual inquiry,* and *feminist participatory research* (see Chapter Two), and their adherents frequently engage in lively debate over which term and corresponding approach best captures the principles and ideological commitments espoused. Such debates have an important role to play, and we are grateful to Peter Reason and Hilary Bradbury whose recent *Handbook of Action Research* (2001) provides a comfortable and welcoming place for such conversations among "family members" to take place. For the purposes of this book, however, we argue that while these different approaches do vary in goals and change theories, they increasingly share a set of core principles and values (Wallerstein, 1999). As summarized by Barbara Israel and her colleagues (1998), the fundamental characteristics of such research are the following (see also Chapter Three):

- It is participatory.
- It is cooperative, engaging community members and researchers in a joint process in which both contribute equally.
- It is a co-learning process.
- It involves systems development and local community capacity building.
- It is an empowering process through which participants can increase control over their lives.
- It achieves a balance between research and action.

With scholars of color and feminist participatory researchers, such as Patricia Hill Collins (2000), bell hooks (1984, 1989), Patricia Maguire (1987, 2001),

M. Brinton Lykes (1997), and Ella Edmonson Bell (2001), we would underscore that CBPR principles should also include prominent attention to the centrality of issues of gender, race, class, and culture, as these interlock and influence every aspect of the research enterprise. Especially in the health field in the United States, where the four-decade Tuskegee study of untreated syphilis in black males remains an indelible reminder of the human costs of unethical "scientific" research and its legacy of distrust in communities of color (Thomas & Crouse Quinn, 2001), issues of race and racism must not be overlooked. With colleagues at the Loka Institute, we share the belief that the racial issues, which too often hover at the periphery of discussions about participatory research, need to be explicitly engaged and brought to center stage (Blair, Cahill, Chopyak, & Cordes, 2000).

The contributors to this volume each bring their own values and assumptions to CBPR, and their different but complementary views provide alternative perspectives on the processes of and forces shaping respectful engagement with communities in combining research with education and action for change. CBPR is used in this book as an overarching name for this orientation to research and praxis, which stresses the principles and values just outlined here and explored in greater detail in subsequent chapters.

Although there has been a greater convergence of principles and values, the majority of participatory and action-oriented approaches to research stem from two separate traditions that fall on opposite ends of a continuum and are discussed in depth in Chapter Two. At one end of the continuum is *action research* in the tradition of Kurt Lewin (1946) and his followers (such as Greenwood & Levin, 1998), for whom the accent is on involving people affected by a problem in practical problem solving through a cyclical process of fact finding, action, and evaluation. As illustrated in Chapter Ten, the term *action research* has more recently been used to reflect an overarching family of "participatory inquiry and practice" approaches (Reason & Bradbury, 2001) including, for example, participatory action research and feminist participatory research (see also Stringer, 1999, and Stringer & Genat, in press). In the United States, however, its most common usage continues to reflect the narrower and often more conservative approaches used in industrial psychology and related applied fields. In this tradition, there is some, but not necessarily extensive, involvement of affected individuals and typically little commitment to broader social change objectives (Brown & Tandon, 1983).

At the other end of this continuum of alternative paradigm research are *participatory research* (PR), *collaborative action research,* and *participatory action research* (PAR) traditions, which have their roots in popular education and related work in the 1970s with and by oppressed peoples in Africa, Asia, and Latin America (Tandon, 1996). Such approaches often developed as a direct counter to the often "colonizing" nature of the research to which they were subjected (Fals-Borda, 1987; Freire, 1982; Swantz, Ndedya, & Masaiganah, 2001). As Budd

Hall (1999, p. 35) has suggested, "participatory research was very largely theorized and disseminated from a social movement or civil society base. Among the original premises were the importance of 'breaking' what we referred to as the 'monopoly over knowledge production' by universities. This was not in the least a form of anti-intellectualism, but was recognition that the academic mode of production was, and remains, in some fundamental way, linked to different sets of interests and power relations than women and men in various social movement settings or located in more autonomous community-based, nongovernmental structures."

As discussed in Chapter Two, feminist participatory research approaches, postmodern, and postcolonial research are among the important variants of and contributors to PR and PAR in this tradition. The accent placed by feminist scholars on the importance of dealing in voices—of having women speak of their own experience and reality in part as a means of understanding power relations—has thus heavily shaped the work of many participatory researchers (including Cornwall & Jewkes, 1995; Lykes, 1997; and Maguire, 1987, 2001). Feminists and postcolonial research traditions have similarly reinforced structural transformation as the ultimate goal of an integrated activity combining "social investigation, educational work, and action" (Hall, 1981, p. 7).

As the contributors to this volume well demonstrate, community based participatory research can and does occur at many places along the continuum from Lewinian action research through participatory research. Yet to really live up to the definition and espoused principles of CBPR for health—principles accenting true partnerships between outside researchers and communities and achieving a balance between research and action toward the goal of ending health disparities—it is the emancipatory end of the continuum that ideally should serve as a "gold standard" for our practice. Particularly for readers in fields like public health and social welfare, with their roots in concerns for social justice, CBPR in this latter sense provides an important goal for which to strive in our collaborative work with communities.

CBPR AND THE FIGHT TO ELIMINATE HEALTH DISPARITIES

In February 1998, President Bill Clinton announced a bold new public health initiative, aimed at eliminating racial and ethnic disparities in health by the year 2010 (U.S. Department of Health and Human Services, 1998). Although calls for the *reduction* of health disparities based on race, ethnicity, and social class have long been a part of national health efforts in the United States, making the actual *ending* of such disparities one of just two national goals of Healthy People 2010 represented an ambitious step forward (U.S. Department of Health and Human Services, 2000).

The need for such a national commitment is underscored in a large body of research documenting profound differences in health and life chances along racial and ethnic lines and along socioeconomic lines (see Amick, Levine, Tarlov, & Walsh, 1995; House & Williams, 2000; Kaplan, Pamuk, Lynch, Cohen, & Balfour, 1996; Krieger, Rowley, Herman, Avery, & Phillips, 1993; Marmot & Wilkinson, 1999). Data from the U.S. Department of Health and Human Services (1998, 2000), for example, showed that Hispanic infants in the United States were continuing to die at twice the rate of white babies, with black babies dying at almost two and a half times the white rate. It documented that diabetes among Hispanics was twice that of the population as a whole, with some Native American tribes having a rate three to five times higher. Finally, these national data revealed that Vietnamese American women were getting cervical cancer at five times the rate or other women and that Asian American men had three to five times the likelihood of other men of getting liver cancer, often related to viral hepatitis.

Recently released data from the National Center for Health Statistics (2002) did reveal an improvement between 1998 and 2000 in the health of racial and ethnic minorities on ten of the seventeen health indicators set by Healthy People 2000. Yet these achievements didn't begin to measure up to those of the nation as a whole, for which significant improvement on sixteen of the seventeen indicators was observed. Troubling trends were also found among particular groups. American Indians and Alaska Natives, for example, saw no improvement in death rates from lung and breast cancer, stroke, or suicide, and improvements in the nation's child poverty rates failed to include Asians and Pacific Islanders. African Americans continued to have the nation's highest cancer death rates, while the overall death rates among the top four cancers increased significantly among Asians and Pacific Islanders (http://www.cdc.gov/mmwr).

The continued racial/ethnic disparities in health have been associated with sociostructural factors such as poverty, racism, minimal public infrastructure, and lack of employment opportunities (Collins & Williams, 1999; Krieger et al., 1993). Particularly disturbing in this regard were the results of the Institute of Medicine's meta-analysis of one hundred studies of racial disparities in health care among people who have insurance (Smedley, Stith, & Nelson, 2002). The study revealed that people of color were significantly less likely than whites to be given appropriate medications for heart disease, undergo needed bypass surgery, or receive kidney dialysis or transplants. Minorities were also significantly less likely to receive the most sophisticated treatments for HIV infections—treatments that could delay the onset of AIDS. Lack of access to care has long been believed to be a major contributor to the race gap in health care access. But the IOM study suggested that subtle racial prejudices and differences in the quality of health plans available to different groups may well play a more important role than was previously recognized in the differential quality of care received.

Environmental factors, such as outdoor air quality and the prevalence of mite allergens, mold, and the like in low-income homes, also, of course, play a role in health disparities. Such factors exacerbate asthma and other conditions in communities of color, which are disproportionately located in poor neighborhoods (Amick et al., 1995; Krieger, 2000). Finally, low social capital, operationalized within epidemiology primarily in terms of horizontal relationships among community members along dimensions such as trust, reciprocity, and civic engagement (Kawachi, Kennedy, Lochner, & Prothrow-Stith, 1997), has been shown to bear a relationship to poverty and health disparities (James, Schulz, & van Olphen, 2001).

Such realities have underscored the importance of creative new approaches that can address health disparities. The creation of the new National Center on Minority Health and Health Disparities within the National Institutes of Health represents an important milestone in this regard, as does the national Campaign to Eliminate Racial and Ethnic Disparities in Health, launched as a partnership between the American Public Health Association and the U.S. Department of Health and Human Services. Large philanthropic organizations, too, have added their weight and their financial support, with the Robert Wood Johnson Foundation, the W. K. Kellogg Foundation, the Rockefeller Foundation, and the California Endowment among those to call for and support ambitious new efforts to eliminate health disparities. Yet as the chapters in this volume underscore, far more needs to be done.

PURPOSES AND GOALS OF THIS BOOK

The reader who has picked up this book hoping to find an extensive scholarly discussion of various critical theories and other perspectives that have helped shape participatory research approaches is likely to be disappointed. For although we review in some detail the historical and conceptual roots of these traditions (see Chapter Two) and emphasize throughout the book themes, such as power relationships and authentic dialogue, that are illuminated through the work of Habermas (1972, 1988), Freire (1970, 1973, 1982), Collins (2000), Maguire (2001), and others, the central purpose of this volume is much more practice-focused. Our goal is to provide a highly accessible text that will stimulate practitioners, students, and academics in health and related fields as they engage—intellectually and, ideally, in practice with community partners—in this alternative approach to collaborative inquiry for action to eliminate health disparities.

As will be discussed in Chapter Two, much of the cutting-edge work in health occurring at the emancipatory end of the AR—PR/PAR continuum today continues to take place in Africa, India, Latin America, and other parts of the Third

World. We therefore are indebted to Korrie De Koning and Marion Martin (1996) for their book, *Participatory Research in Health,* which documents much of this recent activity. Several other excellent volumes have captured the range and depth of participatory research in Third World countries, Australia, and other regions and illuminated earlier participatory research efforts in the United States and Canada (Hall, Gillette, & Tandon, 1982; Park, Brydon-Miller, Hall, & Jackson, 1993; Reason & Bradbury; 2001; Stringer, 1999; Stringer & Genat, in press).

In the United States, this earlier work has included a detailed examination of some of the landmark participatory research conducted by and with the High-lander Research and Education Center in New Market, Tennessee (Lewis, 2001), including early participatory research in the environmental and occupational health in Appalachia more than two decades ago (Merrifield, 1993). The participatory research and organizing of Yellow Creek Concerned Citizens (YCCC) in Middlesboro, Kentucky, stands as one of the classic examples of popular epidemiology in action. In that well-documented case study (Couto, 1987; Merrifield, 1993), residents initiated their own research, tracking the health effects of water pollution in their community, and led effective organizing, political campaigning, and litigation to clean up the creek. But as Ansley and Gaventa (1997, p. 50) point out, they also "were able to remain in charge of their campaign even after legal and technical experts became involved."

The existence of the rich body of literature highlighted here, combined with the importance of paying careful attention to the particular geopolitical and sociohistorical contexts within which participatory research takes place, has led us to focus this book on contemporary CBPR efforts in the United States. We frequently draw on the wisdom of leading PR and PAR scholars and practitioners in the Third World, the United Kingdom, Canada, and elsewhere and believe that many of the skills and conceptual, ethical, and practical issues raised will have relevance beyond U.S. borders. Our central concern, however, is with helping students, scholars, and community members and allies in the United States become more inspired by, comfortable with, and proficient in applying CBPR approaches in their community based work.

Within this context, the contributors to this volume explore such issues as cross-cultural and power dynamics in the CBPR process, with special attention to issues of race and racism; methods and techniques for helping communities identify their strengths and the problems or concerns they wish to explore; collaborative data collection and the involvement of community members in data analysis; issues of rigor and validity in CBPR; special considerations in doing CBPR with hidden populations, youth, and other diverse groups; participatory evaluation; and moving into action so that CBPR efforts can help community members and their outside research partners work collaboratively for social change to end health disparities.

The authors have in common a belief in the power of CBPR, tempered with an awareness of the very real ethical and practical dilemmas that arise in the course of its application. Speaking from both personal experience in the field and a broad understanding of underlying theoretical, methodological, and ethical and value issues, they help us grapple with what it means to engage with communities in CBPR and some of the steps and considerations that underlie ethical and effective engagement. The contributors share as well the formal and informal theories guiding their work, since, in the words of social epidemiologist Nancy Krieger (2000, p. 27), "by clarifying our theories we are likely to enhance our understanding of what kinds of questions we need to ask, and with whom it is we need to think and work, to generate knowledge and action useful in rectifying social inequalities in health."

Finally, the book's contributors provide, through both case studies and an appendix of concrete tools and applications, a host of techniques and methods that may be useful in working collaboratively with communities in different phases of the CBPR process.

A NOTE ON TIMING AND CONTEXT

The timing of this volume is paradoxical, mirroring in many ways the intensified chasm in public health between participatory community based approaches to health problems and narrowly biomedical and, increasingly, genetic approaches. On the one hand, exponential growth in the potential of biotechnology for addressing such diverse health problems as asthma, HIV/AIDS, heart disease, and some cancers has led to an infusion of funds into the already dominant biomedical approach to research. Many schools of public health and related institutions are increasing their emphasis on the "hard sciences," while programs in the behavioral sciences, community health education, and related areas are quietly downsized or terminated (Rothman, 1998). Since the September 11, 2001, terrorist attacks on the World Trade Center and the Pentagon and the subsequent anthrax scare, we have witnessed a major increase in government funds to the Centers for Disease Control and Prevention (CDC) and the Department of Health and Human Services for rebuilding the nation's public health infrastructure. Such funding is a welcome by-product of the September 11 tragedy and its bitter aftermath. Yet without denying the critical need for refurbishing outmoded laboratories and the like, the decision to limit this sizable new stream of funding almost exclusively to laboratory, computer, and other biotechnology infrastructure is unfortunate, for it largely ignores the urgent need for personnel and training to help us better understand and address the social and behavioral determinants of health that figure so prominently in the landscape of today's health and social problems.

Despite the nature of the post–September 11–related funding decisions, however, there has been some evidence of increased concern with support for exploring and attempting to address the social determinants of health and the social protective factors that can promote and improve health on multiple levels. Indeed, when President Clinton announced his initiative to eliminate health disparities, he stressed the importance of approaches that included the broader social, physical, and policy environments, not merely biology and individual behavior (U.S. Department of Health and Human Services, 2000).

Similarly, awareness of the need to understand community dynamics and sociocultural factors and their impact on health has grown dramatically, and appreciation of the need for community-driven research has increased. Recent resources in this area include an Institute of Medicine report on social and behavioral interventions (Smedley & Syme, 2000) and the CDC's *Guide to Community Preventive Services,* which proposes a comprehensive sociocultural environmental framework to be applied to community interventions (http://www.thecommunity guide.org). As noted physician and public health leader Reed Tuckson has pointed out, "Health is the place where all the social forces converge," and for that reason, "the fight against disparities in health is also one against the absence of hope for a meaningful future" (U.S. Department of Health and Human Services, 1998, p. 10). It is a fight that can be won only if our most oppressed communities can be fully engaged as partners in identifying, exploring, and taking action to address the health and social problems they—not we as outsiders—care most deeply about (Minkler, 1997). Such developments have been translated into practice in phenomena like the international Healthy Cities/Healthy Communities network (Norris & Pittman, 2000), the growth of a national, community based movement to study and fight environmental racism (Shepard, 2000), and partnership approaches to the struggle against HIV/AIDS (Schensul, 1999). They are further reflected in the growing momentum for CBPR as a legitimate and valued approach to studying and addressing some of our most intractable health and social problems (Blackwell et al., in press; Green & Mercer, 2001; Minkler, 2000).

In the United States, large and small philanthropic organizations like the W. K. Kellogg Foundation, the Ford Foundation, the Anna B. Casey Foundation, and the Aspen Institute have begun providing substantial support for participatory approaches to CBPR in health and related fields. Seed money for participatory research is also provided through such organizations as the Agency for Health Care Research and Quality (AHRQ). Through its Community Health Scholars Program (2001), the Kellogg Foundation has gone further, committing to training, at the postdoctoral level, a new cadre of researchers with experience in CBPR and a commitment to both scholarly and pedagogical use of this approach in their future academic careers. Although the estimated $45 million[1] now available annually from government and foundation sources to support community based participatory research pales when compared to the nation's $170 billion annual research and development expenditures (Chopyak & Levesque, 2001; Sclove, Scammell, & Holland, 1998), momentum is clearly building for both support and valuing of CBPR as an important alternative approach to more conventional research orientations.

New academic centers and programs dedicated to participatory research and practice have been created in many parts of the United States, and a sample is listed in Appendix H (see also Ansley & Gaventa, 1997). Among these are the Policy Research and Action Group (PRAG), a consortium of four Chicago universities working with the city's community based organizations on locally identified research issues. Three universities—the University of Michigan, the City University of New York, and the University of Washington—are also major partners in the nation's three Urban Health Centers funded by the CDC. Each of these centers emphasizes participatory, community based research approaches to studying and addressing the social determinants of health (see Appendixes C and H). In Little Rock, Arkansas, a school of public health is being created specifically on the model of community based public health with an accent on participatory research. Some law schools, too, are embracing participatory research methods, with Harvard Law School, for example, using collaborative approaches in working with community partners to investigate environmental justice and welfare reform in Massachusetts (Ansley & Gaventa, 1997).

Well beyond the walls of academia, however, community based centers have for decades made critical contributions to the conceptualization and conduct of research of, by, and for communities. From internationally known venues like the Highlander Center in rural Tennessee (Lewis, 2001) to newer organizations like the Applied Research Center in Oakland, California (see Appendix H), such centers have helped underscore the powerful role of community based organizations in "breaking the monopoly" of knowledge creation (Fals-Borda & Rahman, 1991) for social change.

Government agencies, including the CDC and the National Institute of Environmental Health Sciences (NIEHS), have increased their support for CBPR, with the NIEHS funding multimillion-dollar "community-driven research" initiatives that explicitly call for this approach as their modus operandi. The CDC has similarly allocated $13 million in 2002 to support "community based participatory prevention research" to help meet the goals of Healthy People 2010 (http://www.cdc.gov/od/pgo/funding/frantmain.htm). In Vancouver, British Colombia, a set of guidelines for appraising and assessing participatory research in the area of health promotion was developed for the Royal Society of Canada and is being enthusiastically circulated among funding bodies in the United

States as they grapple with how to judge the merits of potential CBPR projects (see George et al., 1998–1999; see also Appendix C).

Decades-old networks and centers for popular education and participatory research, such as the Society for Participatory Research in Asia (Hall, 1999), the Highlander Center in the Southern United States (Lewis, 2001), and the International Participatory Research Network, which began in the mid-1970s (Hall, 1999), are being supplemented by new venues for dialogue and co-learning in many parts of the world. In the United States, the Loka Institute (http://www.loka.org) in Amherst, Massachusetts, has engaged approximately two thousand people as part of its Community Research Network and hosts annual conferences and an active listserv through which participants regularly grapple with ethical and other issues of concern in participatory research. The Seattle-based Campus Community Partnership for Health (http://futurehealth.ucsf.edu/ccph) is a similar network of some one thousand community and campus partners that promotes health through CBPR, as well as through academic service-learning and related avenues.

Many professional journals in the health field have published or plan to publish theme issues or special sections on community based participatory research, including the *Journal of the American Public Health Association,* the *American Journal of Preventive Medicine,* the *Journal of Public Health Management and Practice, Environmental Health Perspectives, Health Education and Behavior,* and the *Journal of General Internal Medicine.*

There remains, of course, a long way to go. As noted, funding for CBPR, though increasing dramatically in recent years, has not kept pace with the financial support available for more traditional research efforts (Sclove et al., 1998). Although participatory research is gaining increased legitimacy in some academic circles (Green et al., 1995; see also Chapter Five and Appendix D), the academy as a whole remains highly skeptical of participatory and action-oriented approaches to scholarship. As Mary Northridge and her colleagues (2000, p. 58) point out, "More often than not, [such research] is accorded a secondary status." The products of such studies are not infrequently rejected out of hand as biased and unscientific (Buchanan, 1999). Pressures for tenure and promotion also present significant challenges for junior faculty who understand the long-term time commitment CBPR requires (Goodman, 2001; see also Appendix D).

Yet despite continuing obstacles, financial, academic, and professional support for participatory research is clearly increasing, both nationally and internationally. Together with growing community demands for research that is participatory, inclusive, and directed at tangible changes in the status quo, such forces underscore the need for a new level of engagement with CBPR as an orientation to research well suited to understanding and addressing complex health and social problems.

ORGANIZATION OF THIS VOLUME

In Chapter Two, Nina Wallerstein and Bonnie Duran situate CBPR and other participatory research approaches historically, conceptually, and in practice through a far-reaching sweep of their major historical and theoretical underpinnings. The roots of much contemporary participatory research in the popular education work of Brazilian educator Paulo Freire (1970, 1973, 1982) are discussed, as are a variety of critical theory, feminist, postmodern, poststructuralist, and postcolonial contributions to the field.

In Chapter Three, Barbara Israel and her academic and community partners share their experiences in developing and following CBPR principles in the University of Michigan's Urban Research Center. Although these authors suggest that each CBPR initiative may seek to come up with its own set of guidelines tailored to local strengths and circumstances, they offer a set of core principles and ethical considerations for the field, including true collaborative and co-learning relationships; empowerment and community capacity building; and research for change, rather than simply for creating new knowledge.

In Part Two, we continue this discussion, grappling further with issues of trust, power, and dialogue as we focus on building relationships with communities and community members on multiple levels. We explore questions related to the roles of outside researchers and of community leadership, the centrality of race or ethnicity and racism, and the difficulties in confronting power differentials based on the interlocking identities of race, class, gender, and professional hierarchy (hooks, 1989).

We begin Part Two with a powerful chapter by Vivian Chávez and colleagues, who examine the multiple dimensions of race and privilege and the context they create for understanding cross-cultural CBPR. The role of historical trauma and internalized oppression in communities of color and the existence of strong social movements within such communities, about which outsiders may have little knowledge, are among the topics explored in Chapter Four.

This book is premised on the assumption that concerned outsiders, including university based researchers and professionals trained in health and related fields, can make useful contributions to community-driven research through engaging in a true CBPR process. In Chapter Five, however, Randy Stoecker takes a step back to ask whether outside academics have a legitimate role to play in participatory research. After examining some of the realities, paradoxes, and challenges frequently confronted by outside researchers, Stoecker offers "guideposts" for their effective and ethical engagement. He further suggests three roles scholars may play—initiator, consultant, and true collaborator—depending on both their abilities and interests and the interests, strengths, and needs of the communities with which they are engaged.

As Roz Lasker and her colleagues have suggested, "Building relationships is probably the most daunting and time-consuming challenge partnerships face" (Lasker, Weiss, & Miller, 2001, p. 192; see also Kreuter, Lezin, & Young, 2000). In Chapter Six, community, university, and health department partners at the Urban Research Center in Seattle, Washington, grapple with the effective formation and functioning of partnerships for CBPR in their efforts to study and address the social determinants of health. The chapter includes a careful look through multiple lenses at the hard questions of what is meant by "community" and "community representation"; issues of power, race, ethnicity, and culture; and the differential benefits of participation for different partners. For each of these problem areas, the authors present illustrations of how Seattle Partners for Healthy Communities has attempted to address the challenges faced and offer lessons for other CBPR partnerships.

Part Three focuses on one of the most important but often neglected processes in CBPR, creating a setting in which community members, rather than outsiders, truly drive decisions around issue selection. In Chapter Seven, Meredith Minkler and Trevor Hancock provide an overview of three core principles that lie at the heart of ensuring community-driven asset identification and issue selection: starting where the people are, building on community strengths, and fostering authentic dialogue. Highlighted are the roles for outside professionals in helping community members identify their strengths and issues, including a diversity of approaches to facilitate this process, such as windshield tours, town hall meetings, community asset and risk mapping, the Delphi technique, and the collaborative development of neighborhood indicators.

In the following chapter, Stephen Fawcett and colleagues at the University of Kansas explore how Internet based tools can be used by community and academic partners to build local capacity and action for CBPR and other community health and development work. A model framework is provided, highlighting core competencies and selected Internet based resources that support them. The chapter then provides an in-depth look at one such Web based resource, the Community Tool Box (http://ctb.ku.edu), and discusses the challenges and benefits of using such resources in CBPR.

In the final chapter of Part Three, Caroline Wang presents a case study with a homeless community in Ann Arbor, Michigan, to document the particular potency of "photovoice" as a tool for communities to identify shared problems and strengths that can in turn lead to collective action for change. Through its use of dialogue and the provision of inexpensive cameras and training in how to "convey their own vision of the world," photovoice is seen as powerfully integrating "community participation, health concerns, and the visual image" (Wang & Burris, 1994, p. 177). Wang explores the advantages and limitations of this approach to issue selection and discusses its potential for use in diverse settings.

Part Four shines a spotlight on some of the knottiest issues in CBPR: the validity and quality of the research and the many difficult ethical and practical issues involved in the implementation of research findings. With regard to validity, feminist researcher Patricia Lather (1993, p. 674) has observed that "validity is a 'limit question' of research, one that repeatedly surfaces, one that can neither be avoided nor resolved, a fertile obsession given its intractability." Many researchers have discovered the value of hiring community members as interviewers for community surveys as a means of increasing response rates. Yet when the next step is taken and community members work in collaborative partnerships with outside researchers on designing research instruments and collecting and analyzing data, hackles frequently rise, along with questions about whether the results can possibly constitute "good" research (Buchanan, 1999; Stringer, 1999). Part Four begins with Hilary Bradbury and Peter Reason's thoughtful examination of a range of issues and "choice points" for improving the quality of action research. Of particular concern to these investigators is "broadening the bandwidth of validity" to include such considerations as whether a project's work is useful and helpful, how well it is grounded experientially, and whether it builds infrastructure so that the work may endure over time.

To further illustrate some of the methodological and ethical issues faced in CBPR and related research traditions, Part Four also presents several in-depth case studies. In Chapter Eleven, Stephanie Farquhar and Steve Wing illustrate unique academic-community partnerships designed to document and expose health problems and related social and environmental racism in rural North Carolina. In the first case study in this chapter, Wing describes how popular epidemiology and sophisticated computer modeling, in close collaboration with community partners, were used to uncover health problems and patterns of environmental racism in the placement of massive hog production operations in low-income, predominantly African American communities. In the second, we learn how Farquhar and her partners used survey research, including more qualitative data collection, to provide dramatic documentation of discriminatory and inadequate emergency environmental and housing policies in the aftermath of Hurricane Floyd. The political fallout of CBPR in these two cases, the problems with charges of bias and "unscientific" research and how they were handled, and the emphasis placed on co-learning by professional and academic team members and their community partners are among the issues highlighted.

Chapter Twelve presents a case study in which members of the disability community in the San Francisco Bay Area and their outside collaborators used CBPR in an effort to broaden the dialogue around a particularly contentious issue in their community: "death with dignity," or physician-assisted suicide legislation. As Pamela Fadem and her colleagues note, although high-level community involvement took place at each stage of the research process, major ethical challenges arose, including the politics of issue selection when the "community" is deeply divided over an issue, insider-outsider issues, and dilemmas over the use of findings.

Despite the difficulties encountered along the way, each of these case studies suggests that authentic partnerships with communities can often result in far richer understandings of a problem area than outsiders could achieve working on their own. Such collaborations can also pave the way for action, while leaving behind a community of people better able to mobilize around, systematically study, and act on their issues in the future.

One of the most important developments in participatory research over the past two decades has been the emergence of new and increasingly popular participatory approaches to evaluation. Such approaches incorporate the principles of empowerment and capacity building while retaining concerns for high-quality inquiry and outcomes (Fetterman, Kaftarian, & Wandersman, 1996; Roe, Bernstein, Goette, & Roe, 1997; Wallerstein, 1999). In the final chapter in Part Four, Jane Springett offers a critical look at participatory evaluation in community health promotion. She considers in particular its relationship to participatory research and the challenges faced in practice related to the multiple and sometimes conflicting roles of the evaluator, questions of how programs are "judged" or "valued," and the contributions of participatory evaluation to program improvement and local capacity development.

Community based participatory research frequently involves collaborations between outside academic or professional researchers and diverse underserved community groups. In Part Five, three theory-driven case studies are presented that explore collaborative research across the divides of class, race and ethnicity, and gender identity. Chapter Fourteen describes the East Side Village Health Worker Partnership in Detroit, Michigan, and its efforts to actively engage neighborhood women, most of whom are single mothers, as lay health workers and CBPR participants in their community. Drawing on feminist and CBPR principles, the project places a heavy emphasis on respect for cultural concerns, time constraints, and health problems the women face while at the same building on their strengths at each phase of the project.

A growing body of participatory action research, particularly in the United States, has involved work with youth (Harper & Carver, 1999; Wang, Morrel-Samuels, Bell, Hutchison, & Powers, 2000). In Chapter Fifteen, Ann Cheatam and Eveline Shen demonstrate both the powerful contributions youth have made as genuine partners in CBPR efforts and the ethical and practical problems that must be faced in working collaboratively with this population. Grounding their case study in the philosophy and methods of Paulo Freire (1970, 1973), the authors analyze a CBPR project involving Cambodian girls in Long Beach, California, who were committed to studying and addressing the high levels of sexual harassment experienced in their school. The early and continued use of "education for critical consciousness" (Freire, 1973) and the high level of youth involvement in the research are described, including successful efforts to use study findings to help secure new policies on the school and district levels.

Conducting research with "hidden populations" presents special challenges for outsider researchers and health care professionals, yet such populations often have both a disproportionate burden of health and social problems and a wealth of internal resources and assets that frequently go unrecognized. In the final chapter in Part Five, Kristen Clements-Nolle and Ari Bachrach describe and analyze the unique participatory methodology employed in the first major epidemiological study of and with a transgender community. The role of community partners in gaining access to this hidden population, in formulating research questions and conducting interviews in gender and culturally sensitive ways that greatly increased the validity and usefulness of findings, and in using findings to promote changes in practice and policy arenas are examined. The extremely high rates of HIV/AIDS, suicide attempts, and other health and social problems uncovered through this study underscore the utility of CBPR approaches to research in populations that are often missed through more traditional approaches to inquiry.

Of the many factors that differentiate CBPR or other participatory research approaches from more traditional outside-expert-driven research is the former's commitment to action as an integral part of the research enterprise. Part Six takes a deeper look at the action component of CBPR, giving particular attention to how CBPR can promote healthy public policy. Makani Themba and Meredith Minkler begin by briefly summarizing two conceptual frameworks for understanding the public policymaking process in the United States. Drawing on a variety of case examples, they discuss and illustrate the roles and entry points for CBPR partners interested in attempting to influence either public policy or policymaking in private sector arenas.

In Chapter Eighteen, Juliana van Olphen and her colleagues provide a detailed case study of the early steps taken in a CBPR project aimed at influencing policy to reduce substance abuse and HIV risk and to facilitate the successful community reintegration of people leaving jail in New York City. The authors describe efforts by community partners and the Center for Urban Epidemiological Studies at the City University of New York to select and study the problem, narrow the specific issue areas, and move to next steps for research and action. They highlight as well the role of unfavorable public policies in widening health disparities and the potential of CBPR for building community capacity and ultimately effecting policy change.

Although policy is most often thought of in broad public policy terms, the potential for improving health through changes in policy at the workplace and in other private sector arenas should not be forgotten. Part Six concludes with

Pam Tau Lee and her colleagues' account of a union-supported CBPR project undertaken by staff and faculty at the Labor Occupational Health Center at the University of California in Berkeley and a group of twenty-five hotel room cleaners, most of them immigrant women. Using risk mapping, focus groups, surveys, and other techniques, the hotel workers and their university partners were able to document high rates of work-related health problems, which the union then successfully used to effect a workload reduction policy in subsequent contract negotiations. The role of the room cleaners in the research, including their active participation at the bargaining table, provides a potent example of high-level collaboration, as well as the impact it can have in bringing about policy change.

The book concludes with nine appendixes designed to provide readers with a variety of tools and applications corresponding to many of the chapter themes and issues raised. Among the instruments included are a sample protocol for community–outside researcher understanding in CBPR, tools for helping communities conduct their own asset and risk mapping, a sample of collaboratively developed neighborhood health indicators, a historical look at federal support for participatory research and related endeavors in the United States, and the Royal Society of Canada's guidelines for appraising the degree to which proposed projects meet the criteria of true participatory action research. The appendixes are designed to help outsider researchers and their community partners put some of the messages central to this volume into practice in their own CBPR efforts.

Community based participatory research is time-consuming and filled with challenges as local communities and their outside research collaborators navigate difficult ethical and practical terrain, addressing issues of power and trust, race, ethnicity, and racism, research rigor, and often conflicting agendas (Chavis, Stucky, & Wandersman, 1983; Cornwall & Jewkes, 1995; Green & Mercer, 2001; Maguire, 2001; Reason & Bradbury, 2001; Stringer, 1999). Yet as the contributors to this volume demonstrate, CBPR holds immense potential for addressing challenging health and social problems, while helping bring about conditions in which communities can recognize and build on their strengths and become full partners in gaining and creating knowledge and mobilizing for change.

Note

1 This figure is undoubtedly conservative and does not include, for example, the $13 million allocated by the CDC in 2002 for the support of participatory research projects aimed at furthering health promotion and disease prevention efforts.

References

Amick, B., Levine, S., Tarlov, A., & Walsh, D. C. (1995). *Society and health.* New York: Oxford University Press.

Ansley, F., & Gaventa, J. (1997, January–February). Researching for democracy and democratizing research. *Change,* pp. 46–53.

Bell, E. E. (2001). Infusing race into the U.S. discourse on action research. In P. Reason & H. Bradbury (Eds.), *Handbook of action research: Participative inquiry and practice* (pp. 48–49). Thousand Oaks, CA: Sage.

Blackwell, A. G., Tamir, H. B., Thompson, M., & Minkler, M. (in press). Community based participatory research: Implications for funders. *Journal of General Internal Medicine.*

Blair, R., Cahill, K., Chopyak, J., & Cordes, C. (2000). *Common problems, uncommon resources: Exploring the social and economic challenges of community based research.* Atlanta: Community Research Network.

Brown, L. D., & Tandon, R. (1983). Ideology and political economy in inquiry: Action research and participatory research. *Journal of Applied Behavioral Science, 19,* 277–294.

Bruce, T. A., & Uranga McKane, S. (2000). *Community-based public health: A partnership model.* Washington, DC: American Public Health Association.

Buchanan, D. (1999). *An ethic for health promotion: Rethinking the sources of human well-being.* New York: Oxford University Press.

Chavis, D. M., Stucky, P. R., & Wandersman, A. (1983, April). Returning basic research to the community: A relationship between scientist and citizen. *American Psychologist, 38,* 424–434.

Chopyak, J., & Levesque, P. (2001, November). *New frameworks for research collaborations: Changing what we mean by research.* Paper presented at the annual meeting of the Society for the Social Studies of Science, Cambridge, MA.

Collins, C., & Williams, D. R. (1999). Segregation and mortality: The deadly effects of racism. *Sociological Forum, 14,* 495–523.

Collins, P. H. (2000). *Black feminist thought: Knowledge, consciousness, and the politics of empowerment* (2nd ed.). New York: Routledge.

Community Health Scholars Program. (2001, June). Definition of CBPR adopted at the spring networking meeting of the Community Health Scholars Program, Ann Arbor, MI.

Cornwall, A., & Jewkes, R. (1995). What is participatory research? *Social Science and Medicine, 41,* 1667–1676.

Couto, R. C. (1987). Participatory research: Methodology and critique. *Clinical Sociology Review, 5,* 83–90.

De Koning, K., & Martin, M. (Eds.). (1996). *Participatory research in health: Issues and experiences* (2nd ed.). London: Zed Books.

Fals-Borda, O. (1987). The application of participatory action research in Latin America. *International Sociology, 2,* 329–347.

Fals-Borda, O., & Rahman, M. A. (1991). *Action and knowledge: Breaking the monopoly with participatory action research.* New York: Apex.

Fetterman, D. M., Kaftarian, S. J., & Wandersman, A. (Eds.). (1996). *Empowerment evaluation: Knowledge and tools for self-assessment and accountability.* Thousand Oaks, CA: Sage.

Freire, P. (1970). *Pedagogy of the oppressed.* New York: Seabury Press.

Freire, P. (1973). *Education for critical consciousness.* New York: Seabury Press.

Freire, P. (1982). Creating alternative research methods: Learning to do it by doing it. In B. L. Hall, A. Gillette, & R. Tandon (Eds.), *Creating knowledge: A monopoly? Participatory research in development.* New Delhi: Society for Participatory Research in Asia.

Gaventa, J. (1981). Participatory action research in North America. *Convergence, 14,* 30–42.

Gaventa, J. (1993). The powerful, the powerless, and the experts: Knowledge struggles in an information age. In P. Park, M. Brydon-Miller, B. L. Hall, & T. Jackson (Eds.), *Voices of change: Participatory research in the United States and Canada* (pp. 21–40). Westport CT: Bergin & Garvey.

George, M. A., Daniel, M., & Green L. W. (1998–1999). Appraising and funding participatory research in health promotion. *International Quarterly of Community Health Education, 18,* 181–197.

Goodman, R. M. (2001). Community-based participatory research: Questions and challenges to an essential approach. *Journal of Public Health Management and Practice, 7*(5), pp. v–vi.

Green, L. W., George, M. A., Daniel, M., Frankish, C. J., Herbert, C. P., Bowie, W. R., & O'Neill, M. (1995). *Study of participatory research in health promotion: Review and recommendations for the development of participatory research in health promotion in Canada.* Vancouver, British Columbia: Royal Society of Canada.

Green, L. W., & Mercer, S. (2001). Can public health researchers and agencies reconcile the push from funding bodies and the pull from communities? *American Journal of Public Health, 91,* 1926–1929.

Greenwood, D., & Levin, M. (1998). *Introduction to action research: Social research for social change.* Thousand Oaks, CA: Sage.

Habermas, J. (1972). *Knowledge and human interests: Theory and practice; communication and the evolution of society* (J. J. Shapiro, Trans.). London: Heinemann.

Habermas, J. (1988). *On the logic of the social sciences.* Cambridge, MA: MIT Press.

Hagey, R. S. (1997). Guest editorial: The use and abuse of participatory action research. *Chronic Diseases of Canada, 18*(2), 1–4.

Hall, B. L. (1981). Participatory research, popular knowledge, and power: A personal reflection. *Convergence, 14,* 6–19.

Hall, B. L. (1992). From margins to center: The development and purpose of participatory action research. *American Sociologist, 23,* 15–28.

Hall, B. L. (1999). Looking back, looking forward: Reflections on the International Participatory Research Network. *Forests, Trees, and People Newsletter, 39,* 3–36.

Hall, B. L., Gillette, A., & Tandon, R. (Eds.). (1982). *Creating knowledge: A monopoly? Participatory research in development.* New Delhi: Society for Participatory Research in Asia.

Harper, G. W., & Carver, L. J. (1999). "Out of the mainstream" youth as partners in collaborative research: Exploring the benefits and challenges. *Health Education and Behavior, 26,* 250–256.

hooks, b. (1984). *From margin to center.* Boston: South End Press.

hooks, b. (1989). *Talking back: Thinking feminism, talking black.* Boston: South End Press.

House, J. S., & Williams, D. R. (2000). Understanding and reducing socioeconomic and racial/ethnic disparities in health. In B. D. Smedley & L. S. Syme (Eds.), *Promoting health: Intervention strategies from social and behavioral research* (pp. 81–124). Washington, DC: Institute of Medicine/National Academy Press.

Israel, B. A., Schulz, A. J., Parker, E. A., & Becker, A. B. (1998). Review of community-based research: Assessing partnership approaches to improve public health. *Annual Review of Public Health, 19,* 173–202.

James, S. A., Schulz, A. J., & van Olphen, J. (2001). Social capital, poverty, and community health: An exploration of linkages. In S. Saegert, J. P. Thompson, & M. R. Warren (Eds.), *Social capital and poor communities* (pp. 165–188). New York: Russell Sage Foundation.

Kaplan, G. A., Pamuk, E. A., Lynch, J. W., Cohen, R. D., & Balfour, J. L. (1996). Inequality in income and mortality in the United States: Analysis of mortality and potential pathways. *British Medical Journal, 312,* 999–1003.

Kawachi, I., Kennedy, B. P., Lochner, K., & Prothrow-Stith, D. (1997). Social capital, income inequality, and mortality. *American Journal of Public Health, 87,* 1491–1498.

Kreuter, M. W., Lezin, N. A., & Young, L. A. (2000). Evaluating community based collaborative mechanisms: Implications for practitioners. *Health Promotion Practice, 1,* 49–63.

Krieger, N. (2000). Social epidemiology and health inequalities: A U.S. perspective on theories and actions. In I. Forbes (Ed.), *Health inequalities: Poverty and policy* (pp. 26–43). London: Academy of Learned Societies for the Social Sciences.

Krieger, N., Rowley, D. L., Herman, A. A., Avery, B., & Phillips, M. T. (1993). Racism, sexism, and social class: Implications for studies of health, disease, and well-being. *American Journal of Preventive Medicine, 9*(6), 82–122.

Lasker, R. D., Weiss, E. S., & Miller, R. (2001). Partnership synergy: A practical framework for studying and strengthening the collaborative advantage. *Milbank Quarterly, 27,* 179–205.

Lather, P. (1993). Fertile obsession: Validity after post-structuralism. *Sociology Quarterly, 34,* 673–693.

Lewin, K. (1946). Action research and minority problems. *Journal of Social Issues, 2,* 34–46.

Lewis, H. M. (2001). Participatory research and education for social change: Highlander Research and Education Center. In P. Reason & H. Bradbury, *Handbook of action research: Participative inquiry and practice* (pp. 124–132). Thousand Oaks, CA: Sage.

Lykes, M. B. (1997). Activist participatory research among the Maya of Guatemala: Constructing meanings from situated knowledge. *Journal of Social Issues, 53,* 725–746.

Maguire, P. (1987). *Doing participatory research: A feminist approach.* Amherst: Center for International Education, University of Massachusetts.

Maguire, P. (2001). Uneven ground: Feminisms and action research. In P. Reason & H. Bradbury (Eds.), *Handbook of action research: Participative inquiry and practice* (pp. 59–69). Thousand Oaks, CA: Sage.

Marmot, M., & Wilkinson, R. G. (Eds.). (1999). *Social determinants of health.* New York: Oxford University Press.

Merrifield, J. (1993). Putting scientists in their place: Participatory research in environmental and occupational health. In P. Park, M. Brydon-Miller, B. L. Hall, & T. Jackson (Eds.), *Voices of change: Participatory research in the United States and Canada* (pp. 65–84). Westport, CT.: Bergin & Garvey.

Minkler, M. (1997). Introduction and overview. In M. Minkler (Ed.), *Community organizing and community building for health* (pp. 3–19). New Brunswick, NJ: Rutgers University Press.

Minkler, M. (2000). Participatory action research and healthy communities. *Public Health Reports, 115,* 191–197.

National Center for Health Statistics. (2002). *Healthy people 2002: Trends in racial and ethnic-specific rates for health status indicators.* Retrieved from http://www.cdc.gov/nchs.

Norris, T., & Pittman, M. (2000). The Healthy Communities Movement and the Coalition for Healthier Cities and Communities. *Public Health Reports, 115,* 118–124.

Northridge, M. E., Vallone, D., Merzel, C., Greene, D., Shepherd, P., Cohall, A. T., & Healton, C. G. (2000). The adolescent years: An academic-community partnership in Harlem comes of age. *Journal of Public Health Management and Practice, 1*(6), 53–60.

Park, P., Brydon-Miller, M., Hall, B. L., & Jackson, T. (Eds.). (1993). *Voices of change: Participatory research in the United States and Canada.* Westport, CT: Bergin & Garvey.

Reason, P., & Bradbury, H. (Eds.). (2001). *Handbook of action research: Participative inquiry and practice.* Thousand Oaks, CA: Sage.

Roe, K. M., Bernstein, C., Goette, C., & Roe, K. (1997). Community building through empowering evaluation: A case study of HIV prevention planning. In M. Minkler (Ed.), *Community organizing and community building for health* (pp. 308–322). New Brunswick, NJ: Rutgers University Press.

Rothman, B. K. (1998). *Genetic maps and the human imagination.* New York: Norton.

Schensul, J. (1999). Organizing community research partnerships in the struggle against AIDS. *Health Education and Behavior, 26,* 266–283.

Schwab, M., & Syme, S. L. (1997). On paradigms, community participation, and the future of public health. *American Journal of Public Health, 87,* 2049–2052.

Sclove, R. E., Scammell, M. L., & Holland, B. (1998). *Community-based research in the U.S.: An introductory reconnaissance, including 12 organizational case studies and comparison with the Dutch Science Shops and the Mainstream American Research System.* Amherst, MA: Loka Institute.

Shepard, P. (2000, March 29–31). Achieving environmental justice objectives and reducing health disparities through community based participatory research and interventions. In *Successful models of community based participatory research.* Final report of the meeting hosted by the National Institute of Environmental Health Sciences, Washington, DC.

Smedley, B. D., Stith, A. Y., & Nelson, A. R. (2002). *Unequal treatment: Confronting racial and ethnic disparities in health care.* Washington, DC: Institute of Medicine/National Academy Press.

Smedley, B. D., & Syme, S. L. (Eds.). (2000). *Promoting health: Intervention strategies from social and behavioral research.* Washington, DC: Institute of Medicine/National Academy Press.

Stringer, E. T. (1999). *Action research* (2nd ed.). Thousand Oaks, CA: Sage.

Stringer, E. T., & Genat, W. (in press). *Action research in health practice.* Upper Saddle River, NJ: Prentice Hall.

Swantz, M.-L., Ndedya, E., & Masaiganah, M. S. (2001). Participatory action research in Tanzania, with special reference to women. In P. Reason & H. Bradbury, *Handbook of action research: Participative inquiry and practice* (pp. 386–395). Thousand Oaks, CA: Sage.

Tandon, R. (1996). The historical roots and contemporary tendencies in participatory research: Implications for health care. In K. De Koning & M. Martin (Eds.), *Participatory research in health: Issues and experiences* (2nd ed., pp. 19–26). London: Zed Books.

Thomas, S. B., & Crouse Quinn, S. (2001). Light on the shadow of the syphilis study at Tuskegee. *Health Promotion Practice, 1,* 234–237.

U.S. Department of Health and Human Services. (1998). *Call to action: Eliminating racial and ethnic disparities in health.* Washington, DC: Author/Grantmakers in Health.

U.S. Department of Health and Human Services. (2000). *Healthy people 2010: Understanding and improving health.* Washington, DC: Government Printing Office.

Wallerstein, N. (1999). Power between evaluator and community: Research relationships within New Mexico's healthier communities. *Social Science and Medicine, 49,* 39–53.

Wang, C. C., & Burris, M. A. (1994). Empowerment through photo novella: Portraits of participation. *Health Education Quarterly, 21,* 171–196.

Wang, C. C., Morrel-Samuels, S., Bell, L., Hutchison, P., & Powers, L. S. (Eds.). (2000). *Strength to be: Community visions and voices.* Ann Arbor: University of Michigan.

Wing, S. (1998). Whose epidemiology, whose health? *International Journal of Health Services, 28,* 241–252.

CHAPTER TWO

The Conceptual, Historical, and Practice Roots of Community Based Participatory Research and Related Participatory Traditions

Nina Wallerstein
Bonnie Duran

If we do our [research] well, reality will appear even more unstable, complex, and disorderly than it does now.
—J. Flax (1987, p. 643)

In the past few decades, a new paradigm of "participatory" research has emerged, raising challenges to the positivist view of science, the construction and use of knowledge; the role of the researcher in engaging society, the role of agency and participation of the community, and the importance of power relations that permeate the research process and our capacity to become a just and more equitable society. By the 1960s, simultaneous crises in academic social theory and in political movements throughout the globe, including peasant, squatter, student, and worker movements—often with military consequences—precipitated the search for new theories and practices of inquiry that would provoke and stimulate the creation of political and economic democracies.

The multiplicity of terms representing this new "participatory research" paradigm, which links applied social science and social activism, has been fairly daunting, and nuances between them are often difficult to decipher (see Chapter One). Some terms, such as *rapid assessment procedures, rapid rural appraisal,* and *participatory rural appraisal,* implemented primarily in developing nations, have represented a methodological emphasis (De Koning & Martin, 1996a). Specific disciplines have produced their own terminology: *classroom action research, critical action research,* and *practitioner research* in the field of education (Kemmis & McTaggart, 2000); *action learning, action science, action inquiry,* and *industrial action research* in the fields of organizational psychology and organizational development (Argyris, Putnam, & Smith, 1985; Torbert, 2001); *cooperative, mutual, or reflective practitioner inquiry* in psychology and human relations (Heron & Reason, 2001; Reason, 1994; Rowan, 2001); *constructivist* or *fourth-generation inquiry* applied to evaluation research (Lincoln, 2001); *emancipatory inquiry* in nursing (Henderson, 1995; Hills, 2001); and *popular epidemiology* in public health (P. Brown, 1992; Wing, 1998). Multiple concepts have come from the community development and social action literature, including *collaborative action research, participatory research, emancipatory* or *liberatory research,* and *dialectical inquiry* (Fals-Borda & Rahman, 1991; Hall, 1992; Hall, Gillette, & Tandon, 1982; Kemmis & McTaggart, 2000; Park, Brydon-Miller, Hall, & Jackson, 1993).

Recently, two terms, *action research* and *participatory action research* (PAR), have begun to be used interchangeably to represent a convergence of principles and values, well-articulated in Chapter Three, in which the community determines the research agenda and jointly shares in the planning, implementation of data collection and analysis, and dissemination of the research (Israel, Checkoway, Schulz, & Zimmerman, 1994; Israel, Schulz, Parker, & Becker, 1998; McTaggart, 1991, 1997; Reason & Bradbury, 2001; Stringer, 1999).

In the past few years, the term adopted in this volume, *community based participatory research* (CBPR), has gained respectability and attention in the health field. Like participatory action research and action research, CBPR takes the perspective that "participatory" research involves three interconnected goals: research, action, and education. As part of collaborative democratic processes, shared principles include a negotiation of information and capacities in both directions: researchers transferring tools for community members to analyze conditions and make informed decisions on actions to improve their lives, and community members transferring their expert content and meaning to researchers in the pursuit of mutual knowledge and application of the knowledge to their communities (Hatch, Moss, & Saran, 1993).

With CBPR emerging as a concept in its own right, a debt remains to the cross-fertilization of "participatory" research endeavors worldwide. As development studies theorist Robert Chambers has noted, it has become difficult to "separate out the innovations, influences and diffusion as if they follow straight lines" because "these sources and traditions have, like flows in a braided stream, intermingled more and more" (1992, p. 2).

Despite this apparent unity, the majority of these terms can be traced to two historical traditions that represent two distinct approaches at opposite ends of a continuum: collaborative utilization-focused research with practical goals of system improvement, sometimes called the *Northern tradition,* and openly emancipatory research, which challenges the colonizing practices of positivist research and political domination by the elites, often called the *Southern tradition* (Brown & Tandon, 1983). Many of the key differences between these two traditions are still applicable, including the role of the community in setting the research agenda, the location of power in the research process, the emphasis on different types of knowledge creation, and the goals of the research, from a continuum of problem solving to societal transformation.

This chapter will articulate the historical roots of these two traditions and discuss the contribution of theories of knowledge; postmodern, poststructuralist, and feminist theories; and theories of power to clarify points of convergence and difference within current theory and practice. The chapter ends with practical approaches for implementing Freirian dialogical education in community based participatory research. Although the best of CBPR contains skills and dimensions from both traditions, this chapter argues that the paramount public health goal of eliminating disparities demands a research practice within the emancipatory perspective that fosters the democratic participation of community members to transform their lives.

HISTORICAL ROOTS

The expression *action research* was coined by Kurt Lewin in the 1940s, as a challenge to bridge the gap between theory and practice and to solve practical problems through an action research cycle involving planning, action, and investigating the results of actions (Lewin, 1948/1997). Lewin rejected the positivist belief that researchers study an objective world separate from the intersubjective meanings understood by participants as they act in their world. In this way, action research not only linked action and research but also assumed an educational mission as part of the problem-solving process (Peters & Robinson, 1984).

Successors to Lewin, considered predominantly to be within the Northern tradition, have adopted the challenge of practical problem solving and developed collaborative methodologies to bring together stakeholders, primarily in organizational settings, such as work sites or schools, to solve problems at the small group or system level (Chisholm & Elden, 1993). In education, for example, teachers have been encouraged to become researchers in their classrooms to tackle questions previously left to academics (Stringer, 1999).

This tradition most broadly emanates from the sociological theory of Talcott Parsons and his predecessors, who view social progress as rational decision making based on applying ever-increasing scientific knowledge to world problems. With an emphasis on practitioners acting as coequals to the research process, action science researchers from organizational development and social psychology have often worked in a consensus model, assuming that management and workers together create quality improvement (Brown & Tandon, 1983). The assumption has been that problems could be solved through social engineering, new knowledge produced, and transformational leadership inspired to create a self-reflective community of inquiry (Argyris & Schön, 1974; Greenwood, Whyte, & Harkavy, 1993).

Although this approach can be abused through management manipulation, humanistic psychology researchers have created a cooperative inquiry strand, which adopts a firm belief in human agency—that people can choose how they live through a process of reflexive inquiry. This strand insists on researcher and community member reciprocity, with no parties excluded or alienated from the research process as they exchange ideas and actions (Rowan, 2001).

Since the early 1970s, the tradition of participatory research, arising within Latin America, Asia, and Africa and known collectively as the Southern tradition, received much of its impetus from the structural crises of underdevelopment, the radical critiques by social scientists of existing theory, liberation theology, and the search for new practice by the adult education and development fields in how best to work with communities vulnerable to globalization by the dominant society.

An outflow of education and social science academics from universities to work with land movements and community-based organizations transformed the concept that knowledge emanated from the academy and created an openness to popular and existential knowledge learned from experience, or *vivencia,* from the Latin American philosopher José Ortega y Gasset (Fals-Borda, 1991). Exiled Brazilian philosopher Paulo Freire, through the publication of *Pedagogy of the Oppressed* (1970) and other banned writings during the Latin American military dictatorships in the 1970s, influenced the transformation of the research relationship from viewing communities as objects of study to viewing community members as subjects of their own experience and inquiry. Freire's notion was that reality was not an objective truth or facts to be discovered but "includes the ways in which the people involved with facts perceive them. . . . The concrete reality is the connection between subjectivity and objectivity, never objectivity isolated from subjectivity" (1982, p. 29).

Rather than viewing research as neutral, participatory research intellectuals adopted the goals and commitment to critical consciousness, emancipation, and social justice as they challenged their own roles in communities with the ideology that "self-conscious people, those who are poor and oppressed, will progressively transform their environment by their own praxis" (Rahman, 1991, p. 13). Intellectuals were to be catalysts and supports of educational processes but not the vanguard of social change (Hall et al., 1982).

By 1976, institutions outside of academia began to take the lead, with the creation of the Participatory Research Group by the International Council of Adult Education in Toronto and its network of centers in India, Tanzania, the Netherlands, and Latin America (Hall, 2001). Other nodes of activity in the same tradition included the Collaborative Action Research Group's work with Aborigines in Australia (Kemmis & McTaggart, 2001) and the Highlander Center in Tennessee, the oldest adult education and social change center in the United

States (Bell, Gaventa, & Peters, 1990; Horton, 1990). The first World Symposium of Action Research was held in Cartegena, Colombia, in 1977, with the eighth held twenty years later, again in Cartegena, with two thousand delegates from sixty-one countries (Fals-Borda, 2001).

The Southern tradition, originating in Marxist social theory, has viewed social progress through mass participation in challenging inequitable distribution of resources. This tradition has more recently incorporated post-Marxist approaches that highlight the noneconomic, cultural, and social oppression of mainstream knowledge production (Said, 1994). In both research and political terms, participatory research therefore challenges the material production of power in communities and the knowledge production of power through its dominant academic discourse.

By 1985, Fals-Borda had started using the term *participatory action research* to emphasize the role of action in the research process, but with no references to the Northern approach, he remained grounded in the emancipatory participatory research tradition. Likewise, organizational development theorist William Foote Whyte had published in 1991 a book titled *Participatory Action Research* but included no references to the Southern tradition.

In the past decade, traditions and common principles have undergone a rapprochement, though overt and subtle differences remain. Constructivist-focused evaluators, for example, have shared values of transforming the relationship between the researcher and the researched and expanding the dimensions of knowing and a mandate for action, though they have often seen their role first as utilization-focused rather than as having a political agenda (Lincoln, 2001).

It is difficult to place each term used by various disciplines on the continuum between the problem-solving utilitarian and the emancipatory traditions because the actual research practice may vary with the local context, history, and ideology of the stakeholders. In general, however, action science and related traditions grounded in the Lewinian model would be found at one end of the continuum, with cooperative and mutual inquiry moving closer to the middle. The participatory research and PAR approaches associated with Freirian methods and the Southern tradition would be clustered at the other end. Understanding and dissecting the issues, however, within the core concepts of participation, knowledge, power, and praxis will enable each of us to reflect on our own practice and discover where we fall on this continuum.

CORE CONCEPTS AND NEW THEORIES

To adhere to the emancipatory tradition in CBPR, we need to examine or "problematize" four key concepts in our practice: the role of participation of the community and researcher, the types and use of knowledge produced by the research, the context of power dynamics, and the goals of praxis, or the social action-conscientization-reflection cycle. To situate these concepts in the Southern tradition, we will include contributions from political economy, critical, postmodern, poststructuralist, postcolonial, and feminist theory.

Participation

Habermas observed that "in the process of enlightenment, there can only be participants" (1974, p. 40). If we adopt Habermas's succinct statement in our work to create a democratic society, the core question remains, What do we mean by "participation"? Who is participating, for whom are we participating, in what spheres are we participating, to what ends or goals are we participating, and perhaps most important of all, who or what is limiting participation in shaping our lives? In other words, where does the power lie? (Bopp, 1994; Cornwall & Jewkes, 1995; Gaventa & Cornwall, 2001; Rifkin, 1996).

For community based participatory research, in particular, we need to ask, "If all research involves participation, what makes research participatory?" (Cornwall & Jewkes, 1995, p. 1668). In the health field, such questions become particularly crucial as international conferences since Alma Ata (1977) through Ottawa (1986) and Jakarta (1996) have declared the importance of community participation to improve health conditions. With health viewed as a resource originating from people within their social context rather than from the health care system, participation is seen as critical to reduce dependency on health professionals, to ensure cultural sensitivity of programs, to facilitate sustainability of change efforts, and to enhance health in its own right (Jewkes & Murcott, 1998).

Despite the decades of value-based rhetoric of participation in development studies, public health, and participatory research, only relatively recently have researchers begun to question if the reality of participation reflects the ideal. Some have questioned the authenticity of the participatory process (Tandon, 1988) or viewed participation in a more limited fashion, as in the use of rapid rural appraisal to engage community members as informants (Cornwall & Jewkes, 1995). Others have suggested that participation is a developmental emergent process that requires nurturing beyond the initial intentions (Goodman, 2001; Greenwood et al., 1993).

The most important issue for community based participatory researchers is the relationship between outside researchers and community members (Brown & Vega, 1996). Habermas offers insights into these relationships through his theorizing about modernity (Habermas, 1987). To Habermas, capitalist societies have created two distinct worlds: the *systems world* of highly differentiated legal, economic, and political systems and the *life world,* the resource in which individuals form their identity and reproduce their culture.

As the life world has increasingly become colonized by the systems world, people begin to define themselves by their role within systems. They become objects—clients and consumers—rather than subjects or democratic members of civil society who reproduce themselves as social and cultural beings. The manifestation of this colonization is seen in anomie, powerlessness, dysfunctional behaviors, increases in mental and physical disease, and the overall decline of civil society. For CBPR, outside researchers may unwittingly become part of this dynamic, as our universities often reinforce community member roles as clients and consumers.

Even within a CBPR practice that recognizes the importance of establishing relationships beyond that of expert and client, the actual practice between outside researchers and community members remains complex and involves making transparent the power differences, recognized or not. This includes who represents the community at the community level and who represents findings to the external world, as well as the very basic question of which realities are revealed in the research process and which realities will remain hidden as part of the natural participation of community members (Scott, 1990).

Although CBPR researchers expect that building collaborative relationships with community members will be sufficient to surmount any differences, power differentials can and often do remain substantial. Academic researchers almost always have greater access to resources, scientific knowledge, research assistants, and time than small community based organizations (Chataway, 1997). In a participatory evaluation study of healthy communities in New Mexico, lack of recognition of the power differences between communities and the evaluator inhibited collaboration and restricted use of research findings (Wallerstein, 1999).

One of the principles of CBPR involves recognizing that both outside researchers and community members have needs and agendas, which may sometimes be shared and other times be divergent or conflicting, especially if professional researchers pursue their career advancement at the expense of the community (Fine, 1994; Huberman, 1991; Lather, 1986). For example, community members might be more interested in job development that research projects may bring to a community than in the knowledge production itself. In practice, this principle is highly complex, starting with the concern about who decides the research agenda.

Increasingly, CBPR researchers interested in genuine partnership face communities, previously colonized by researchers, that are now demanding their rights to determine what research is done and who will do it (De Bruyn, Chino, Serna, & Fullerton-Gleason, 2001). Historically, "helicopter research" in Indian Country, for example, was epitomized by the researcher flying in and taking information without leaving anything in return (Deloria, 1992). If CBPR practitioners fail to recognize the validity of these historical issues, they might be denied entry or have their research undermined through overt or hidden forms of resistance. In some tribal communities, institutional review boards directly control (and deny) access to researchers who are not fulfilling community needs, including the ability to publish findings. Good CBPR practice therefore demands a recognition of historic or current oppression and assurance that all parties will materially benefit from the knowledge produced (Duran & Duran, 1999; Duran, Duran, Brave Heart, & Davis, 1998; see also Appendix E).

Nevertheless, the contribution of CBPR researchers should not be undervalued. They may know of funding opportunities and have expertise to offer about important health issues. They may also face their own challenges for academic tenure and promotion, which can be made difficult in the context of building long-term relationships with communities (Goodman, 2001). Negotiation of a mutual code of collaborative working relationships and ethics (see Chapter Three) therefore becomes critical for adopting a participatory partnership (Fawcett, 1991; Gitlin & Russell, 1994; Perkins & Wandersman, 1990). Recently, researchers have developed instruments to evaluate the extent to which their research would serve the community and the extent of community participation in the research itself (George, Daniel, & Green, 1998; Brown & Vega, 1996; see also Appendixes A, C, and D). These instruments, coupled, with codes of ethics developed with and by local tribes and communities (Macaulay et al., 1998; see also Appendix E), provide a welcome opportunity to ensure that communities are a driving force in their own research. Codes of ethics may also need to be renegotiated periodically as different research stages generate different levels of excitement, buy-in, or concerns of possible abuse of findings.

Who represents the community remains a key issue in participation. Often service providers are asked to serve on community advisory boards, yet they may or may not represent their constituents (Jewkes & Murcott, 1998). As Aiwa Ong has stated, there is a First World in every Third World community (Ong, 1991). If stakeholders reflect people who have the power base of the First World, are they appropriate to fully represent local community residents (Green & Mercer, 2001)? As expressed throughout this book, CBPR represents the view that community members themselves need to be brought into the research process as decision-making participants. Participatory mechanisms range from least to most powerful, from community members who provide information input to being involved as focus group facilitators or interviewers to participating in data analysis and interpretation as advisory groups to actual decision-making authority, such as institutional review boards or partnership boards. The relationships, which favor the community most, are those that place funding in the community lead agencies, which then subcontract to researchers (Duran & Duran, 1999).

A provocative new book, *Participation: The New Tyranny?* (Cooke & Kothari, 2001), challenges the field of developmental studies in its wholesale adoption of the technologies and ideologies of participation. The authors argue that communities are too often viewed naively, concealing power relations and masking biases within communities, such as those based on ethnicity, gender, caste, or age, or between facilitators and community participants, between donors and beneficiaries, and in the discourse of participation itself.

Three tyrannies are proposed: the *tyranny of decision making,* in which legitimate decision-making processes are overridden by development experts; the *tyranny of the group,* where group dynamics may reinforce the individuals in the community already in power; and the *tyranny of methods* such as participatory rural appraisal (PRA). An approach like PRA ideally uses dialogue and often visualization processes with local people to "document and acknowledge local knowledge" (De Koning & Martin, 1996b, p. 2), enriching our understanding of community strengths and health needs that may in turn contribute to problem solving. Yet the prominence of these methods may obscure the need for analysis of larger institutional structures and policies that often override local determinants of well-being (Francis, 2001). These are important challenges and remind those of us working in the field that CBPR is not "reified out there, but constructed by a cadre of . . . professionals, be they academics, practitioners or policy makers, whose ability to create and sustain this discourse is indicative of the power they possess" (Cooke & Kothari, 2001, p. 15).

Unlike these authors, however, we take a more optimistic stand, that reflexivity within ourselves and with our community collaborators can inspire a continual cycle of learning about our successes and about our failures. As Rifkin (1996) states, participation should not be seen as a magic bullet but as a complex and iterative process, which can change, grow, or diminish, based on the unfolding of power relations and the historical and social context of the research project. Ultimately, the issue is how differences are negotiated so that the research perspective does not supercede community perspectives or colonize the community in its intent or its outcomes.

Theories and Use of Knowledge

The creation and use of knowledge are inherently the motivating force behind all research, yet like participation, CBPR raises the questions of knowledge defined by whom, about whom, and for what purpose (Cornwall & Jewkes, 1995; Gaventa & Cornwall, 2001; Hall, 1992; Tandon, 1988). Although positivist research paradigms have legitimized researcher interpretation of knowledge creation as a neutral and value-free activity, CBPR researchers have often drawn from critical theory, interpretive, and postmodern approaches to research. These approaches offer more reflexive and pluralistic (including both qualitative and quantitative) modes of inquiry and explore the dialectic between researcher and what's being researched (Denzin & Lincoln, 2000; Poland, 1996; Reason, 1994).

CBPR critiques of positivists' search for objective truths have been pointed, stating that traditional inquiry discounts experiential knowledge, reinforces passivity of the subjects, and obscures other voices (Gaventa & Cornwall, 2001). In relation to public health theory, positivism has been criticized: not only is it "*not* the only method for gaining valid knowledge, but it is a powerful ideology that thwarts the field's interests in alleviating suffering and promoting social justice" (Buchanan, 1998, p. 440). A reductionist approach, for example, which identifies lack of information as a proximal risk factor for ill health, may do more harm than good by directing attention away from inequitable social processes that determine access to education.

The emancipatory traditions of CBPR have drawn on critical social theory, which views knowledge as historically and socially constructed and mediated through perspectives of the dominant society. Critical theorist Jürgen Habermas's ideas of knowledge production are particularly relevant for CBPR and can be seen as three distinct aims of research (1971; Kemmis, 2001). *Empiricoanalytic reason* supports the aim of technical, instrumental control over problems and material and economic reproduction, which is a rationale for the Northern tradition of utilitarian problem solving to make systems work better. *Practical reason* is normative in that actors orient their actions to common values of their cultural and social environment, rather than as solitary actors. *Practical reason* aims to reproduce the social and cultural spheres of individuals and can inform both the Northern and Southern traditions. For example, reflection on community values in CBPR can produce an appreciation for history and tradition or a questioning of the need for cultural change.

Critical or emancipatory reason reflects the research aim to go beyond existing power struggles, such as ethnic and religious strife, to understand why a situation has come about based on human actions and what the future could be—central organizing principles of the Southern tradition (Habermas, 1971; Kemmis & McTaggart, 2000).

Whereas all three kinds of knowledge may be useful for improving health and social conditions, Habermas's call for critical emancipatory knowledge challenges both outside researchers and community members to go beyond their existing and conventional worldviews to make room for new social relations while not losing their cultural identities in the process. Emancipatory reason demands critical reflection and action for researchers and community members to recognize issues of concern, to understand how current discourse and social practice have been historically constructed, and to come to consensus through the course of dialogue and involvement with social movements about what new practices, discourse patterns, or social actions can be undertaken (Kemmis, 2001; Kemmis & McTaggart, 2000).

Freire provides the psychosocial understanding of how emancipatory knowledge can lead to having the power to make change. As people engage in dialogue with each other about their communities and the larger social context, their own internal representation—how they think and ascribe meaning—about their social world changes; their relationships to each other become strengthened; and ultimately, their ability to reflect on their own values and choices is affected.

These three dimensions have been called the "power of competence, connection, and confidence" (Park, 2001, p. 87).

Power Relations

Although knowledge is a major source of power and control, other material and institutional power relations are also central for understanding the dynamic relationships between researchers and communities. In addition to a two-tiered approach of the power relationships between researchers and communities, CBPR is situated within a much broader context of power relations, including the societal context in which the research takes place, the origins of the research, and the purpose of the research itself. CBPR researchers who hope to act on the most important problems in society, such as disparities based on race, class, gender, and other socially constructed domains, need to produce knowledge that clarifies and seeks to change the maldistribution of power and resources.

In addressing imbalances of power in society, participatory researchers may be aided by political economy—a broad, multidisciplinary framework that emphasizes how the structure of the economy and society affects the lives (and the health) of individuals (Alford & Friedland, 1985). Political economy assumes that resources are allocated not according to merit or relative efficiency but on the basis of power. In the area of health and health care, it suggests that the behavior and dynamics of visible and behind-the-scenes players can be understood only in relation to their power and class position in society (Minkler, Wallace, & McDonald, 1994–1995; Navarro, 1984).

Gaventa (1980) and Gaventa and Cornwall (2001) have presented four dimensions of power in CBPR, analyzing how power is exercised and who is excluded. The pluralist liberal democratic view assumes that power is a product of an open system of equal competing agendas. Who wins and who loses is based on knowledge or resources, and lack of participation is seen as a function of apathy or choice (Dahl, 1969). Individuals with this perspective, also called situational power, make decisions according to the existing rules of the game, representing in some ways a reflection of the Northern tradition.

The second view argues that there is a hidden face to power in which some actors and issues are kept from open discussion through a mobilization of bias by elites and powerful organizations against their interests (Bachrach & Baratz, 1962). Dominant knowledge or resources may establish rules that simply discredit other knowledge bases.

Stephen Lukes (1974) raises a third, and more insidious, dimension of power that excludes grievances by preventing conflicts from even surfacing because of its systemic and structural nature. Certain interests are favored without need for conscious decisions or manipulation of policy (Minkler et al., 1994–1995; Wallace, Williamson, Lung, & Powell, 1991). On this level, internalized oppression (see Chapter Four for more detail) or other hegemonic and ideologic means of control contribute to the development of a culture of silence, where people have a restricted view of their own possibilities.

All three of these dimensions represent, in Foucault's framework (1977), a repressive view of power, which is seen as a resource that individuals have or don't have. Repressive power may be exercised through direct and indirect control over people's opportunities to better education, employment, and living conditions, which together favor certain interests or classes of people over others. Emancipatory CBPR uncovers these mechanisms of control, biases, and internalized representations of reality as a key strategy for change.

Foucault (1979) has best articulated a fourth perspective of power as productive and relational. Rather than repressive power being monolithic or a resource to be possessed, he conceptualizes power as built into a web of discourses and practices found in institutions, communities, and families that are exercised through actions in a multiplicity of relationships. These power relationships are inherently unstable and therefore open to challenge.

Productive power has both negative and positive attributes. On the one hand, productive power may produce discourses that can marginalize or stereotype communities, as in fundamentalist tracts portraying women as patriarchally dominated housewives and mothers. On the other hand, productive power as an emancipatory CBPR discourse challenges communities to reshape their self-view away from clients or consumers toward democratic community participants and research collaborators.

For Foucault, knowledge symbolizes power. "There is no power relation without the correlative constitution of a field of knowledge, nor any knowledge that does not presuppose and constitute at the same time power relations" (1977, p. 27). Repressive power, as expressed through the "regimes of truth," which also permeate public health institutions and research discourse, can circumscribe how communities may respond to researchers.

As power, however, knowledge also opens the possibility of communities challenging existing limits and reconceptualizing new practices (Foucault, 1980; Gaventa & Cornwall, 2001). As Deveaux (1999, p. 242) has noted, "Where there is power, there is resistance." As communities gain power in the research relationship and researchers lose power, community members may also expand their capabilities to bring about change in an unjust world (Le Compte, 1995).

In CBPR, as noted earlier, the relationship between researchers and communities requires trust and mutual commitment over time. These relationships don't take place in a vacuum. Rather, they are subject to overall power relations in society, the history of research in the community, the immediate issues facing the community, and the origins of this particular research and the ability to negotiate relationships between the CBPR researchers and community representatives. CBPR practice therefore must be about asking questions and examining the power dynamics that exist when some people speak and others are silent.

In a valuable analysis of community dialogue, James Scott (1990) has outlined public and hidden discourse (see Chapter Four). In relation to research, public transcripts are the official language of what outside researchers bring to the table and what communities offer in return. Public transcripts may not be fully revelatory, however. For example, community members may seem to be participating but are in fact responding in ways that they think will please the researchers. Hidden transcripts may remain outside the purview of what is observed by the outside research team or represent a form of resistance that is also unobserved in the public space. As noted in Chapter Four, there is a critical need for balance in CBPR relationships between maintaining safety for expression on the one hand and respecting silence on the other.

In the postmodern perspective, CBPR researchers would situate themselves by their gender, race, class, and status positions in relation to the researched. This exposure of one's own stance establishes the outside researcher as only one player in the telling and interpretation of stories and disrupts the researcher-community imbalance of power (Buroway et al., 1991). If the goal is to create reciprocity, then both outside researchers and community members become, in the words of singer Chris Williamson, "the changer and the changed" (Lather, 1986, p. 263).

In CBPR, there is never a perfect equilibrium of power. All research efforts undergo cycles of participation and questioning by community members, bringing greater or lesser participation and greater or lesser buy-in. In times of frustration, community members may retreat to hidden discourse, expressing concerns in private, ridiculing experts (especially if they speak languages different than the outside researchers), or simply pretending greater willingness to participate. In more open times, public discourse may represent more sharing and even access to otherwise hidden discourse. This dialectic of collaboration and resistance between research partners and community participants presents a continual challenge.

Emerging theories of feminism, poststructuralism, and postcolonialism offer conceptual innovation into theories of power and authority in their applicability to CBPR.

CONTRIBUTIONS OF FEMINISM, POSTSTRUCTURALISM, AND POSTCOLONIALISM

Feminist participatory researchers add critical dimensions to our understanding of the theory and practice of CBPR. In early critiques, they challenged the exclusion of women through the use of universal language of "the oppressed" and the lack of attention to gender differences of participation in data collection and analysis (Maguire, 1987).

Over the past forty years, feminism has shifted from studying women as a universal construct to "theorizing gender" culturally and historically, with shifting identities of class, race and ethnicity, sexual orientation, and other differences (Collins, 2000; Hesse-Biber, Gilmartin, & Lydenberg, 1999; Maguire, 2001; Olesen, 2000). Gender is seen as central in power relations, with different mechanisms that can silence women, such as censorship, intimidation, marginalization, or trivialization (Devault & Ingraham, 1999; Maguire, 2001).

Poststructuralism focuses on the ways that language, discourse, and narratives construct reality and our view of social institutions, such as academia, public health, or medicine, and how these constructions are resisted by communities. Postcolonialism takes this further by focusing on how race became the primary organizing principle of European colonization. To counter the civilizing mission of dominant portrayals of the "Other," CBPR research, within a postcolonial tradition, seeks to uncover and privilege community explanations and narratives of the condition of their lives (Duran & Duran, 1995; Walters & Simoni, 2002). The role of the outside researcher may therefore be largely to weaken the power of the dominant discourse and create spaces for competing community discourses to emerge.

In CBPR, poststructuralist, postcolonialist, and feminist theory share certain methods and goals: analyzing personal lives in relation to the structures (both overt and hidden) that might control people's lives; celebrating strengths, not just emphasizing victimization; restructuring the power relations within the research process; and working for goals of social justice (Maguire, 2001).

Issues within feminism and within racism (discussed in detail in Chapter Four), such as how women (or women of color) construct their identities in a particular context, elucidate the complexities of CBPR in understanding communities and change processes (Edmondson Bell, 2001). African American women, for example, as detailed in Patricia Hill Collins's work (2000), can appear to conform to societal roles in public spaces yet adopt opposing roles in other contexts, such as church, family, or community. In complex ways, they are resisting stories of themselves as the Other; constructing new stories based on other identities, such as sisterhood or motherhood, an expression of Foucaultian productive power; and remaining silent or not about the extent to which dominant society depends on them (Collins, 1999, 2000; Fine, Weis, Weseen, & Wong, 2000).

"Post-" theories have challenged the right of researchers to privilege their interpretations and thereby silence the community (Fine et al., 2000; Mohanty, 1988; Spivak, 1988). For CBPR, interpretation of data often falls to the outside researcher; participatory data analysis is very difficult to achieve. Often with qualitative data, the mountain of transcripts is daunting, and the iterative processes needed are time-consuming. Yet if undertaken, participatory data analysis of both qualitative and quantitative data not only improves external validity of the data but forces a different approach to publication as well.

Michelle Fine (1994) articulates three researcher stances in relation to community voices and their publication: (1) "ventriloquy," when researchers describe the Other as empirical truth, never using the word *I* in their texts or connecting themselves (by gender, race, or class) to their analysis of the data; (2) "voices," when researchers speak for the Other, recording people's words and stories without a critical analysis of the context or history of people's experience; and (3) "activist feminist research," when researchers develop a negotiated stance, being explicit about their position and identity, and interrupting "Othering" in the text through dialogue with the Other in interpretation and portrayal of knowledge.

This third stance (which postmodernists adopt) cautions against simply portraying multiple community voices, because some voices may be more powerful than others or may reflect internalized oppression rather than fostering an emancipatory perspective illuminating oppressive conditions (Fine, 1994; Le Compte, 1995). Fine et al. (2000) calls for us as outside (or trained) researchers to be wary of research intended to "help the Other" and encourages us to engage in the difficult task of negotiating representation with the community as we situate ourselves and our community partners in all phases of the research process.

In sum, feminism, poststructuralism, and postcolonialism provide useful lenses to broaden our understanding of the core concepts in CBPR: participation, production of knowledge, and power, as discussed earlier in this chapter; and praxis, as discussed next.

PAULO FREIRE AND PRAXIS

Although community based participatory research rests solidly on critical theory and postmodern revolutions in academia and on our understanding of the complexities of participation, knowledge, and power relations, this orientation to research also cannot exist without its practical applications in the community. Reality dictates that research is not divorced from its effects on communities: CBPR research, whether focused on etiology, explanatory models, or direct community improvement, always takes an intervention activist approach. To explore the actualities of CBPR practice and methodologies, therefore, it is helpful to return to Brazilian educator Paulo Freire, a major source of inspiration from the Southern emancipatory tradition.

Freire's starting point of concern for the powerless is reflected in his initial work teaching literacy in the *favelas* and *barrios* with the marginalized poor, who had what he termed a naive or magical consciousness that they could not be actors in their own fate. Using emotionally and socially charged words and pictures, Freire (1970, 1982) generated dialogue to facilitate transformation to conscientization (or critical consciousness) and praxis (action based on critical reflection) on how to improve their lives. Exiled from Brazil at the time of the military coup in 1964, Freire fled to Chile until exiled once again; he worked for the World Council of Churches until he was able to return to Brazil by the early 1990s.

To Freire (1970), the purpose of education is human liberation, which means that people are the subjects of their own learning, not empty vessels filled by the knowledge of experts. To promote the learner as subject, Freire proposes a listening-dialogue-action approach (Wallerstein, 1992). The first step is listening to the generative themes or issues of community members in order to create a *structured dialogue* in which everyone participates as co-learners to jointly construct a shared reality of themselves as individuals in their social context. Individuals must not only be involved in efforts to identify their problems but also to engage in conscientization to analyze the societal context for these problems. *Conscientização* in Portuguese connotes both critical consciousness and conscience and personal engagement with the knowledge (Freire, 1970; Park, 2001).

The goal of dialogue and conscientization is *praxis,* the ongoing interaction between reflection and the actions people take to promote individual and social change. It is only through actions and encountering resistance to social actions that people truly shape their knowledge of how the world works, linking their cognitive intellectual understanding with the visceral and emotional.

Much of the creativity of the Freirian approach, also called *popular* or *empowerment education,* has been in the development of codes (sometimes called triggers or discussion catalysts) that codify the generative themes into a physical form (using pictures, videos, role-playing, and so on) so that participants can "see" their reality with new eyes and consequently develop alternative ways of thinking and acting. Multiple dialogue and communication methodologies, such as photodocumentary research (see Chapter Nine); Agosto Boal's Theater of the Oppressed to characterize conditions; and video portrayals of research results, rather than written reports, are all expressions of this approach (Bell et al., 1990; Sohng, 1996). A Freirian structured questioning approach facilitates dialogue based on the triggers, which can benefit the participatory process, especially during the research interpretation phase (Arnold, Burke, James, Martin, & Thomas, 1995; Hope & Timmel, 1984; Nadeau, 1996; Vella, 1995; Wallerstein, 1994).

Worldwide, popular or empowerment education has been widely applied in the fields of adult and health education and community development. In the United States, the Highlander Research and Education Center has been an inspiration for the past sixty years in its history of participatory education, research, and labor, civil rights, voting rights, youth, and environmental organizing (Horton, 1990; Lewis, 2001).

For their underlying importance to CBPR, Freire's writings reinforce a deep belief in humanity and people's role in making change:

> To be a good [participatory researcher] means above all to have faith in people; to believe in the possibility that they can create and change things. It is also necessary to love . . . , to be convinced that the fundamental effort of community . . . education, is toward the liberation of people, never their "domestication." This liberation begins to the extent that men [and women] reflect on themselves and their condition in the world—the world in which and with which they find themselves. To the extent that they are more conscientized, they will insert themselves as subjects into their own history [Freire, 1971, p. 62].

In *Teaching to Transgress,* bell hooks (1994) builds on Freire and Thich Nhat Hanh to challenge us to examine the mutual process of "engaged pedagogy," or in our case, engaged CBPR. Rather than expecting only that community members become immersed in the creation of their history, CBPR research is a process in which outside researchers also become transformed. When we bring our own narratives or interpretations, "it eliminates the possibility that we can function as all-knowing silent interrogators" (p. 21).

Freire returns to this theme of researcher engagement in a dialogue book with Ira Shor in his discussion of the risks and fears of transformation, acknowledging that resistance may be real, "but if you don't risk, you don't create anything. Without risking for me, there is no possibility to exist" (Shor & Freire, 1987, p. 61). Concerns about becoming liberatory researchers may be based on our own previous socialization as researchers; our fears (often unspoken) that we *won't* be seen as experts; our fears or expectations that we *will* be seen as experts; or in some circumstances, fear of repression.

In a grand tour of participatory action research, Kemmis and McTaggart (2000) provide a taxonomy within which to view the study of practice in communities: as individual behavior studied objectively through the point of view of behaviors and performances, as individual behavior studied subjectively through personal meanings, as group behavior studied objectively through social interactions or systems, and as socially structured behaviors studied subjectively through analysis of discourse and historical tradition. They call for transcending "either-or dichotomies" for a critical social science engaged in a "reflexive-dialectical view of subjective-objective relations and connections" (p. 576)—in other words, a praxis of our own actions and theorizing as we engage in similar reflection with communities.

In a summary of key participatory research features, Kemmis and McTaggart (2000) further call for an eclectic and complex research practice that draws from

Marxist critical theory, applied utilitarian problem solving, and poststructuralist and feminist approaches, which promote our understandings of personal and collective agency under specific local and global historical conditions. Ultimately, they situate CBPR in its emancipatory tradition in its aim to work with communities to "release themselves from the constraints of irrational, unproductive, unjust, and unsatisfying social structures that limit their self-development and self-determination" (p. 597). Freirian methodologies can be helpful in pointing researchers and communities to the dialogical processes that facilitate these complex understandings.

Issues of participation, knowledge creation, power, and praxis are not abstract phenomena but rather authentic tensions that get enacted both in academia and in community settings. If, for example, we are not honest about our own power bases, as researchers with education, resources, skills, and privilege possibly due to race or ethnicity, gender, sexual orientation, or other identities, there is little hope to transform power dynamics. We need to understand how our personal biographies inform our ability to interpret the world, both in understanding the problems and in visioning community strengths. We also need to remember that we likely will not have full access to the phenomena being studied, though we must be open to mutual learning with community members and to the notion of the community as an educator whose knowledge can greatly enrich our understanding.

A major challenge for those of us in the field lies in the potential limits of CBPR given the realities of globalization, the imposition of Western cultural and economic hegemony on the rest of the world, and the difficulties for local communities in making meaningful change. Scaling up has become a buzzword in world institutions seeking to bring lessons from small communities to nation-states (Gaventa & Cornwall, 2001). Can CBPR be scaled up when so much depends on relationship building and commitment to collaborative work over time? Can realities be transformed at the local level that enhance health and contribute to a more equitable society? While these questions are important, we must ensure that critiques and challenges of CBPR don't play into conservative strategies that dismiss the role of communities participating in change (or that, conversely, leave the work of change to local communities without adequate government support).

Another major challenge is in recognizing the potential consequences of our research. As we produce negotiated versions of community "truths" from our investigations, these meanings may in turn supersede the very perspectives we worked to uncover. In a dynamic world, this is cause for both grave concern and for celebration. In many ways, CBPR relies on what N. Scott Momaday captured so beautifully: "We are what we imagine. Our very existence consists in our imagination of ourselves" (cited in Vizenor, 1978, p. vi).

Ultimately, CBPR is about knowledge creation and the value of practical and critical reason for understanding power dynamics, for recognizing the interconnections between the personal and social and between life worlds and system worlds, and for identifying the barriers and facilitators of human agency and participation toward the goals of action and social change. This can be a daunting and contradictory task but one full of promise and hope as we engage with community to promote democracy in a more just society.

References

Alford, R., & Friedland, R. (1985). *Powers of theory.* New York: Oxford University Press.

Argyris, C. Putnam, R., & Smith, D. M. (1985). *Action science: Concepts, methods, and skills for research and intervention.* San Francisco: Jossey-Bass.

Argyris, C., & Schön, D. (1974). *Theory and practice: Increasing professional effectiveness.* San Francisco: Jossey-Bass.

Arnold, R. Burke, B. James, C. Martin, D., & Thomas, B. (1995). *Educating for a change.* Toronto: Between the Lines.

Bachrach, P. & Baratz, M. S. (1962). The two faces of power. *American Political Science Review, 56,* 947–952.

Bell, B. Gaventa, J., & Peters, J. (Eds.). (1990). *We make the road by walking: Conversations on education and social change—Myles Horton and Paulo Freire.* Philadelphia: Temple University Press.

Bopp, M. (1994). The illusive essential evaluating participation in non-formal education and community development processes. *Convergence, 27,* 23–45.

Brown, D., & Tandon, R. (1983). Ideology and political economy in inquiry: Action research and participatory research. *Journal of Applied Behavioral Science, 19,* 277–294.

Brown, L., & Vega, W. (1996). A protocol for community-based research. *American Journal of Preventive Medicine, 12*(4), 4–5.

Brown, P. (1992). Popular epidemiology and toxic waste contamination: Lay and professional ways of knowing. *Journal of Health and Social Behavior, 22,* 267–281.

Buchanan, D. (1998). Beyond positivism: Humanistic perspectives on theory and research in health education. *Health Education Research, 13,* 439–450.

Buroway, M., Burton, A., Ferguson, A., Fox, K. J., Gamson, J., Gartrell, N., et al. (1991). *Ethnography unbound: Power and resistance in the modern metropolis.* Berkeley: University of California Press.

Chambers, R. (1992). *Rural appraisal: Rapid, relaxed and participatory.* Discussion Paper No. 311. Brighton, England: Institute for Development Studies.

Chataway, C. (1997). An examination of the constraints on mutual inquiry in a participatory action research project. *Journal of Social Issues, 4,* 747–766.

Chisholm, R., & Elden, M. (1993). Features of emerging action research. *Human Relations, 46,* 275–297.

Collins, P. H. (1999). Learning from the outsider within. In S. Hesse-Biber, C. Gilmartin, & R. Lyderberg (Eds.), *Feminist approaches to theory and methodology* (pp. 155–178). Oxford: Oxford University Press.

Collins, P. H. (2000). *Black feminist thought: Knowledge, consciousness, and the politics of empowerment* (2nd ed.). New York: Routledge.

Cooke, B. & Kothari, U. (Eds.). (2001). *Participation: The new tyranny?* London: Zed Books.

Cornwall, A., & Jewkes, R. (1995). What is participatory research? *Social Science and Medicine, 41,* 1667–1676.

Dahl, R. (1969). The concept of power. In R. Bell, D. Edwards, & H. Wagner (Eds.), *Political power: A reader in theory and research.* New York: Free Press.

De Bruyn, L., Chino, M., Serna, P., & Fullerton-Gleason, L. (2001). Child maltreatment in American Indian and Alaska Native communities: Integrating culture, history, and public health for intervention and prevention. *Child Maltreatment, 6*(2), 89–102.

De Koning, K., & Martin, M. (Eds.). (1996a). *Participatory research in health: Issues and experiences* (2nd ed.). London: Zed Books.

De Koning, K., & Martin, M. (1996b). Participatory research in health: Setting the context. In K. De Koning & M. Martin (Eds.). *Participatory research in health: Issues and experiences* (2nd ed., pp. 1–18). London: Zed Books.

Deloria, V. (1992). *God is red: A native view of religion.* Golden, CO: North American Press.

Denzin, N. K., & Lincoln, Y. S. (Eds.). (2000). *Handbook of qualitative research* (2nd ed.). Thousand Oaks, CA: Sage.

Devault, M., & Ingraham, C. (1999). Metaphors of silence and voice in feminist thought. In M. Devault, *Liberating method* (R. Bell, D. Edwards, & H. Wagner, Eds.; pp. 175–186). Philadelphia: Temple University Press.

Deveaux, M. (1999). Feminism and empowerment. In S. Hesse-Biber, C. Gilmartin, & R. Lydenberg (Eds.), *Feminist approaches to theory and methodology* (pp. 236–256). Oxford: Oxford University Press.

Duran, B., & Duran, E. (1999). Assessment, program planning, and evaluation in Indian Country: Toward a postcolonial practice. In R. M. Huff & M. V. Kline (Eds.), *Promoting health in multicultural populations: A handbook for practitioners* (pp. 291–311). Thousand Oaks, CA: Sage.

Duran, E., & Duran, B. (1995). *Native American postcolonial psychology.* Albany: State University of New York Press.

Duran, E., Duran, B., Brave Heart, M.Y.H., & Davis, S. (1998). Healing the American Indian soul wound. In Y. Danieli (Ed.), *International handbook of multigenerational legacies of trauma.* New York: Plenum Press.

Edmondson Bell, E. (2001). Infusing race into the U.S. discourse on action research. In P. Reason & H. Bradbury (Eds.), *Handbook of action research: Participative inquiry and practice* (pp. 48–58). Thousand Oaks, CA: Sage.

Fals-Borda, O. (1991). Some basic ingredients. In O. Fals-Borda & M. A. Rahman (Eds.), *Action and knowledge: Breaking the monopoly with participatory action research* (pp. 3–13). New York: Apex.

Fals-Borda, O. (2001). Participatory (action) research in social theory: Origins and challenges. In P. Reason & H. Bradbury (Eds.), *Handbook of action research: Participative inquiry and practice* (pp. 27–37). Thousand Oaks, CA: Sage.

Fals-Borda, O., & Rahman, M. A. (Eds.). (1991). *Action and knowledge: Breaking the monopoly with participatory action research.* New York: Apex.

Fawcett, S. (1991). Some values guiding community research and action. *Journal of Applied Behavior Analysis, 24,* 621–636.

Fine, M. (1994). Working the hyphens. In N. K. Denzin & Y. S. Lincoln (Eds.), *Handbook of qualitative research* (pp. 70–82). Thousand Oaks, CA: Sage.

Fine, M., Weis, L., Weseen, S., & Wong, L. (2000). In N. K. Denzin & Y. S. Lincoln (Eds.), *Handbook of qualitative research* (2nd ed., pp. 107–132). Thousand Oaks, CA: Sage.

Flax, J. (1987). Postmodernism and gender relations in feminist theory. *Signs: Journal of Women and Culture in Society, 12,* 621–643.

Foucault, M. (1977). *Discipline and punish: The birth of the prison.* London: Allen Lane.

Foucault, M. (1979). *The history of sexuality* (Pt. 1). London: Allen Lane.

Foucault, M. (1980). *Power/knowledge: Selected interviews and other writings, 1972–1977* (C. Gordon, Ed.). New York: Pantheon Books.

Francis, P. (2001). Participatory development at the World Bank: The primacy of process. In B. Cooke & U. Kothari (Eds.), *Participation: The new tyranny?* (pp. 72–87). London: Zed Books.

Freire, P. (1970). *Pedagogy of the oppressed.* New York: Seabury Press.

Freire, P. (1971). To the coordinator of the culture circle. *Convergence, 4*(1), 61–62.

Freire, P. (1982). Creating alternative research methods: Learning to do it by doing it. In B. L. Hall, A. Gillette, & R. Tandon (Eds.), *Creating knowledge: A monopoly?* (pp. 29–37). Toronto: Participatory Research Network.

Gaventa, J. (1980). *Power and powerlessness: Quiescence and rebellion in an Appalachian valley.* Urbana: University of Illinois Press.

Gaventa, J., & Cornwall, A. (2001). Power and knowledge. In P. Reason & H. Bradbury (Eds.), *Handbook of action research: Participative inquiry and practice* (pp. 70–79). Thousand Oaks, CA: Sage.

George, M., Daniel, M., & Green, L. (1998). Appraising and funding participatory research in health promotion. *International Quarterly of Community Health Education, 18,* 181–197.

Gitlin, T., & Russell, R. (1994). Alternative methodologies and the research context. In A. Gitlin (Ed.), *Power and method: Political activism and educational research* (pp. 181–202). New York: Routledge.

Goodman, R. (2001). Community-based participatory research: Questions and challenges to an essential approach. *Journal of Public Health Management Practice, 7*(5), v–vi.

Green, L. W., & Mercer, S. (2001). Can public health researchers and agencies reconcile the push from funding bodies and the pull from communities? *American Journal of Public Health, 91,* 1926–1938.

Greenwood, D., Whyte, W., & Harkavy, I. (1993). Participatory action research. *Human Relations, 46,* 175–191.

Habermas, J. (1971). *Knowledge and human interests* (J. Shapiro, Trans.). Boston: Beacon Press.

Habermas, J. (1974). *Theory and practice* (J. Viertel, Trans.). London: Heinemann.

Habermas, J. (1987). *The theory of communicative action: Vol. 2. Lifeworld and system: A critique of functionalist reason* (T. McCarthy, Trans.). Boston: Beacon Press.

Hall, B. L. (1992). From margins to center: The development and purpose of participatory research. *American Sociologist, 23,* 15–28.

Hall, B. L. (2001). I wish this were a poem of practices of participatory research. In P. Reason & H. Bradbury (Eds.), *Handbook of action research: Participative inquiry and practice* (pp. 171–178). Thousand Oaks, CA: Sage.

Hall, B. L., Gillette, A., & Tandon, R. (1982). *Creating knowledge: A monopoly?* New Delhi: Society for Participatory Research in Asia.

Hatch, J., Moss, N., & Saran, A. (1993). Community research: Partnership in black communities. *American Journal of Preventive Medicine, 9*(6), 27–31.

Henderson, D. (1995). Consciousness raising in participatory research: Method and methodology for emancipatory nursing inquiry. *Advanced Nursing Science, 17*(3), 58–69.

Heron, J., & Reason, P. (2001). The practice of cooperative inquiry: Research "with" rather than "on" people. In P. Reason & H. Bradbury (Eds.), *Handbook of action research: Participative inquiry and practice* (pp. 179–188). Thousand Oaks, CA: Sage.

Hesse-Biber, S., Gilmartin, C., & Lydenberg, R. (Eds.). (1999). *Feminist approaches to theory and methodology.* New York: Oxford University Press.

Hills, M. (2001). Using cooperative inquiry to transform evaluation of nursing students' clinical practice. In P. Reason & H. Bradbury (Eds.), *Handbook of action research: Participative inquiry and practice* (pp. 340–347). Thousand Oaks, CA: Sage.

hooks, b. (1994). *Teaching to transgress.* New York: Routledge.

Hope, A., & Timmel, S. (1984). *Training for transformation* (Vols. 1–3). Harare, Zimbabwe: Mambo Press.

Horton, M. (1990). *The long haul: An autobiography.* Garden City, NY: Doubleday.

Huberman, M. (1991). Linkage between researchers and practitioners: A qualitative study. *American Educational Research Journal, 27,* 363–391.

Israel, B. A., Checkoway, B., Schulz, A. J., & Zimmerman, M. A (1994). Health education and community empowerment: Conceptualizing and measuring perceptions of individual, organizational, and community control. *Health Education Quarterly, 21,* 149–170.

Israel, B. A., Schulz, A. J., Parker, E. A., & Becker, A. B. (1998). Review of community-based research: Assessing partnership approaches to improve public health. *Annual Review of Public Health, 19,* 173–202.

Jewkes, R., & Murcott, A. (1998). Community representatives: Representing the "community"? *Social Science Medicine, 46,* 843–858.

Kemmis, S. (2001). Exploring the relevance of critical theory for action research: Emancipatory action research in the footsteps of Jürgen Habermas. In P. Reason & H. Bradbury (Eds.), *Handbook of action research: Participative inquiry and practice* (pp. 91–102). Thousand Oaks, CA: Sage.

Kemmis, S., & McTaggart, R. (2000). Participatory action research. In N. K. Denzin & Y. S. Lincoln (Eds.), *Handbook of qualitative research* (2nd ed., pp. 567–605). Thousand Oaks, CA: Sage.

Lather, P. (1986). Research as praxis. *Harvard Educational Review, 56,* 257–277.

Le Compte, M. (1995). Some notes on power, agenda, and voice: A researcher's personal evolution toward critical collaborative research. In P. McLaren & J. Giarelli (Eds.), *Critical theory and educational research* (pp. 91–112). Albany: State University of New York Press.

Lewin, K. (1997). *Resolving social conflicts and field theory in social science.* Washington, DC: American Psychological Association. (Original work published 1948)

Lewis, H. (2001). Participatory research and education for social change: Highlander research and education center. In P. Reason & H. Bradbury (Eds.), *Handbook of action research: Participative inquiry and practice* (pp. 356–362). Thousand Oaks, CA: Sage.

Lincoln, Y. S. (2001). Engaging sympathies: Relationships between action research and social constructivism. In P. Reason & H. Bradbury (Eds.), *Handbook of action research: Participative inquiry and practice* (pp. 124–132). Thousand Oaks, CA: Sage.

Lukes, S. (1974). *Power: A radical view.* London: Macmillan.

Macaulay, A., Delormier, T., McComber, A., Cross, E., Potvin, L., Paradis, G., Kirby, R., Saad-Haddad, C., & Derosiers, S. (1998). Participatory research with native community of Kahnawake creates innovative code of research ethics. *Canadian Journal of Public Health, 89,* 105–108.

Maguire, P. (1987). *Doing participatory research: A feminist approach.* Amherst: University of Massachusetts, Center for International Education.

Maguire, P. (2001). Uneven ground: Feminisms and action research. In P. Reason & H. Bradbury (Eds.), *Handbook of action research: Participative inquiry and practice* (pp. 59–69). Thousand Oaks, CA: Sage.

McTaggart, R. (1991). Principles for participatory action research. *Adult Education Quarterly, 41,* 168–187.

McTaggart, R. (1997). *Participatory action research: International contexts and consequences.* Albany: State University of New York Press.

Minkler, M., Wallace, S., & McDonald, M. (1994–1995). The political economy of health: A useful theoretical tool for health education practice. *International Quarterly of Community Health Education, 15,* 111–125.

Mohanty, C. (1988). Under Western eyes: Feminist scholarship and colonial discourses. *Feminist Review, 30,* 60–88.

Nadeau, D. (1996). *Counting our victories: Popular education and organizing.* New Westminster, British Columbia, Canada: Repeal the Deal Productions.

Navarro, V. (1984). Medical history as justification rather than explanation: A critique of Starr's "Social transformation of American medicine." *International Journal of Health Services, 14,* 511–528.

Olesen, V. (2000). Feminisms and models of qualitative research. In N. K. Denzin & Y. S. Lincoln (Eds.), *Handbook of qualitative research* (2nd ed., pp. 158–174). Thousand Oaks, CA: Sage.

Ong, A. (1991). *The ethnography of resistance.* Berkeley: University of California Press.

Park, P. (2001). Knowledge and participatory research. In P. Reason & H. Bradbury (Eds.), *Handbook of action research: Participative inquiry and practice* (pp. 81–90). Thousand Oaks, CA: Sage.

Park, P., Brydon-Miller, M., Hall, B. L., & Jackson, T. (Eds.). (1993). *Voices of change: Participatory research in the United States and Canada.* Westport, CT: Bergin & Garvey.

Perkins, D. D., & Wandersman, A. (1990). You'll have to work to overcome our suspicions: The benefits and pitfalls of research with community organizations. *Social Policy, 21,* 32–41.

Peters, M., & Robinson, V. (1984). The origins and status of action research. *Journal of Applied Behavioral Sciences, 20,* 113–124.

Poland, B. (1996). Knowledge development and evaluation in, of, and for healthy community initiatives: Part 1. Guiding principles. *Health Promotion International, 11,* 237–247.

Rahman, M. A. (1985). The theory and practice of participatory action research. In O. Fals-Borda (Ed.), *The challenge of social change* (pp. 107–132). Beverly Hills, CA: Sage.

Rahman, M. A. (1991). The theoretical standpoint of PAR. In O. Fals-Borda & M. A. Rahman (Eds.), *Action and knowledge: Breaking the monopoly with participatory action research* (pp. 13–24). New York: Apex.

Reason, P. (1994). Three approaches to participative inquiry. In N. K. Denzin & Y. S. Lincoln (Eds.), *Handbook of qualitative research* (pp. 324–339). Thousand Oaks, CA: Sage.

Reason, P., & Bradbury, H. (Eds.). (2001). *Handbook of action research: Participative inquiry and practice.* Thousand Oaks, CA: Sage.

Rifkin, S. (1996). Paradigms lost: Toward a new understanding of community participation in health programmes. *Acta Tropica, 61,* 79–92.

Rowan, J. (2001). The humanistic approach to action research. In P. Reason & H. Bradbury (Eds.), *Handbook of action research: Participative inquiry and practice* (pp. 114–123). Thousand Oaks, CA: Sage.

Said, E. (1994). *Culture and imperialism.* New York: Vintage Books.

Scott, J. (1990). *Domination and the arts of resistance: Hidden transcripts.* New Haven, CT: Yale University Press.

Shor, I., & Freire, P. (1987). *A pedagogy for liberation: Dialogues on transforming education.* Westport, CT: Bergin & Garvey.

Sohng, S.S.L. (1996). Participatory research and community organizing. *Journal of Sociology and Social Welfare, 23*(4), 77–97.

Spivak, G. (1988). Can the subaltern speak? In L. Nelson (Ed.), *Marxism and the interpretation of culture* (pp. 271–313). Urbana: University of Illinois Press.

Stringer, E. T. (1999). *Action research* (2nd ed.). Thousand Oaks, CA.: Sage.

Tandon, R. (1988). Social transformation and participatory research. *Convergence, 21*(2), 5–18.

Torbert, W. R. (2001). The practice of action inquiry. In P. Reason & H. Bradbury (Eds.), *Handbook of action research: Participative inquiry and practice* (pp. 250–260). Thousand Oaks, CA: Sage.

Vella, J. (1995). *Training through dialogue: Promoting effective learning and change in adults.* San Francisco: Jossey-Bass.

Vizenor, G. (1978). *Word arrows: Indians and whites in the new fur trade.* Minneapolis: University of Minnesota Press.

Wallace, S., Williamson, J., Lung, R., & Powell, L. (1991). A lamb in wolf's clothing? The reality of senior power and social policy. In M. Minkler & C. Estes (Eds.), *Critical perspectives on aging: The political and moral economy of growing old* (pp. 95–114). Amityville, NY: Baywood.

Wallerstein, N. (1992). Powerlessness, empowerment, and health: Implications for health promotion programs. *American Journal of Health Promotion, 6,* 197–205.

Wallerstein, N. (1994). Empowerment education applied to youth. In A. Matiella (Ed.), *The multicultural challenge in health education* (pp. 153–176). Santa Cruz, CA: ETR Associates.

Wallerstein, N. (1999). Power between evaluator and community: Research relationships within New Mexico's healthier communities. *Social Science and Medicine, 49,* 39–53.

Walters, K., & Simoni, J. (2002). Reconceptualizing Native women's health: An "indigenist" stress-coping model. *American Journal of Public Health, 92,* 520–524.

Whyte, W. (1991). *Participatory action research.* Thousand Oaks, CA: Sage.

Wing, S. (1998). Whose epidemiology, whose health? *International Journal of Health Services, 28,* 241–252.

CHAPTER THREE

Critical Issues in Developing and Following Community Based Participatory Research Principles

Barbara A. Israel
Amy J. Schulz
Edith A. Parker
Adam B. Becker
Alex J. Allen III
J. Ricardo Guzman

There is increasing research evidence that a disproportionate burden of morbidity and mortality exists within communities with few economic and social resources and communities of color, as noted in Chapter One (House & Williams, 2000; Kaplan, Pamuk, Lynch, Cohen, & Balfour, 1996; Krieger, Rowley, Herman, Avery, & Phillips, 1993; Lillie-Blanton, Parsons, Gayle, & Dievler, 1996; Marmot & Wilkinson, 1999). Addressing these disparities in health status is a major challenge for researchers, practitioners, community leaders, and the affected communities. Historically, within such communities, research has rarely benefited and sometimes actually harmed the people involved (Hatch, Moss, Saran, Presley-Cantrell, & Mallory, 1993; Thomas & Quinn, 1991), and interventions have often not been successful in improving health and well-being (Institute of Medicine, 1997; Mittelmark, Hunt, Heath, & Schmid, 1993; Steuart, 1993; Susser, 1995). In addition, for the most part, research has been conducted in ways that systematically exclude some people from having influence and power over the research process

Note: Portions of this chapter were adapted from "Review of Community-Based Research: Assessing Partnership Approaches to Improve Public Health," by B. A. Israel, A. J. Schulz, E. A. Parker, & A. B. Becker, 1998, *Annual Review of Public Health, 19,* pp. 173–202. Adapted with permission of the publisher. The authors thank Sue Andersen for her valuable assistance in the preparation of this manuscript.

(Fals-Borda & Rahman, 1991; Gaventa 1993; Hall, 1992; Hatch et al., 1993; Israel, Schulz, Parker, & Becker, 1998; Maguire, 1996; Wallerstein, 1999). To reduce these health disparities, there is a need to address fundamental questions such as these: What is the purpose of research? Who benefits from research? How are the results of research used? How can research contribute to reducing health disparities? and What role does research play in intervention and policy change and in knowledge generation?

There have been increasing calls and growing funding support for the use of more participatory approaches to research as one strategy for considering these questions (Green et al., 1995; Hatch et al., 1993; Israel et al., 1998; Labonté, 1997; Mittelmark et al., 1993). However, these more participatory approaches vary in the extent to which they address basic inequalities in both the content and process of conducting the research and applying the knowledge gained to change efforts. Specification of key principles of participatory research processes, referred to here as community based participatory research (CBPR), can serve as guidelines for those interested in this approach. However, it is also crucial to recognize that there are numerous issues that arise in every given local context and research partnership that need to be considered when developing and adhering to such CBPR principles. The purpose of this chapter is to present a set of community based participatory research principles based on an integration of the literature and the collective experiences of the authors, who have worked together on several CBPR efforts. In addition, we use case examples from our work, with a CBPR partnership, the Detroit Community-Academic Urban Research Center (URC),[1] to illustrate and discuss critical issues in the adoption and following of these principles. Throughout the chapter, we emphasize the importance of flexibility, constant reflection, and critical analysis in applying and adapting these principles in different contexts.

COMMUNITY BASED PARTICIPATORY RESEARCH: DEFINITION AND KEY PRINCIPLES[2]

Community based participatory research in public health is a partnership approach to research that equitably involves, for example, community members, organizational representatives, and researchers in all aspects of the research process. The partners contribute "unique strengths and shared responsibilities" (Green et al., 1995, p. 12) to enhance understanding of a given phenomenon and the social and cultural dynamics of the community, and integrate the knowledge gained with action to improve the health and well-being of community members (Hatch et al., 1993; Schulz, Israel, Selig, & Bayer, 1998).

The following nine principles or characteristics seek to capture key elements of this approach based on the present state of knowledge in the field. These principles will continue to evolve as further community based participatory research is conducted and evaluated. They are presented with the recognition that the extent to which any research endeavor can achieve any one or a combination of these principles will vary depending on the context, purpose, and participants involved in the process. Each principle may be located on a continuum, with the principle as described here representing an ideal goal toward which to strive (Cornwall, 1996; Green et al., 1995). Although they are presented here as distinct items, community based participatory research is an integration of these elements.

1. *CBPR recognizes community as a unit of identity.* The concept of community as an aspect of collective and individual identity is central to community based participatory research (Israel et al., 1998). Units of identity—for example, membership in a family, friendship network, or geographic neighborhood—are all socially constructed dimensions of identity, created and re-created through social interactions (Hatch et al., 1993; Steuart, 1993). Community is characterized by a sense of identification and emotional connection to other members, common symbol systems, shared values and norms, mutual (although not necessarily equal) influence, common interests, and commitment to meeting shared needs (Israel, Checkoway, Schulz, & Zimmerman, 1994; Klein, 1968; Sarason, 1984; Steuart, 1993). Communities of identity may be centered on a defined geographic neighborhood or a geographically dispersed group with a sense of common identity and shared fate (such as a racial or ethnic group or gay men and lesbians). Furthermore, a city or other geographic area may not be a community in this sense of the term but rather an aggregate of individuals who do not share a common identity or may contain several different overlapping communities of identity within its boundaries. Community based participatory approaches to research attempt to identify and to work with existing communities of identity and to strengthen a sense of community through collective engagement (Israel et al., 1994). Communities of identity contain many individual and organizational resources but may also benefit from skills and resources available from outside of the immediate community of identity. Thus community based participatory research efforts may involve individuals and groups who are not members of the community of identity. Such partnerships may include representatives from health and human service organizations, academia, community based organizations, and community members at large.

2. *CBPR builds on strengths and resources within the community.* Community based participatory research seeks to identify and build on strengths, resources, and relationships that exist within communities of identity to address their communal health concerns (Israel et al., 1998; McKnight, 1994; Steuart, 1993). These resources may include skills and assets of individuals (McKnight, 1994), networks of relationships characterized by trust, cooperation, and mutual

commitment (Israel & Schurman, 1990), and mediating structures within the community such as churches and other organizations where community members come together (Berger & Neuhaus, 1977). Community based participatory research explicitly recognizes and seeks to support or expand social structures and social processes that contribute to the ability of community members to work together to improve health.

3. *CBPR facilitates collaborative, equitable partnership in all phases of the research,* involving an empowering and power-sharing process that attends to social inequalities. In CBPR, all parties participate and share control over all phases of the research process, including problem definition, data collection, interpretation of results, and application of the results to address community concerns (De Koning & Martin, 1996; Green et al., 1995; Hatch et al., 1993; Israel, Schurman, Hugentobler, & House, 1992; Israel et al., 1998; Park, Brydon-Miller, Hall, & Jackson, 1993; Stringer, 1996). These partnerships focus on issues and concerns identified by community members (De Koning & Martin, 1996; Green et al., 1995; Hatch et al., 1993; Israel et al., 1998; Petras & Porpora, 1993; Singer, 1993) and create processes that enable all parties to participate and share influence in the research. Recognizing that socially and economically marginalized communities often have not had the power to name or define their own experience, researchers involved with CBPR acknowledge the inequalities between themselves and community participants and the ways that inequalities among community members may shape their participation and influence in collective research and action (Blankenship & Schulz, 1996; Maguire, 1987). Attempts to address these inequalities involve explicit attention to the knowledge and expertise of community members and an emphasis on creating an empowering process that includes sharing information, decision-making power, resources, and support among members of the partnership (Israel et al., 1994; Israel et al., 1998; Labonté, 1994; Martin, 1996).

4. *CBPR promotes co-learning and capacity building among all partners.* Community based participatory research is a co-learning process that facilitates the reciprocal transfer of knowledge, skills, and capacity (De Koning & Martin, 1996; Freire, 1973; Israel et al., 1994; Israel et al., 1998; Nyden & Wiewel, 1992; Singer, 1993; Stringer, 1996). For example, researchers can learn from community members' administrative and management skills and from their "local theories"— understandings commonly held about the community and broader social context (Elden & Levin, 1991), and community members acquire further skills in how to conduct research. Emphasis here is on enhancing the capacity of all partners involved, which will both improve the effectiveness of the CBPR effort and be applicable to other endeavors that partner organizations are involved in as well.

5. *CBPR integrates and achieves a balance between research and action for the mutual benefit of all partners.* Community based participatory research seeks

to build a broad body of knowledge related to health and well-being while also integrating and balancing that knowledge generation with community and social change efforts that address the concerns of the communities involved (Green et al., 1995; Israel et al., 1994; Israel et al., 1998; Maguire, 1987; Park et al., 1993; Singer, 1993). Information is gathered to inform action, and new understandings emerge as participants reflect on actions taken. If agreed on by the partners involved (see Chapter Nine), CBPR may not always incorporate a direct action component, but there is a commitment to the translation and integration of research results with community change efforts with the intention that all partners involved will benefit (De Koning & Martin, 1996; Green et al., 1995; Petras & Porpora, 1993; Schulz, Israel, et al., 1998).

6. *CBPR emphasizes local relevance of public health problems and ecological perspectives that recognize and attend to the multiple determinants of health and disease.* Community based participatory research addresses public health problems that are of local relevance to the community involved and considers the concept of health from a positive model (Antonovsky, 1979; Hancock, 1993) that emphasizes physical, mental, and social well-being (World Health Organization, 1946). It also emphasizes an ecological model of health (Gottlieb & McLeroy, 1994; Hancock, 1993; Israel et al., 1994, Israel et al., 1998; Stokols, Allen, & Bellingham, 1996) that, as defined by Bronfenbrenner (1990), considers and encompasses the individual, the immediate contexts within which he or she lives (such as family or social network), and the larger contexts in which these are embedded (such as community or society). Accordingly, such approaches recognize and attend to, for example, biomedical, social, economic, cultural, and physical environmental factors as determinants of health and disease. Given this attention to multiple units of practice and the complex set of determinants of health and disease, CBPR efforts strive to achieve broad-scale social changes aimed at eliminating health disparities.

7. *CBPR involves systems development through a cyclical and iterative process.* Community based participatory research involves systems development in which a system (for example, a partnership) develops the competencies to engage in a cyclical, iterative process that includes partnership development and maintenance, community assessment, problem definition, development of research methodology, data collection and analysis, interpretation of data, determination of action and policy implications, dissemination of results, action taking (as appropriate), specification of learnings, and establishment of mechanisms for sustainability (Altman, 1995; Israel et al., 1994; Israel et al., 1998; Stringer, 1996; Tandon, 1981).

8. *CBPR disseminates findings and knowledge gained to all partners and involves all partners in the dissemination process.* Community based participatory research seeks to disseminate findings and knowledge gained to all partners involved, in language that is understandable and respectful, and "where

ownership of knowledge is acknowledged" (Bishop, 1994, p. 186; Gaventa, 1993; Hall, 1992; Israel et al., 1998; Schulz, Israel, et al., 1998). The ongoing feedback of data and use of results to inform action are integral to this approach (Israel, Schurman, & Hugentobler, 1992; Schulz, Parker, et al., 2002). This dissemination principle also includes the involvement of all partners as coauthors and reviewers of publications and copresenters at meetings and conferences.

9. *CBPR involves a long-term process and commitment.* Given the negative experiences of many communities with research projects, and in order to genuinely follow the principles described so far, community based participatory research involves a long-term process and commitment on the part of all partners (Centers for Disease Control and Prevention and Agency for Toxic Substances and Disease Registry, 1997; Hatch et al., 1993; Israel, Schurman, Hugentobler, & House, 1992; Mittelmark et al., 1993). To establish and maintain the trust required to successfully conduct CBPR efforts and to accomplish the aims of reducing health disparities, this long-term commitment has to extend beyond a single research project or funding period. There needs to be a commitment to continue to work together even if funding is not available. While there is no set time frame for what "long-term" means, the emphasis in CBPR remains on the development of relationships and commitments that extend beyond any one funding period. Some goals, such as modifying local policies that affect, for example, the presence of environmental risks in a local community, may take a decade or more to realize. Although a specific partnership may reach a point at which it decides not to continue as a partnership, there should be a commitment to the relationships that exist between the individuals and organizations involved and agreement that they will continue to collaborate with and support each other as needed and as desired.

ISSUES IN DEVELOPING AND FOLLOWING CBPR PRINCIPLES

A number of publications in the literature have examined the challenges and facilitating factors in conducting community based participatory research (including Green et al., 1995; Israel et al., 1998; Israel et al., 2001; Lantz, Viruell-Fuentes, Israel, Softley, & Guzman, 2001; Schell & Tarbell, 1998; Schensul, 1999) and have discussed the key components of equitable community-researcher partnerships (Baker, Homan, Schonhoff, & Kreuter, 1999; Israel, Schurman, & Hugentobler, 1992; Koné et al., 2000; Labonté, 1997; Lasker, Weiss, & Miller, 2001; Northridge et al., 2000; Schensul, 1999). The purpose of this section is to discuss critical issues that specifically arise when trying to adopt and follow the nine CBPR principles presented earlier, providing cases examples from our own efforts. Drawing from the literature and our experiences, some of these issues are put forth as recommended strategies, while others raise questions that need to be considered for which there is no one suggested strategy or resolution. In all instances, we suggest that these are important topics for CBPR partnerships to reflect on and address.

1. *No one set of community based participatory research principles is applicable for all partnerships.* While we strongly support and work to apply the CBPR principles presented here, we recommend equally strongly that this set of principles not be adopted as is and imposed on other partnerships. Although we suggest that some core values underlying these principles may be applicable in most situations, all of these principles are not going to be applicable in all settings or in all cultures and communities. Furthermore, in keeping with CBPR approaches, any such principles must be "owned" by the specific group and therefore need to be adapted, taking into account the local context of each partnership. It is important not to assume that everyone will understand and agree to a set of principles developed by others. Furthermore, the very process of a partnership jointly developing its principles provides an opportunity for much needed dialogue and sharing of perspectives that helps build trust and establish relationships.

Several of us were involved in developing an initial set of CBPR principles as part of a community based public health (CBPH) initiative funded by the W. K. Kellogg Foundation that involved representatives from academia, health agencies, and community based organizations in Detroit and Flint, Michigan (Schulz, Israel, et al., 1998). This process of developing the principles took over a year and a half, involving multiple constituencies in numerous meetings, negotiations, and revisions before the final principles were adopted by all the partners involved. Several years later, when the Detroit Community-Academic Urban Research Center partnership was established, these original principles were distributed and discussed over several URC board meetings. The final principles adopted by the URC were an adaptation of those initially developed by the CBPH partnership. One addition, for example, was the inclusion of language that placed greater emphasis on both knowledge generation and action that benefits the community.

While the time spent to discuss and adopt the CBPR principles was much shorter for the URC partnership due to a preexisting set of principles to begin our conversations, it took the URC partnership longer to internalize and own the principles. The internalization of the principles began to happen only as we engaged in particular CBPR projects in which we faced implementing the principles on a day-to-day basis. As new URC-affiliated projects are organized and new partners are added to CBPR project-related steering committees, the principles are discussed and adapted as appropriate (Maciak, Guzman, Santiago, Villalobos, & Israel, 1999). Further, some of the language in the principles that sounded good to CBPR partners initially did not really have meaning until they faced particular decision points. Thus as participants gain additional insights, the understanding of the principles changes over time, and they need to be revisited and revised accordingly. Developing a set of CBPR principles therefore needs to occur within the context of a specific partnership and to be viewed as fluid and evolving.

2. *Who is the "community" in a community based participatory research partnership?* The CBPR principles developed and implemented will vary in any given partnership, depending on how the "community" is defined and who is around the table representing the defined community (Israel et al., 1998; Koné et al., 2000). Recognizing that no single answer is applicable in all situations, partnerships need to discuss a number of critical questions, such as the following: Who is the community? Who represents the community? Who has influence in the community, and how, if at all, are they involved? Who decides who the community partners will be in a CBPR effort? Are the community partners involved as individuals or as representatives of community based organizations (CBOs)? If as individuals, do community members have a constituency that they represent and report to? If community members are representatives of community based organizations, what is the connection or link between the CBO and the community in which they work? How "grassroots" are the community members and CBOs involved? Who are the representatives and participants involved in the partnership, and how do they compare to members of the community in terms of class (income and education level), gender, and race or ethnicity? Who has the time, resources, skills, and flexibility to sit on boards and committees and attend meetings and review documents as necessary? Who is defined as "outside" the community and not invited to participate?

The Detroit URC and affiliated projects are primarily involved in two communities that qualify as both geographic communities and communities of identity (Israel et al., 1998; Koné et al., 2000). East Side Detroit is predominantly African American, and Southwest Detroit is the area of the city in which the largest percentage of Latinos reside. It was initially decided that the community partners would be community based organizations that are highly respected by the community in which they operate and that individual staff would serve on the URC board as representatives from their organization (Israel et al., 2001). To the extent possible, individuals were selected to serve on the board who held positions of leadership within the organization or were appointed by the leadership. Thus board members work in the communities involved but some do not actually live in these communities. In addition, if an individual leaves the organization, he or she no longer serves on the board and is replaced by another individual appointed by the organization.

Members of the board, even those who are from and still reside within the community, are sometimes somewhat different from community members at large, primarily in terms of education level and income. In the latter instance, it is important to recognize that such differences do not mean that the persons are no longer "community members." Those of us in academia and health agencies need to be careful not to impose a definition of what it means to be "from the community." Even within marginalized communities, not all members are going to be poor or have little formal education, and it is often those with more formal education and income who are best situated to participate in CBPR efforts, while at the same time having the inside view of what it is like to live in the community (Steuart, 1993). The evaluation of the first four years of the URC board's efforts found that the community partners perceive that they understand and can represent at the URC board level the communities in which they reside and work. However, they also recognize the need for participation of additional community based organizations on specific project-related steering committees (Lantz et al., 2001).

As another example, the East Side Village Health Worker Partnership, one of the URC-affiliated projects, also has a steering committee composed of individuals who represent community based organizations (Parker, Schulz, Israel, & Hollis, 1998; Schulz, Parker, et al., 1998). However, a decision was made early on to add several groups with long-standing and close ties in the community. In addition, several years into the project, both the steering committee and the Village Health Workers themselves—individuals who are considered natural helpers within the community to whom other community members turn to for advice and support—decided that there was not enough interaction between the two groups, and they agreed to add two Village Health Workers as members of the steering committee.

In another URC-affiliated project, Community Action Against Asthma (CAAA; Parker et al., 2002), the community partners are again primarily representatives from community based organizations, but the steering committee decided early on that there was also a need to include a community member who is a parent of a child with asthma, the focus of the project. While we still consider this a viable strategy, it is important to note that just as no one organization can represent the "community," no one individual can represent a specific subpopulation. In this situation, it is also important to consider how to ensure that every individual is treated with respect and listened to, especially if representing what might be referred to as a stigmatized group (such as substance users or gang members) who may be the focus of a CBPR effort. Furthermore, it is important to reflect on whether some groups are being excluded from being around the table and to address this issue accordingly.

3. *All partners involved need to decide what it means to have a "collaborative, equitable partnership" and how to make that happen.* Perhaps one of the most critical principles of community based participatory research is its emphasis on creating and sustaining partnerships in which all members share control

of the decision-making process. As an ideal to strive for, this is a core value of CBPR, but how does a CBPR effort ensure equity and shared influence and control? Every partnership needs to ask itself whether members are true "partners" or just "part" of the "partnership"—in other words, are all partners ready and able to share power? This requires considerable time and attention by all involved. Yet such attention to the partnership process may be frustrating for some, particularly if it is perceived to draw time and energy away from the accomplishment of the specific objectives of the CBPR effort (Israel et al., 2001; Lantz et al., 2001).

The Detroit Urban Research Center has engaged in a number of strategies to define and try to achieve a collaborative, equitable partnership. Although it is beyond the scope of this chapter to elaborate on these, a few examples are provided (see Israel et al., 2001, for a more in-depth discussion). Not only did the URC board discuss and adopt a set of CBPR principles, but we engaged in a process of developing operating norms and procedures that would help us adhere to these principles (Israel et al., 2001). One of the procedures adopted that has been identified by community partners as contributing to shared influence and control is the use of consensus decision making applying a 70 percent rule, rather than using a majority vote approach to decision making. The use of consensus requires that the board openly discuss, debate, and revise as appropriate any major decisions it faces. Consensus decision making takes considerable time and has been known to hamper decision making in other situations (Johnson & Johnson, 2000). However, the slight variation used by the URC board, referred to as the 70 percent rule, requires that all partners (100 percent) have to buy into a decision with at least 70 percent of their support. This approach has enabled board members to thoroughly examine issues and consider multiple perspectives prior to making a decision, giving everyone the opportunity to express opinions, influence the decisions made, and develop support for decisions reached without the expectation that everyone will be in complete agreement on all decisions (Israel et al., 2001).

Another approach that the URC takes is to work toward shared distribution of resources for the partners involved, including direct and indirect costs associated with grants (Israel et al., 2001; Lantz et al., 2001). While the core funding and some of the URC-affiliated project funds go primarily to the university, in several projects one of the community based organizations is the fiduciary and lead organization, and in all instances the community partner organizations receive modest financial compensation. The board also reviews the budget for the core funding and influences decisions on budget-related matters. This is an area that has the potential to create conflicts in a partnership and requires ongoing consideration (Israel et al., 1998; Lantz et al., 2001). It is important to recognize that not all partner organizations may have the interest in or capability to manage large-scale projects and that this may be an area in which to focus capacity-building efforts. In addition, there are other ways to distribute the benefits and rewards for participating in CBPR projects that need to be explored by a partnership (for example, the provision of technical assistance and educational opportunities as desired or attendance and presentation at professional meetings).

It is also important to acknowledge that while shared influence and control are a goal and equity is a basic premise of CBPR, there are other real inequities among partners that are more difficult to erase (especially in terms of race, gender, and class). These inequities can and most likely do get played out to some extent even in a process that strives for equity among partners. If partners acknowledge and discuss these inequities, they may be better able to see how they affect the work of the partnership. Such an understanding can then lead to more effective processes for reducing the impact that power imbalances may have on the relationships among group members and the work of the partnership. For example, in the East Side Village Health Worker Partnership (see Chapter Fourteen), we have had numerous discussions at meetings, retreats, and informally, involving steering committee members (both researchers and representatives from community based organizations) and village health workers regarding how race, class, gender, and other inequities influence our work and the communities with whom we work. At times these inequities have been used for the mutual benefit of the partners involved. For example, there have been situations where community partners have requested a university colleague to attend a meeting to "enhance their credibility," and university partners have made similar requests of community partners.

4. *Participation in all phases of the research does not mean that everyone is involved in the same way in all activities.* Another core value of CBPR is that all partners participate in all phases of the research process. Here again, it is important for CBPR partnerships to determine what that means for them, realizing that it may not mean that everyone is involved in the same way in all issues and activities. For example, in the East Side Village Health Worker Partnership, the steering committee played a major role in developing a conceptual framework of a stress process, designing a survey instrument and how it should be administered, interpreting the results of the survey, and applying the results to establish and implement intervention strategies (Schulz, Israel, et al., in press; Schulz, Parker, et al., 1998; Schulz, Parker, et al., 2002). The steering committee was not, however, involved in the actual process of data entry and data analysis of the survey questionnaire. It has been our experience that given the time demands and technical aspects of these two processes, different levels of involvement may be appropriate for different partners, while also recognizing that this may be an area where community partners are interested in enhancing their skills. However, it is crucial that the results of data analyses be fed back in ways that are understandable and useful and that all partners engage in the

process of interpreting the data, which might include requesting that additional analyses be conducted. Given the multiple skills and expertise of the partners involved and the multiple demands on their time, choices need to be made on how best to draw on the diverse capabilities and interests that exist. Given that this often means that the researchers are making some choices (have some power) in terms of what data get analyzed and what results are fed back, there is an even greater need for self-critique and self-reflection among those partners who are taking the lead in these various components of a project. In a related example, day-to-day project management may be most appropriately the responsibility of paid staff (for example, writing minutes of meetings, developing and sending mailings, coordinating project-related travel and presentations). However, it is crucial that partners are not excluded from major decisions, such as determining priority issues to address and budget expenditures.

5. *Establish procedures for dissemination.* A number of questions related to the dissemination of CBPR findings need to be addressed. Who are the coauthors of publications and copresenters at professional meetings? How is it decided who they are? What are their roles and responsibilities? What happens when only one partner is invited to present or submit an article? What are the priority publication outlets (journal articles, popular press), and who makes those decisions? How is a balance reached between time spent developing reports to feed back results within the community and writing peer-reviewed publications? Here again, there is no one answer to these questions that will work for all partnerships. Rather, a partnership needs to engage in a process of developing procedures that will help ensure that the dissemination principle is followed.

A year into the Community Action Against Asthma project, the University of Michigan partners were receiving numerous requests to present papers at professional meetings. Based on our experiences with the URC as a whole, we knew we wanted to make joint presentations (a university and a community partner) to the extent possible. We also began to identify the numerous publications that would be possible and recognized the need to map out a publication strategy. The CAAA steering committee established a dissemination subcommittee, made up of an equal number of university and community partners, and met over several months to draft dissemination procedures. These were brought to the steering committee and adopted after a number of revisions. These procedures spell out, for example, how participants will be selected as coauthors and copresenters and what the expectations are for these roles. These procedures were subsequently reviewed by the URC board itself and several other project-related steering committees and have been adapted for their use. The development and application of such procedures across the projects has greatly expanded our discussion of these issues and has enhanced how we have dealt with them.

While we recommend that written dissemination procedures be established, it is important that these not be perceived as formal or rigid. Flexibility and a willingness to respond quickly as requests arise that may not fit within the specified parameters are necessary. We also consider these to be evolving procedures that need to be revisited and revised as determined by each particular partnership. The adoption of these procedures has occurred at different stages in our different projects, ranging from five years into a project to within the first six months of a newly developing effort. Although it may be ideal to address these questions during the early phases of a project, many of the issues may not seem relevant or compelling until a partnership has had to face them directly. What is most important here is to view this as an ongoing topic of conversation and deliberation, making changes as needed along the way.

6. *Recognize and value priorities identified by the community.* Although community based participatory research emphasizes the importance of examining and addressing the social determinants of health, at multiple levels of practice (individual, family, community), we need to be careful that researchers do not impose that approach on the partnership. Understandably, community partners may initially be most interested in addressing specific, tangible issues that seem more amenable to change than trying to address broad-scale policies associated with social determinants of health. Indeed, there is an extensive literature in the community organizing field that indicates that an essential component of effective organizing efforts is winning tangible, small-scale changes in a relatively short period of time (Minkler, 1997; Minkler & Wallerstein, 1997). As noted by Meredith Minkler and Cheri Pies (1997), one of the key ethical precepts of community organizing and community building is self-determination, that is, "starting where the people are" (Nyswander, 1956). This is also a major principle of community based participatory research, with its emphasis on the local relevance of public health problems and community involvement in all aspects of the research process. Importantly, the choice here does not have to be either-or. Rather, although a CBPR effort begins by addressing specific priority issues identified by the community, over time, as part of the research and intervention process, the partnership can engage in dialogue aimed at gaining a better understanding of the role of and what can be done to affect the social determinants of the specific issue selected.

As discussed in Chapter Fourteen, the East Side Village Health Worker Partnership uses a stress process model as a conceptual framework to address the social determinants of health on Detroit's East Side (Parker et al., 1998; Schulz, Parker, et al., 1998; Schulz, Parker, et al., 2002). Although the model was included in the initial grant proposal, in which there was not much community involvement, it was never presented to the community per se. Instead, a locally defined stress process model was developed by the steering committee over a series of meetings (Schulz, Parker, et al., 1998). Based on this stress process model and subsequent in-depth interviews and survey questionnaires conducted with community members, the Village Health Workers prioritized the issues that they wanted to address. These included strengthening socially supportive relationships, enhancing relationships with the police, increasing safety for children, improving accessibility and appropriateness of health services, and fostering environments conducive to diabetes management and prevention. While each of these issues has underlying social determinants, the initial strategies in which the partnership engaged have emphasized short-term activities aimed at addressing these concerns (Halloween parties for children, "pamper me" events for women, participating in Police Week). These successful events have led to an increased sense of community competence, and through ongoing conversations with the Village Health Workers and steering committee members, some participants also seem ready to engage in broader-scale policy and social changes (Schulz, Parker, et al., 2002).

7. *Work with the cultural diversity of the partners involved.* Community based participatory research partnerships are likely to involve partners from diverse cultural backgrounds, with respect to ethnicity or race, gender, social class, sexual orientation, community or academic role, and academic discipline. The multiple perspectives involved requires the development of a common language, trust, mutual respect, understanding of the cultural context, and the recognition that participants may have different goals, agendas, experiences with, and degrees of commitment to CBPR, conflicting loyalties, and multiple demands on their time and what they can contribute to the CBPR effort (Israel et al., 1998; Israel et al., 2001; Koné et al., 2000; Lantz et al., 2001; Northridge et al., 2000). As noted, consideration also has to be given to how structural inequities contribute to the cultural differences that exist within CBPR partnerships. Although the development of cultural competency is particularly germane for researchers working in community settings, as the following examples indicate, there are also important differences within and across communities of identity that need to be considered.

The Community Action Against Asthma project was the first URC-affiliated project to simultaneously involve participants from both East Side and Southwest Detroit and also to involve researchers from the disciplines of environmental health science as well as health behavior and health education. Initially, some of the researchers who had less experience with CBPR were perceived by the community partners as being somewhat aloof and interested only in their research findings and not in the community members themselves. In addition, some of the Latino community partners from Southwest Detroit interpreted some of the comments from East Side partners, a predominantly African American community, as being stereotypical and discriminatory toward Latinos. During the early phases of the project, the steering committee discussed the need to engage in a cultural competency training workshop. For a number of reasons, it took time to make arrangements for such a workshop, and subsequently the steering committee decided that they were better suited to address these issues within the group itself. Since that time, the issue has risen again and continues to be an important topic of conversation and reflection within the steering committee, and it is not yet clear what will be the most effective means of ensuring that the cultural diversity that exists is respected and celebrated (Parker et al., 2002).

In another example, during the early phases of the East Side Village Health Worker Partnership, a number of village health workers expressed concerns to the Detroit-based African American project staff that they were not clear about the motives of the university-based white staff and did not trust what "they" were doing. The VHWs also felt that the Detroit-based staff was becoming too closely aligned with the university-based staff. The VHWs requested a meeting with only the Detroit-based staff to address their concerns. Over time, the trust and mutual respect has grown among the VHWs, the Detroit-based staff, and the university participants. In working with diverse cultures, it is important to recognize that we all bring with us historical and present-day experiences and that we have to pay attention to and allow time for partners to see and move beyond broad social stereotypes and prejudices.

It is also useful to point out that these differences occur across research disciplines, as well as between researchers and community members. For example, there have been several occasions when the environmental scientists and social scientists involved in CAAA have used the same words with very different meanings. In one instance, the term *qualitative data* was used by the environmental scientists to refer to any data that are not calibrated by a machine, meaning that the results of a closed-ended survey was considered qualitative data. In the social sciences, however, *qualitative data* refers to a different research paradigm involving open-ended data collection approaches. Similarly, the use of the term *scale* by a social scientist at a meeting discussing the results of a factor analysis and the formation of indices from a survey questionnaire caused some confusion among the environmental health scientists, who use the term *scale* to refer to an instrument that measures substances in the environment. The recognition of these language differences has provided some levity and humor to our conversations and a commitment to work on an ongoing basis to develop a mutually understandable language.

8. *Develop processes and procedures for ensuring that CBPR principles are followed.* As a CBPR partnership establishes trust and a track record of successfully conducting research and interventions, there are likely to be other researchers and community organizations that want the partnership to work with them in response to, say, a funding agency's particular call for proposals or a community's specifically identified problem. However, the rationale for reaching out to the partnership may not be in the partnership's or community's

best interest. For example, some researchers may see working with the partnership as a way to get "access to subjects," and some community based organizations may see the partnership as a mechanism to obtain "access to resources." It is important that partnerships develop a process and procedures for disseminating their CBPR principles to potential collaborators and ensuring that new projects adhere to these principles. Such procedures may be perceived by others as gatekeeping mechanisms that "keep others out." Communicating that the principles can provide a means to "open the gate" remains an ongoing challenge.

The URC board has procedures for distributing the principles and reviewing requests for new projects (Israel et al., 2001). In brief, a subcommittee (or sometimes the entire board) reviews a written (or oral) submission of the request. If the subcommittee decides to move the request forward, it is brought to the full board for consideration and may include a presentation by the interested parties. Given that the preferred procedure adopted by the board occurs over several meetings, we have also developed a process for a more expedited review that involves the use of e-mail and conference calls as necessary to ensure that the full board has participated in the decision making. Although these procedures have worked quite well for the board and have resulted in a number of in-depth conversations around the principles and what they mean, at times the process has upset colleagues wanting to work with the URC. In one instance, a faculty member not affiliated with the URC requested a letter of support for a grant proposal from a faculty member who is involved and did not understand the need to wait and get approval from the URC board. In another case, a community based organization interested in joining one of the CBPR projects did not understand why a community partner could not make that happen.

9. *The size of the partnership needs to be decided by and appropriate for the community involved.* A question that we are frequently asked is, "What is the most appropriate or effective number of partners to include in a community based participatory research effort?" No firm answer can be found in the literature—or in our experience. The specific context and goals have to be considered, and the initial partners involved have to decide what is most appropriate in their particular situation. Based on our own experience, we recommend that a CBPR partnership start small, beginning with partner organizations from only one or two communities of identity (Israel et al., 2001). Such an approach has the advantage of building on existing relationships and trust and the likelihood of identifying mutually agreed goals while also recognizing the considerable research evidence that the most effective size for problem-solving groups is eight to twelve members (Johnson & Johnson, 2000). If there are preestablished, long-standing relationships in the community of identity, a partnership might be effective with a somewhat larger initial number of partners. Furthermore, it is also important to realize that there are limits to the skills, resources,

and time available from members in smaller groups, and thus there may be a need to have a slightly larger core group (ideally not more than twelve to sixteen partner organizations), as well as to identify other mechanisms to involve additional persons.

In our own work, we often use what could be considered a Venn diagram approach to participation, in which at the center of a series of overlapping circles is a core group of partners involved as the members of and the decision-making group for the CBPR partnership. In addition, there is often a need for specific work groups or action teams in which other individuals or organizations are invited to participate along with members from the core group (members of the outer, nonoverlapping part of the circle). For example, the REACH Detroit Partnership has a steering committee made up of representatives of the eleven core partner organizations and also two work groups (Family/Health Care System and Social Support/Community) that guide the specific intervention and research components, and these include both members from the partner organizations and others who have needed expertise. Another approach that we use could more closely be represented using a concentric circle diagram, in which the core partners in the CBPR effort are represented in the center circle and other organizations are invited to participate in a more limited way in the outer circle. For example, in the Community Action Against Asthma project, the steering committee, which is the core decision-making body, is composed of representatives from thirteen partner organizations. In addition, we are establishing a more loosely affiliated interorganizational network consisting of organizations with similar interests in environmental triggers of asthma. The organizations in this network will be kept informed of the work of the project, and some organizations will be involved in specific community organizing efforts as they seem appropriate.

In general, therefore, we recommend that the core group of CBPR partners remain fairly small, recognizing that there are multiple approaches to expanding to include others as needed. Importantly, this issue of partnership size needs to be recognized as fluid and evolving and as a critical topic for consideration by the partnership. In an existing partnership that is considering adding new members, it is helpful to develop a set of criteria for membership in which the partners discuss and agree on the needs of the partnership that new members would help meet; the expectations, roles, and responsibilities of new members; and the procedures for adding new members. While it is useful to spell out such criteria and procedures in writing, we caution against being too formal and rigid, as that could undermine the very strength of a community-driven participatory process.

10. *Recognize that CBPR principles alone do not dictate research design and methodology.* There is some confusion in the field that suggests that community based participatory research approaches by definition dictate what types of

research design and methods are appropriate. What is important here is that there is no one design or method appropriate for all CBPR efforts. Instead, each partnership has to decide what works best for its research question and intervention goal in its particular community context. For example, although qualitative methods provide in-depth understanding of a given phenomenon and give voice to those who are often not listened to, CBPR partnerships and communities may also be interested in knowing how widespread opinions are on a given issue. With the East Side Village Health Worker Partnership, in addition to conducting group dialogues and in-depth interviews on the stress process, we also conducted a random sample survey with community residents (Schulz, Parker, et al., 1998).

In addition, from a research design perspective, while the use of a "control group" that receives no direct benefit from the research is neither appropriate nor, we would suggest, ethical in the context of CBPR, there are other viable designs. For example, the Community Action Against Asthma project involves a staggered intervention design in which half of the children (and their households) enrolled in the project were randomly selected to receive the intensive phase of the intervention during the first year and the second half were selected to receive the intervention during the second year of the project. This will allow us to evaluate the intervention effects comparing wave 1 and wave 2 participants, a fairly standard research design. Although this was agreed on by the partners involved, it is important to note that many participants assigned to wave 2 were troubled by the delay in receiving the intervention and the multiple requests to provide data during the first year in which they did not receive any direct benefits.

11. *Conduct ongoing evaluation to assess the extent to which CBPR principles are followed.* To develop and maintain an effective CBPR partnership and to enhance our understanding of the factors that contribute to this effectiveness, it is necessary to conduct an ongoing evaluation of the extent to which and in what ways the CBPR principles are being followed (Israel et al., 2001; Parker et al., 2002; Schulz et al., in press). Such an evaluation needs to be an integral part of the partnership, in which members are involved in all aspects of the evaluation and in which the results are fed back on a regular basis and used to make changes in how the partnership operates, as appropriate.

Since the beginning of the Urban Research Center, an evaluation has been conducted to assess URC board members' perceptions and experiences of the board's activities, processes, and progress, including accomplishments, adherence to CBPR principles, challenges, and facilitating factors (Israel et al., 2001; Lantz et al., 2001). An evaluation subcommittee of the board guides this assessment, which includes multiple data collection methods (including in-depth interviews with board members conducted at two points in time and annual mailed closed-ended survey questionnaires completed by board members). Each year, the results of this evaluation have been fed back and discussed at URC board meetings and have contributed to an enhanced understanding of the CBPR principles adopted and how to effectively follow them (Israel et al., 2001; Lantz et al., 2001). In addition to this evaluation of the overall URC board, a number of the affiliated projects engage in a similar ongoing assessment of their partnerships (Parker et al., 2002; Schulz, Israel, & Lantz, in press; Schulz et al., 2002).

As discussed throughout this chapter, in order to address the growing disparities in health status between marginalized communities and those with greater social and economic resources, more equitable approaches to research are needed that involve action as well as knowledge generation that is beneficial to and reflective of the communities involved. Community based participatory research is one approach that engages diverse partners in strategies aimed at obtaining multiple perspectives in order to address community-identified concerns. Although our set of community based participatory research principles can be used as guidelines by those interested in this approach, we reiterate that no one set of principles is appropriate for all communities and all situations. Similarly, we want to emphasize that there is not just one approach to CBPR. As partnerships consider the issues raised here, each partnership will develop its own approach to inquiry and change, along with principles that are appropriate to working together in their specific context. What is crucial is the long-term commitment to reducing fundamental inequalities that exist throughout the systems in which we live and work.

Notes

1. The Detroit Community-Academic Urban Research Center (URC) was established in 1995 as part of the Urban Research Centers Initiative of the Centers for Disease Control and Prevention (CDC), Grant No. U48/CCU515775. The Detroit URC develops, implements, and evaluates interdisciplinary, collaborative, community based participatory research and intervention projects that aim to improve the health and quality of life for residents of the Southwest and East Side of Detroit. The Detroit URC is a partnership among the University of Michigan Schools of Public Health and Nursing, the Detroit Health Department, and eight community based organizations (Butzel Family Center, Community Health and Social Services Center, Detroit Hispanic Development Corporation, Friends of Parkside, Kettering/Butzel Health Initiative, Latino Family Services, Southwest Counseling and Development Services, and Warren Conner Development Coalition), Henry Ford Health System, and the CDC. The experiences of the URC board and affiliated projects have greatly contributed to the ideas presented here.

2. This discussion includes excerpts and revised portions from the original set of CBPR principles presented by Israel et al. (1998), pp. 177–180.

References

Altman, D. G. (1995). Sustaining interventions in community systems: On the relationships between researchers and communities. *Health Psychology, 14,* 526–536.

Antonovsky, A. (1979). *Health, stress, and coping: New perspectives on mental and physical well-being.* San Francisco: Jossey Bass.

Baker, E. A., Homan, S., Schonhoff, R., & Kreuter, M. W. (1999). Principles of practice for academic/practice/community research partnerships. *American Journal of Preventive Medicine, 16*(3), 86–93.

Berger, P. L., & Neuhaus, R. J. (1977). *To empower people: The role of mediating structures in public policy.* Washington, DC: American Enterprise Institute for Public Policy Research.

Bishop, R. (1994). Initiating empowering research? *New Zealand Journal of Educational Studies, 29,* 175–188.

Blankenship, K. M., & Schulz, A. J. (1996, August). *Approaches and dilemmas in community-based research and action.* Presented at the annual meeting of the Society for the Study of Social Problems, New York.

Bronfenbrenner, U. (1990). *The ecology of human development: Experiments by nature and design.* Cambridge, MA: Harvard University Press.

Centers for Disease Control and Prevention/Agency for Toxic Substances and Disease Registry. (1997). *Principles of community engagement.* Atlanta: Centers for Disease Control and Prevention, Public Health Practice Program Office.

Cornwall, A. (1996). Towards participatory practice: Participatory rural appraisal (PRA) and the participatory process. In K. De Koning & M. Martin (Eds.), *Participatory research in health: Issues and experiences* (pp. 94–107). London: Zed Books.

De Koning, K., & Martin, M. (1996). *Participatory research in health: Issues and experiences.* London: Zed Books.

Elden, M., & Levin, M. (1991). Cogenerative learning: Bringing participation into action research. In W. F. Whyte (Ed.), *Participatory action research* (pp. 127–142). Newbury Park, CA: Sage.

Fals-Borda, O., & Rahman, M. A. (1991). *Action and knowledge: Breaking the monopoly with participatory action research.* New York: Apex.

Francisco, V. T., Paine, A. L., & Fawcett, S. B. (1993). A methodology for monitoring and evaluating community health coalitions. *Health Education Research, 8,* 403–416.

Freire, P. (1973). *Education for critical consciousness.* New York: Continuum.

Gaventa, J. (1993). The powerful, the powerless, and the experts: Knowledge struggles in an information age. In P. Park, M. Brydon-Miller, B. L. Hall, & T. Jackson (Eds.), *Voices of change: Participatory research in the United States and Canada* (pp. 21–40). Westport, CT: Bergin & Garvey.

Gottlieb, N. H., & McLeroy, K. R. (1994). Social health. In M. P. O'Donnell & J. S. Harris (Eds.), *Health promotion in the workplace* (pp. 458–493). Albany, NY: Delmar.

Green, L. W., George, M. A., Daniel, M., Frankish, C. J., Herbert, C. P., Bowie, W. R., & O'Neill, M. (1995). *Study of participatory research in health promotion: Review and recommendations for the development of participatory research in health promotion in Canada.* Vancouver, British Columbia: Royal Society of Canada.

Hall, B. L. (1992). From margins to center: The development and purpose of participatory research. *American Sociologist, 23*(4), 15–28.

Hancock, T. (1993). The healthy city from concept to application: Implications for research. In J. K. Davies & M. P. Kelly (Eds.), *Healthy cities: Research and practice* (pp. 14–24). New York: Routledge.

Hatch, J., Moss, N., Saran, A., Presley-Cantrell, L., & Mallory, C. (1993). Community research: Partnership in black communities. *American Journal of Preventive Medicine, 9*, 27–31.

House, J. S., & Williams, D. R. (2000). Understanding and reducing socioeconomic and racial/ethnic disparities in health. In B. D. Smedley & S. L. Syme (Eds.), *Promoting health: Intervention strategies from social and behavioral research* (pp. 81–124). Washington, DC: Institute of Medicine/National Academy Press.

Institute of Medicine. (1997). *Improving health in the community: A role for performance monitoring.* Washington, DC: National Academy Press.

Israel, B. A., Checkoway, B., Schulz, A. J., & Zimmerman, M. A. (1994). Health education and community empowerment: Conceptualizing and measuring perceptions of individual, organizational, and community control. *Health Education Quarterly, 21*, 149–170.

Israel, B. A., Lichtenstein, R., Lantz, P. M., McGranaghan, R. J., Allen, A., Guzman, J. R., et al. (2001). The Detroit Community-Academic Urban Research Center: Lessons learned in the development, implementation, and evaluation of a community-based participatory research partnership. *Journal of Public Health Management and Practice, 7*(5), 1–19.

Israel, B. A., Schulz, A. J., Parker, E. A., & Becker, A. B. (1998). Review of community-based research: Assessing partnership approaches to improve public health. *Annual Review of Public Health, 19*, 173–202.

Israel, B. A., & Schurman, S. J. (1990). Social support, control, and the stress process. In K. Glanz, F. M. Lewis, & B. K. Rimer (Eds.), *Health behavior and health education: Theory, research, and practice* (pp. 179–205). San Francisco: Jossey-Bass.

Israel, B. A., Schurman, S. J., & Hugentobler, M. K. (1992). Conducting action research: Relationships between organization members and researchers. *Journal of Applied Behavioral Science, 28*, 74–101.

Israel, B. A., Schurman, S. J., Hugentobler, M. K., & House, J. S. (1992). A participatory action research approach to reducing occupational stress in the United States. In

V. Di Martino (Ed.), *Preventing stress at work: Conditions of work digest* (Vol. 2, pp. 152–163). Geneva: International Labor Office.

Johnson, D. W., & Johnson, F. P. (2000). *Joining together: Group theory and group skills* (7th ed.). Boston: Allyn & Bacon.

Kaplan, G. A., Pamuk, E. A., Lynch, J. W., Cohen, R. D., & Balfour, J. L. (1996). Inequality in income and mortality in the United States: Analysis of mortality and potential pathways. *British Medical Journal, 312,* 999–1003.

Klein, D. C. (1968). *Community dynamics and mental health.* New York: Wiley.

Koné, A., Sullivan, M., Senturia, K. D., Chrisman, N. J., Ciske, S. J., & Krieger, J. W. (2000). Improving collaboration between researchers and communities. *Public Health Reports, 115,* 243–248.

Krieger, N., Rowley, D. L., Herman, A. A., Avery, B., & Phillips, M. T. (1993). Racism, sexism, and social class: Implications for studies of health, disease, and well-being. *American Journal of Preventive Medicine, 9*(6), 82–122.

Labonté, R. (1994). Health promotion and empowerment: Reflections on professional practice. *Health Education Quarterly, 21,* 253–268.

Labonté, R. (1997). Community, community development, and the forming of authentic partnerships: Some critical reflections. In M. Minkler (Ed.), *Community organizing and community building for health* (pp. 88–102). New Brunswick, NJ: Rutgers University Press.

Lantz, P. M., Viruell-Fuentes, E., Israel, B. A., Softley, D., & Guzman, J. R. (2001). Can communities and academia work together on public health research? Evaluation results from a community-based participatory research partnership in Detroit. *Journal of Urban Health, 78,* 495–507.

Lasker, R. D., Weiss, E. S., & Miller, R. (2001). Partnership synergy: A practical framework for studying and strengthening the collaborative advantage. *Milbank Quarterly, 79,* 179–205.

Lillie-Blanton, M. P., Parsons, E., Gayle, H., & Dievler, A. (1996). Racial differences in health: Not just black and white, but shades of gray. *Annual Review of Public Health, 17,* 411–448.

Maciak, B. J., Guzman, J. R., Santiago, A., Villalobos, G., & Israel, B. A. (1999). Establishing LA VIDA: A community-based partnership to prevent intimate violence against Latina women. *Health Education and Behavior, 26,* 821–840.

Maguire, P. (1987). *Doing participatory research: A feminist approach.* Amherst: University of Massachusetts, Center for International Education.

Maguire, P. (1996). Considering more feminist participatory research: What's congruency got to do with it? *Qualitative Inquiry, 2,* 106–118.

Marmot, M., & Wilkinson, R. G. (Eds.). (1999). *Social determinants of health.* New York: Oxford University Press.

Martin, M. (1996). Issues of power in the participatory research process. In K. De Koning & M. Martin (Eds.), *Participatory research in health: Issues and experiences* (pp. 82–93). London: Zed Books.

McKnight, J. L. (1994). Politicizing health care. In P. Conrad & R. Kern (Eds.), *The sociology of health and illness: Critical perspectives* (4th ed., pp. 437–441). New York: St. Martin's Press.

Minkler, M. (Ed.). (1997). *Community organizing and community building for health.* New Brunswick, NJ: Rutgers University Press.

Minkler, M., & Pies, C. (1997). Ethical issues in community organization and community participation. In M. Minkler (Ed.), *Community organizing and community building for health* (pp. 120–136). New Brunswick, NJ: Rutgers University Press.

Minkler, M., & Wallerstein, N. (1997). Improving health through community organization and community building. In K. Glanz, F. M. Lewis, & B. K. Rimer (Eds.), *Health behavior and health education: Theory, research, and practice* (2nd ed., pp. 241–269). San Francisco: Jossey-Bass.

Mittelmark, M. B., Hunt, M. K., Heath, G. W., & Schmid, T. L. (1993). Realistic outcomes: Lessons from community-based research and demonstration programs for the prevention of cardiovascular disease. *Journal of Public Health Policy, 14,* 437–462.

Northridge, M. E., Vallone, D., Merzel, C., Greene, D., Shepard, P., Cohall, A. T., & Healton, C. G. (2000). The adolescent years: An academic-community partnership in Harlem comes of age. *Journal of Public Health Management and Practice, 6,* 53–60.

Nyden, P. W., & Wiewel, W. (1992). Collaborative research: Harnessing the tensions between researcher and practitioner. *American Sociologist, 24,* 43–55.

Nyswander, D. (1956). Education for health: Some principles and their application. *California Health, 14,* 65–70.

Park, P., Brydon-Miller, M., Hall, B. L., & Jackson, T. (Eds.). (1993). *Voices of change: Participatory research in the United States and Canada.* Westport, CT: Bergin & Garvey.

Parker, E. A., Israel, B. A., Brakefield-Caldwell, W., Keeler, G., Ramirez, E., Rowe, Z., & Williams, M. (2002). *Community Action Against Asthma: Examining the partnership process of a community-based participatory research project.* Unpublished manuscript.

Parker, E. A., Schulz, A. J., Israel, B. A., & Hollis, R. (1998). Detroit's East Side Village Health Worker Partnership: Community-based health adviser intervention in an urban area. *Health Education and Behavior, 25,* 24–45.

Petras, E. M., & Porpora, D. V. (1993). Participatory research: Three models and an analysis. *American Sociologist, 24,* 107–126.

Sarason, S. B. (1984). *The psychological sense of community: Prospects for a community psychology.* San Francisco: Jossey-Bass.

Schell, L. M., & Tarbell, A. M. (1998). A partnership study of PCBs and the health of Mohawk youth: Lessons from our past and guidelines for our future. *Environmental Health Perspectives, 106,* 833–840.

Schensul, J. J. (1999). Organizing community research partnerships in the struggle against AIDS. *Health Education and Behavior, 26,* 266–283.

Schulz, A. J., Israel, B. A., & Lantz, P. M. (in press). Evaluating group dynamics within community-based participatory research. *Evaluation and Program Planning.*

Schulz, A. J., Israel, B. A., Parker, E. A., Lockett, M., Hill, Y. R., & Wills, R. (in press). Community based participatory research: Integrating research with action to reduce health disparities. *Public Health Reports.*

Schulz, A. J., Israel, B. A., Selig, S. M., & Bayer, I. S. (1998). Development and implementation of principles for community-based research in public health. In R. H. MacNair (Ed.), *Research strategies for community practice* (pp. 83–110). New York: Haworth Press.

Schulz, A. J., Parker, E. A., Israel, B. A., Allen, A., De Carlo, M., & Lockett, M. (2002). Addressing social determinants of health through community-based participatory research: The East Side Village Health Worker Partnership. *Health Education and Behavior, 29,* 326–341.

Schulz, A. J., Parker, E. A., Israel, B. A., Becker, A. B., Maciak, B. J., & Hollis, R. (1998). Conducting a participatory community-based survey: Collecting and interpreting data for a community intervention on Detroit's East Side. *Journal of Public Health Management and Practice, 4*(2), 10–24.

Schulz, A. J., Williams, D. R., Israel, B. A., Becker, A. B., Parker, E. A., & James, S. A. (2000). Unfair treatment, neighborhood effects, and mental health in the Detroit metropolitan area. *Journal of Health and Social Behavior, 41,* 314–332.

Singer, M. (1993). Knowledge for use: Anthropology and community-centered substance abuse research. *Social Science and Medicine, 37,* 15–25.

Steuart, G. W. (1993). Social and cultural perspectives: Community intervention and mental health. *Health Education Quarterly,* Suppl. 1, S99–S111.

Stokols, D., Allen, J., & Bellingham, R. L. (Eds.). (1996). Translating social ecological theory into guidelines for community health promotion. *American Journal of Health Promotion, 10,* 282–298.

Stringer, E. T. (1996). *Action research: A handbook for practitioners.* Thousand Oaks, CA: Sage.

Susser, M. (1995). The tribulations of trials: Intervention in communities. *American Journal of Public Health, 85,* 156–158.

Tandon, R. (1981). Participatory evaluation and research: Main concepts and issues. In W. Fernandes & R. Tandon (Eds.), *Participatory research and evaluation* (pp. 15–34). New Delhi: Indian Social Institute.

Thomas, S. B., & Quinn, S. C. (1991). The Tuskegee Syphilis Study, 1932 to 1972: Implications for HIV education and AIDS risk education programs in the black community. *American Journal of Public Health, 11,* 1498–1505.

Wallerstein, N. (1999). Power between evaluator and community: Research relationships within New Mexico's healthier communities. *Social Science and Medicine, 49,* 39–53.

World Health Organization. (1946). *Constitution.* New York: Author.

POWER, TRUST, AND DIALOGUE

Working with Communities on Multiple Levels in Community Based Participatory Research

As Angela Cornwall and Rachel Jewkes (1995) suggest, participatory research is fundamentally about "the who question"—who defines the problem? And who generates, analyzes, represents, owns, and acts as a result of the information? The central issues in how we answer these questions are ultimately issues of power and control. In Part Two, we continue to surface these issues, with a related set of questions that serve as threads that run throughout the book. These questions include the following:

- Who is the "community"?

- What roles can (or should) outsider researchers play in CBPR?

- How do we create processes that help build community leadership without making people "strangers in their own communities"?

- How can we openly confront and attempt to address power differentials based on race, class, gender, and professional hierarchy?

- How can race and racism in particular be addressed more centrally in CBPR?

The continued centrality of race/ethnicity and racism in the social fabric of the contemporary United States and of interlocking oppressions based on race/ethnicity, class, and gender (hooks, 1989) make a special focus on these topics critical to any in-depth look at CBPR for health. Chapter Four examines the difficult issues of race/ethnicity, racism, and white privilege that must be confronted when community based participatory research involves communities of color. Camara Jones's (2000) three-tiered model of racism is presented, providing an important context for understanding the possible dynamic interactions between these tiers (institutionalized, personalized, and institutionalized racism) within CBPR practice. The intimate interdependence between racism and power is then examined, with special attention to Michael Foucault's (1977) differentiation between *repressive power*—power that limits the opportunity structures for people of color—and *productive power*, power that through the creation of norms, truths, and knowledge both enables dominant control and provides the opportunity for subordinate communities to challenge power structures and bring about change. Concepts such as historical trauma and hidden and public transcripts, the critical role of language in cultural translation, and the important yet often unspoken role of white privilege in the CBPR relationship are each explored and illustrated in this chapter. The authors then examine how understanding racism in all of its forms can help CBPR partners, regardless of their own race/ethnicity, build "alliances across differences." Such alliances will by definition be uncomfortable at times. Yet as Vivian Chávez and her colleagues conclude, in this very discomfort, and in embracing "the conflict that characterizes cross-cultural work" (Gutierrez & Lewis, 1997, p. 220), CBPR partners will be better positioned to dance—and continually learn to dance—in the multicultural context that characterizes so much of our work.

As Richard Couto (1987) has argued, although a core function of participatory research is to surface and validate the community's knowledge, "in practice, this is very difficult to do without some person, outside the community, with professional credentials, lending assistance or credence to local knowledge and claims about its validity" (p. 85). Issues of power, potential conflict, and development of partnerships once again are deeply embedded in this reality.

In Chapter Five, sociologist Randy Stoecker describes three contrasting roles that outside academics may play in community based participatory research—the roles of initiator, consultant, and collaborator. Determining which of these roles may be most appropriate in a given CBPR effort requires key questions to be addressed from the onset: What is the project attempting to do? What skills does the outside academic bring to the project and the partnership? And how much participation does the community actually need and want? "Guideposts" for the effective and ethical engagement of outside academics in CBPR are offered in this chapter, as is a perspective on how the outsider roles may change over the life of the project as community needs, capacities, and desires grow and change. Finally, the author reminds us that doing participatory research is in fact not an end in itself but a means to an end—community-driven social change.

In the final chapter in this part, we broaden the lens through which CBPR relationships are examined as community members and their university and health department collaborators at the Urban Research Center in Seattle, Washington, take a hard look at such partnerships. Drawing on both their personal experiences and insights and their earlier research exploring community perceptions, Marianne Sullivan and colleagues present a diversity of perspectives on the meaning of community and community representation, the differential reward structure for participation in CBPR, issues of power and conflict, and the often intertwined issues of race/ethnicity and culture that surface in the course of such research. By presenting illustrative problems that arose in each issue area and following each with a discussion of how Seattle Partners for Healthy Communities attempted to address the challenges faced, the chapter offers a host of useful lessons and insights for others engaged in such partnerships.

References

Cornwall, A., & Jewkes, R. (1995). What is participatory research? *Social Science and Medicine,* 41, 1667–1676.

Couto, R. (1987). Participatory research: Methodology and critique. *Clinical Sociology Review,* 5, 83–90.

Foucault, M. (1977). *Power and knowledge: Selected interviews and other writings* (C. Gordon, Ed.). New York: Pantheon.

Gutierrez, L. M., & Lewis, E. A. (1997). Education, participation, and capacity building in community organizing and women of color. In M. Minkler (Ed.), *Community organizing and community building for health* (pp. 216–229). New Brunswick, NJ: Rutgers University Press.

hooks, b. (1989). *Talking back: Thinking feminism, talking black.* Boston: South End Press.

Jones, C. P. (2000). Levels of racism: A theoretic framework and a gardener's tale. *American Journal of Public Health,* 90, 1212–1215.

CHAPTER FOUR

The Dance of Race and Privilege in Community Based Participatory Research

Vivian Chávez
Bonnie Duran
Quinton E. Baker
Magdalena M. Avila
Nina Wallerstein

Dancing provides a provocative analogy for exploring the interplay of race/ethnicity, racism, and privilege that often goes unacknowledged in community based participatory research (CBPR). Like dancing, CBPR has the potential for making research partners feel exhilarated, awkward, controlled, and free. The dance involves being aware of differences and respecting that while some people appear to be "natural" dancers, others need more time and instruction as they experiment with movement. Dancers complement each other's steps, sometimes leading, sometimes following; they are aware of each other, navigating the dance floor while trying not to step on each other's toes. And when toes do get stepped on, they must be self-reflective enough to learn from the experience and not be defensive, to decide whether to continue dancing or to take a seat, and to know that these dynamic processes are normal and inevitable, however rewarding or hurtful they may be.

Dancing, like CBPR, comes in a myriad of forms and styles, depending on the dance partner's style, interest, and background music played. However, because the dance takes place in the United States, and our country is, perhaps more than any other industrialized country in the world, distinguished by the size and diversity of its racial and ethnic populations (Smelser, Wilson, & Mitchell, 2000), dancing takes on a racialized character. Dancers from different cultures must learn each other's movements, rhythms, and meanings. To dance is to express our social and cultural context without imposing an absolute "correct way" to dance.

Admittedly, dancing may not be the best analogy for CBPR, as it doesn't begin to capture the issues of pain and structural oppression that are a part of racism and privilege and therefore often at play in research relationships. Nevertheless, dancing goes back as far in history as research and curiosity. In the words of Zora Neale Hurston, "Research is formalized curiosity. It is poking and prying with purpose. It is a seeking that s/he who wishes may know the cosmic secrets of the world and they that dwell therein" (Walker, 1979, p. 49).

The construct of race/ethnicity, though problematic, is used throughout this chapter because of its historical importance in the American psyche. Furthermore, the trilogy of race/ethnicity, racism, and white privilege is underscored throughout this chapter not because it is more important than other dimensions, such as social class or gender, but because it has often been neglected in CBPR and other areas of research. Race is not a biological construct that reflects innate differences but rather a social construct that captures the impact of racism. As such, the variable "race" measures a combination of social class, culture, and genes (Lin & Kelsey, 2000). As a rough though imperfect proxy for socioeconomic status, race captures the social classification that governs the distribution of risks and opportunities in a race-conscious society such as the United States (Jones, 2000, 2001). The meaning of race in the United States cannot be seen simply as an objective fact or treated as an independent variable (Omi, 2000). Contemporary immigration to the United States is a factor in the changing meaning of race. Between 1971 and 1995, the United States officially admitted just over 17 million immigrants, who are residing in various neighborhoods and communities all over the country (Camarillo & Bonilla, 2000). As Michael Omi comments, "The massive influx of new immigrant groups has destabilized specific concepts of race, led to a proliferation of identity positions, and challenged prevailing modes of political and cultural organization" (2000, p. 245).

This chapter will build on the principles of CBPR (see Chapter Three) to examine the hard issues of race and ethnicity, racism, and white privilege that every community based participatory researcher, whether white or a person of color, should consider when doing CBPR with communities of color. We begin with an overview of a useful framework for understanding racism that addresses institutional and personally mediated racism, as well as internalized oppression. We then discuss the powerful role of language and the potential errors that arise in translating cultural constructs in research and practice. Third, we explore the concept of white privilege (Cooper, 1989; Hurtado, 1996; Krieger, Williams, & Zierler, 1999; McIntosh, 1998) and how this power imbalance often obstructs the trust and community-building aspects of participatory research. We conclude with suggestions for building alliances across difference and offer a set of recommendations CBPR researchers can draw on in attempting to better address issues of race, racism, and privilege that often hover at the periphery of participatory research (Blair, Cahill, Chopyak, & Cordes, 2000).

FRAMEWORK OF OPPRESSION AND RACISM

Although most often talked about in relation to the oppressed (such as women, the poor, and people of color), race, class, and gender are part of the whole fabric of experience for all groups (Stoller & Gibson, 1999). These variables exist within interlocking hierarchies that create systems of privilege as well as disadvantage (Andersen & Collins, 1995; Stoller & Gibson, 1999). The complexity of social relations, social issues, and social justice is infused with race, class, and gender (Andersen & Collins, 1995). These processes are dynamic and change by time and place, with individual vulnerability to oppression increasing to the degree that the interlocking systems of oppression increase. That is, the less power a person has in society, the more "at risk" that person is for health and social problems (Garrett, 2000; Hogue, Hargraves, & Collins, 2000). The emphasis on the intersection of these multiple systems of inequality explains how people can simultaneously experience oppression along one dimension (class) and privilege along another (gender)—for example, a wealthy white woman or a poor Latino male. The primary roots of oppression worldwide are economic, social, cultural, and gender inequalities reproduced by an institutionalized system of power imbalance between and among groups of people (Kim, Irwin, Gershman, & Millen, 1999; Marmot & Wilkinson, 1999). Although oppression may look similar across cultures and generations, its mechanisms are historically and locally determined and change over time and place, depending on domination and resistance.

Some scholars and activists have defined racism as "prejudice plus power" (Omi, 2000); others posit racism as a life-threatening illness (James, 1994; Krieger, Rowley, Herman, Avery, & Phillips, 1993; Williams, 1997). Recognizing the multiple mechanisms of oppression and drawing on the work of Jones (2001), Omi (2000), Sherover-Marcuse (1986), Tilley (1990), Foucault (1980), and others, we offer three interrelated theories of how racism and privilege may manifest in community based participatory research projects. These are a three-tiered framework for racism, an analysis of power as repressive versus productive, and an understanding of discourse in communities, which may be public or hidden to the researcher.

Three-Tiered Framework for Racism

Camara Jones (2000) has developed a framework for understanding racism as institutionalized, personally mediated, and internalized. *Institutionalized* racism manifests itself in both material conditions and access to power. Examples include differential access to quality education, adequate housing, gainful employment, appropriate medical facilities, and a clean environment. With regard to power, institutionalized racism includes differential access to information, including one's own history, resources, and voice, and representation in government and the media. *Personally mediated* racism refers to prejudice, discrimination, stereotypes, and judgments based on assumptions about the abilities, motives, and intentions of others according to their race. As Jones (2001, p. 300) notes, this "is what most people think of when they hear the word *racism.* . . . It manifests as lack of respect, suspicion, devaluation, scapegoating, and dehumanization."

Internalized racism does not need an outside judge of character. It is characterized by people's own belief in the negative messages they receive about their race/ethnicity. The core of this perspective is that "an oppressive society recreates itself in its victims' hearts" (Sherover-Marcuse, 1986, p. 4). Internalized oppression addresses subjectivity, questions of power, and the part each person plays in the evolution of his or her own life story. It acknowledges that oppression does not come only from an external intersection of multiple systems of inequality; the enemy is also within.

The interaction of institutionalized racism, personally mediated racism, and internalized racism produces a racial climate that can manifest itself in community based participatory research in the following manner. In many major U.S. cities, whites have fled to suburbia, abandoning the inner city to turf battles among different racial minorities for housing, public services, and economic development (Omi, 2000). Racial segregation of neighborhoods, created through institutionalized policies or norms, have limited educational or employment opportunities for communities of color. With more than 80 percent of whites living in virtually all-white neighborhoods and nearly nine in ten white suburbanites living in communities with fewer than 1 percent African Americans, this degree of isolation can lead to a skewed perception of what other people experience and a reinforcement of personally mediated stereotypes. This skewed perception is bolstered by images, descriptions, and depictions fostered by cultural institutions such as the mass media. After all, if one doesn't know many African Americans or doesn't personally experience discrimination, and the only knowledge comes from second- or thirdhand sources, it is more likely that one will find the notion of widespread mistreatment unbelievable. Finally, the isolation of people of color can lead to internalized racism, whereby people internalize their lack of opportunities as self-blame.

These three levels of racism may also be played out in the relationship between researchers and communities. First, on the institutional level, structural factors inform the class and ethnic makeup of the CBPR collaborators. Given differential access by race to goods, services, and opportunities in society, CBPR often involves university researchers who are white working in communities of color where social and health problems are identified. People and communities of color are those being studied, not those doing the studying. Clarence Spigner (2000, p. 259) extends this point further, noting contradictions within CBPR itself: "The research establishment is overwhelmed by well-meaning non-minorities who recognize racism and its consequences on health, but only greater representation of people-of-color in the health establishment can ameliorate the inherent contradictions of 'participatory democracy' fundamental to the process of community based participatory research." As Marianne Sullivan and her colleagues (2001; see also Chapter Six) suggest, diversifying academic research faculty and other forms of institutional change must be seen as important goals of CBPR if we are to successfully overcome this problem. However, while it is crucial to take steps in this direction, it is important to note that institutionalized racism works to establish the dominant culture and its way of doing things, including traditional forms of research as the yardstick that measures and establishes credibility.

On the second level, personally mediated racism may manifest in stereotypical projections between public health professionals as outsiders and community members as insiders. When the outsider does not share the lived experiences of community members, assumptions and preconceived ideas about each other are often made (Hatch, Moss, Saran, Presley-Cantrell, & Mallory, 1993; Perkins & Wandersman, 1990). In the case of the outside researchers, these assumptions tend to focus on finding deficits rather than community resources because the framework in health and human service systems charges its workers to assess problems rather than recognize solutions (McKnight, 1995). This deficit model promotes the idea that solutions must come from outside the community, a view supported as well by those looking for someone to come in and "save" the community from itself.

Third, on the level of internalized oppression and racism, researchers of color face their own experiences with racism and privilege as "outsider-insiders." People of color involved in CBPR may not be able to identify their community's assets due to feelings of internalized oppression that make them undervalue community resources. Before one can name the gifts, talents, and resources in a community, the community members themselves have to believe these exist. Finally, internalized oppression may also lead community residents to value white researchers and dismiss educated members of their own community as well as the learning and teaching available in communities of color from the residents themselves.

Repressive and Productive Power

To understand racism more clearly, it is important to understand the multiple ways that power is manifest in both the dominant society and subordinate communities. Foucault differentiates between power that represses others and power that produces "Others." Repressive power structures, like institutional forms of racism, operate through direct control over people's opportunities to education, employment, living conditions, and other factors that contribute to health or disease. Productive power, exercised by mainstream institutions including those of public health, creates and reproduces the symbols and hierarchies of structural power that normalize and mask repressive relationships—for example, believing that "research" must be carried out in the conventional manner taught by professional experts at major universities. Repressive and productive power is not monolithic, however; it is built into a web of relationships and practices found in institutions, communities, and families, which are inherently unstable and therefore susceptible to challenge (Foucault, 1980).

Productive power as expressed by subordinate communities offers the possibility of challenging oppressive structures, through the capacity of communities to bring about outcomes and effects in the world (Tilley, 1990, p. 287). This community productive power, emanating from lived experience, is the origin of race/ethnicity-centered interventions and indigenous theories of health and illness, which represent a counterhegemonic challenge to outside definitions of community problems and solutions. In other words, if hegemony is the claim that the dominant culture controls the ideological sectors of society—culture, religion, education, and the media—in a manner that disseminates values to reinforce its position (Scott, 1985), then counterhegemony is the interruption of this practice from the grassroots perspective.

One example of counterhegemonic theory is the concept of historical trauma, which has gained popularity among Native American community based health practitioners and consumers (Brave Heart & De Bruyn, 1998; Duran, Duran, & Brave Heart, 1998). The theory of historical trauma posits that traumatic assaults on past generations, most notably the colonization of the Americas, created a psychological and physical health effect on the descendents of those affected. The historic events of the colonization are in part important root causes of both high rates of physical and psychological health disparities and of weak mainstream political will to ameliorate them.

Community based participatory researchers working in communities of color, and particularly in native communities, would be well advised to be conversant with historical trauma and related theories. The advantage of engaging with such approaches is that they speak directly to the lived experience of individuals and groups and may therefore be more widely accepted as the basis for research and intervention emanating from the community.

Hidden and Public Transcripts

The relationship between community members and outside researchers in CBPR is based on dialogue, mutual respect, and sharing of lived realities (Ansley & Gaventa, 1997; Cornwall & Jewkes, 1995; Israel, Schulz, Parker, & Becker, 1998). However, though researchers may believe they have access to community norms and ideas, they may only have access to what is considered public. James Scott (1985) theorizes that there are four levels of community dialogue: public discourse, hidden transcripts, coded defiance, and open defiance. Public discourse is the official, institutionalized language for health that takes as its basis the authority of public health systems. Hidden transcripts, by contrast, are characterized by subordinates gathering outside the gaze of power and constructing a sharply critical political and cultural discourse. As Makani Themba suggests (1999), much rap music is an example of a form of hidden transcript that provides members of an oppressed group with a critical venue for "expressing rage at the status quo as well as holding a candid discussion of social issues" (p. 22). There may be many hidden transcripts in any given community, and outsiders rarely have access to all of these. Coded counterhegemonic discourse is the use of disguise and anonymity, which subordinate groups will use as an avenue for the veiled expression of hidden transcripts in public discourse. In the case of CBPR, where researchers and community members have entered into collaborative understanding, open expression of conflict may be rare. Yet among themselves, as noted in Chapter Two, community researchers of color may express defiance, make jokes, and express tensions not safe to bring up in the presence of their white counterparts from university or professional environments.

With internalized oppression, community partners in research may often self-censor and conform to what is presented. They may nod their heads and say yes in resignation—when the heart feels no—as a result of having been led to believe that they are "deficient" and dare not challenge. When community research participants feel that they are not truly equal partners, the range of allowable forms of self-expression is limited. Community based ethnographic research on substance abuse and substance abusers (Bourgois, Lettiere, & Quezada, 1997) describes how community members who are paid to participate in studies anticipate what the researcher wants and may speak those words in order to maintain the relationship and not disturb the peace: "Street addicts usually do not want to appear stupid or offensive to a friendly interviewer. In fact they usually have at least a partially internalized society's normalizing judgments and are depressed, ashamed, or ambivalent about their marginality. . . . He liked the researcher administering the interview protocol, so he tried to respond in what he thought was a socially appropriate manner" (p. 166).

This interaction involves a dialectic of resistance between outside research partners and community participants with very real ethical dilemmas involved in speaking truth to power. There may be fear of speaking out about personal and community oppression because of the risks involved in creating stereotypes and misinformation, which then may be generalized to all communities of color. Furthermore, people from communities of color learn very early not to reveal true information to white people because they do not believe that whites want to hear the "truth" or because they fear that the "truth" will not be heard. As Scott (1985) has aptly pointed out, "The greater the disparity in power between dominant and subordinate and the more arbitrarily it is exercised, the more the public transcript of subordinated will take on a stereotyped, ritualistic cast" (p.11).

Community based participatory research must go beyond the surface issues of making research questions culturally and linguistically appropriate and relevant. Research participants have obvious and compelling reasons to seek refuge behind "public transcripts" when in the presence of power. Similarly, outside researchers often adopt a "public transcript" in the presence of "subordinates" that consists of expected gestures and words. As subordination requires a credible performance of humility and deference, so domination requires a credible performance of mastery and power.

CBPR must be about asking questions and examining the power dynamics that exist when some people speak and others are silent. Drawing on Freire's (1970) work, CBPR can transform the culture of silence among oppressed groups. Community members take risks in sharing their personal stories and speaking with outside researchers. Even in CBPR, time constraints sometimes lead outside or university researchers to stop the telling of a community story without knowing its importance and opt for more closed-ended matters. This way of conducting research silences community members and impedes their full participation in the research process. In addition, it limits the information gathered to whatever the outside researcher thinks is relevant. This in turn leads to research results and interventions that lack an authentic community "voice." Solutions are consequently developed with incomplete and inadequate information from a limited outside researcher's perspective. Cynthia Chataway (1997), a white female university researcher, also notes that doing all the talking and presenting of opinions and facts may get in the way of participatory research. She suggests that withholding information can allow space for the "other" to speak and act to bring a balance of power to the relationship that forces the other to speak outside of the public transcript. Chataway's description of silencing herself to avoid dominating the research relationship is an important one for CBPR researchers who are outside or university members of the team to consider. However, a word of caution: withholding information can in some cases be manipulative. The important issue is that outside researchers must learn to value what community participants have to say, listen to everyone in a meaningful way, and not speak as the "expert." Once again, a dance is involved; balancing silence and speaking creates the space for community members to express themselves.

LANGUAGE: TRANSLATING CULTURE

How do you say *empowerment* in Spanish? What does empowerment mean for African Americans? The answers to these questions are crucial in CBPR because the concept of empowerment is an important goal. Practitioners have been grappling with questions about translating *empowerment* and communicating cultural constructs since the first time this word appeared in the literature (Erzinger, 1994). The question of how to say *empowerment* in Spanish matters to CBPR researchers concerned about the development of culturally and linguistically relevant data collection. Data collection instruments rely not only on literal translations but also on a deeper translation of meaning, concepts, and cultural constructs. Empowerment operationalized from a multicultural perspective is played out in a range of ways that challenge researchers to make evident the need to remember the first principle of CBPR (see Chapter Three): *local relevance and attention to the social, economic, and cultural conditions that influence health status.* The issue of empowerment raises the question of whether many public health concepts are relevant, meaningful, and translatable across cultures. For example, since collectivism, or family- or group-centeredness, is a sociobehavioral orientation in many communities of color (Aguirre-Molina, Molina, & Zambrana, 2001; Braithwaite & Taylor, 2000; Spigner, 2000), are the constructs of individually focused health education theories applicable to people who identify with more collective, cooperative models? The answer to this question matters, as it may affect every step of the research process, from problem definition to instrument development, data collection, and analysis, as well as dissemination of research findings.

A key principle of CBPR is the notion that *research must be produced, interpreted, and disseminated to community members in clear, useful, and respectful language.* Nonetheless, academia has its own language and assumptions that often clash with those of the majority of the people in the communities where research is conducted. As professionally trained outside researchers, we often take for granted knowledge of words, acronyms, and concepts that are familiar to us, assuming that others who don't understand will ask for an explanation. The commitment to disseminate research and communicate back with the community where the data were gathered requires that CBPR researchers go outside the usual boundaries of academic convention. Often the frame of reference for disseminating research findings is guided by "acceptable" standards of academia, such as publication in peer-reviewed journals or presentation at professional meetings (see Chapters Five and Six). However, even with community members involved, specialized professional language often prescribes how health issues and community needs should be introduced and studied, findings posed and disseminated, and strategies recommended. To be true to the principles of CBPR, projects must be designed in which research is only a piece of the work to be undertaken. Successful CBPR projects acknowledge the role of history; specifically, that the relationship between researchers and community members begins not with the project itself but centuries ago, with the advent of slavery and other forms of exploitation.

Another important point at the nexus of language and culture is how researchers of color are often expected to serve as translators, ventriloquists, and spokespersons (Trinh, 1989). Often researchers of color are not in the role of primary investigator but act in a secondary capacity to bridge the gap between communities of color and institutions of research, bringing knowledge across in both directions. Researchers who speak the language of the community become privy to the hidden transcripts in communities of color and might come across information that on both ethical and practical grounds may best be kept confidential. It is important to respect that relationships are primary and integral to the goals of CBPR. A researcher who learns and publishes information that should have remained confidential can cause considerable conflict and pain within the community if and when this breach of confidence comes to light. It will also make it far more difficult to establish that level of trust again in that community and thus limit access to crucial information and data. The abuse of trust in communities has been a recurring reality that must be taken seriously if outside researchers are committed to a long-term relationship (Braithwaite & Taylor, 2000, Hatch et al., 1993; Perkins & Wandersman, 1990). The violation of trust historically affects questions of accountability. And this brings to bear a significant question: To whom is the outside researcher accountable?

WHITE PRIVILEGE

Although there are multiple sources of overlapping privilege, it is especially important in the United States to confront the experience of privilege that goes with being of the dominant race (Cooper, 1989; Hurtado, 1996; Krieger et al., 1999; McIntosh, 1998; Omi, 2000). The experience of the dominant group often serves as the point of reference, the "norm," and is compared with that of people who are disadvantaged along a continuum of oppression and powerlessness (McIntosh, 1998).

Experiences of bias and discrimination mask the ways in which systems of privilege work. The racialization process for whites is evident on college campuses as white students encounter a heightened awareness of race that calls their own identity into question (Omi, 2000). Research on white Americans suggests that they do not experience their ethnicity as a definitive aspect of their social identity unless they work or live in diverse communities. Omi (2000, p. 257) remarks, "Whites tend to locate racism in color consciousness and find its absence in color-blindness. In so doing, they see the affirmation of difference and racial identity among racially defined minority students as racist. Black students, by contrast, see racism as a system of power, and correspondingly argue that they cannot be racist because they lack power."

In essence there seem to be "two languages of race" (Blauner, 1994), one in which members of communities of color see the centrality of race in history and everyday experience and another in which whites see race as a peripheral reality and do not perceive themselves as racist.

Unconscious racism—being able to ignore issues surrounding race—is a key aspect of white privilege (McIntosh, 1998). Being white, male, and of the middle or upper class provides unearned advantages. White privilege, however, is independent of feelings of racism. Whereas in the past, white privilege was asserted through blatantly racist acts and political policies, today the mechanisms of white privilege are more complex and firmly entrenched. Even when they may perceive a lack of "racist feelings," whites may reproduce the system of white privilege in several ways: (1) by feeling that they are only getting what is due to them, what they deserve (meritocracy) (Mills, 1998); (2) by mistaking prevalent white culture as culturally neutral; (3) by not recognizing that their privilege is not automatically shared or conferred on others; and (4) by not having to contend with internalized oppression (Cooper, 1989; Hurtado, 1996; Kivel, 1996; Krieger et al., 1999; McIntosh, 1998).

The advantage of not having to deal with race is denied to people of color who are constantly reminded of our "disadvantaged status." Jerry Tello tours the country giving seminars on cultural competency and systems change for health and human services personnel. He notes that it is vital that people of color not forget where they came from. "The minute you forget and get comfortable, someone will remind you," whether it is with the innocent question "Where are you from?" or more poignantly "Who are you here with?" or "Why are you here?" Similarly, Paulo Freire (1973) expressed early on his concern that leadership training and by extension professional or academic training in research makes people of color "strangers in their own community."

For professionally trained researchers who are white or otherwise advantaged, privilege is one of the most important and difficult arenas in CBPR to address, as it in part defines who we understand ourselves to be. The outcomes and mechanisms of institutionalized racism are easier to uncover because they are not personal. To look internally at privilege conferred due to education, race, sexual orientation, gender, or institutional affiliation means a long-term commitment to engage in deep inner work researchers may not be prepared to do.

PARTNERSHIPS: BUILDING ALLIANCES ACROSS DIFFERENCES

Hugh Vasquez, Nell Myhand, and Allan Creighton, authors of *Celebrating Diversity, Building Alliances* (2002), emphasize the hope in the momentum being built that has created an increased demand for justice. People are willing to find ways of working together with partners who may be different from themselves to see justice happen. They underscore that it is in human nature to want to be close to people and break down all the divisions that exist among us. The first step is the desire to examine what the systemic and personal barriers are. Makani Themba (1999) adds to the hopefulness with a reality test. "Racism" she says, "is like the gorilla in the living room. It's running through the place making noises and everyone is trying to sit politely and ignore it" (p. 157). Themba also notes that the privileges and pain associated with racism make it vital to remember that racism is a system that is much larger than the sum of the individuals who it affects. In order to address racism, she notes, we have to understand its systemic nature and learn how to build new, less comfortable alliances. Similarly, as Lorraine Gutierrez and Edith Lewis (1997) suggest, we must "recognize and embrace the conflict that characterizes cross-cultural work" (p. 220).

The larger context in which the dance of racism and privilege takes place makes it necessary that we continue to work against structural or institutionalized racism because as long as it is present, any CBPR is severely limited in what it can hope to achieve. As Camara Jones (2000, p. 1214) points out, "Institutionalized racism is the most fundamental of the three levels [of racism] and must be addressed for important change to occur." The dance analogy suggests that CBPR is not only about dancing; it is also about continuously "learning to dance" while accepting the invariability of continued mistakes along the way. The failure to dance—that is, failing to address racism and privilege—will inevitably lead to power imbalances and lack of coordination between white researchers and community researchers. "Power imbalances often stand in the way of developing effective working relationships grounded in trust" (Sullivan et al., 2001, p. 136).

RECOMMENDATIONS FOR RESEARCH AND PRACTICE

In addition to the suggestions implicit in the basic principles of CBPR, such as having community partners involved in all phases of the research process, the following set of recommendations, drawn from a variety of sources (Chávez et al., in press; Duran & Duran, 1999; Jones, 2001; Omi, 2000; Spigner, 2000; Themba, 1999; Wallerstein, 1999), puts special emphasis on reducing racism and privilege in CBPR.

- Acknowledge the diversity within racial and ethnic groups. Expand data collection to include questions on ancestry, migration history, and language. Researchers need to be attentive to the increasing heterogeneity of racial/ethnic groups and rethink the nature and types of research questions asked.
- Acknowledge that race is a social construct, not a biologic determinant, and model race as a contextual variable in multilevel analyses.

- Address the present-day existence and impacts of racism (institutionalized, personally mediated, and internalized) not only as variables to measure but also as lived experiences within the research process. The complex nature of race relations in the post–civil rights era United States requires that we move beyond discussions of race and racism as a "black-white" phenomenon to encompass multiple racial and ethnic groupings.

- Examine the role of racism in diminishing the health of the entire population, not just the health of members of low-income communities of color. Emphasize the "intersectionality" of race, gender, age, and class to examine how different categories engage with racism and with each other.

- Encourage people from communities of color to pursue higher education. They will bring new perspectives to CBPR and will raise new questions. Institutional change, such as diversifying academic research faculty, is an important goal of CBPR.

- Use the research process and outcomes to mobilize and advocate for change to reduce disparities and enhance race relations.

- Listen, listen, and listen. Pay close attention to both hidden and public transcripts, and speak about white privilege and racism.

- Accept that outsiders cannot fully understand community and interpersonal dynamics. Do not, however, let this stop you from taking part in the "dance."

- Recognize that privilege, especially white privilege, is continually operating to some degree and creating situations of power imbalance. Such an understanding is crucial in honest, ongoing communication that builds trust and respect.

- Build true multicultural working relationships, and in a partnership mode, develop guidelines for research data collection, analysis, publication, and dissemination of research findings.

CBPR attempts to change the paradigm in which research is conceived and operationalized. Racism and privilege are major factors that challenge this paradigm shift. Understanding the roots of oppression and its relationship to trust and community building are part of the dance that is indispensable to doing this work. So is addressing the challenge of true equal partnerships in CBPR in a world of injustice. Having as collaborators working-class people of color who consider themselves equal partners and are considered equal partners in the research process requires ongoing effort.

The effort to understand racism and all its consequences is work done in the context of relationships. To empower a community, we must become a community, supporting and challenging each other as we implement culturally competent, power- and race-sensitive inquiry. Dancing forward, following the flow of the dance of race and privilege in community based participatory research, outside researchers must become comfortable with not always taking the lead but dancing side by side with the community and sometimes following the community's lead.

References

Aguirre-Molina, M., Molina, C., & Zambrana, R. (Eds.). (2001). *Health issues in the Latino community.* San Francisco: Jossey-Bass.

Andersen, M. L., & Collins, P. H. (1995). *Race, class, and gender: An anthology* (2nd ed.). Belmont, CA.: Wadsworth.

Ansley, F., & Gaventa, J. (1997, January-February). Researching for democracy and democratizing research. *Change,* pp. 46–53.

Blair, R., Cahill, K., Chopyak, J., & Cordes, C. (2000). *Common problems, uncommon resources: Exploring the social and economic challenges of community based research.* Atlanta: Community Research Network.

Blauner, B. (1994). Talking past each other: Black and white languages of race. In F. Pincus & H. Ehrlich (Eds.), *Race and ethnic conflict: Contenting views on prejudice, discrimination, and ethno-violence* (pp. 18–28). Boulder, CO: Westview Press.

Bourgois, P., Lettiere, M., & Quezada, J. (1997). Social misery and the sanctions of substance abuse: Confronting HIV risk among homeless heroin addicts in San Francisco. *Social Problems, 44,* 155–173.

Braithwaite, R., & Taylor, S. (2000). *Health issues in the black community.* San Francisco: Jossey-Bass.

Brave Heart, M.Y.H., & De Bruyn, L. M. (1998). The American Indian holocaust: Healing historical unresolved grief. *American Indian and Alaska Native Mental Health Research, 2,* 60–82.

Camarillo, A. M., & Bonilla, F. (2000). Hispanics in a multicultural society: A new American dilemma? In N. J. Smelser, W. J. Wilson, & F. Mitchell (Eds.), *America becoming: Racial trends and their consequences* (Vol. 1, pp. 103–134). Washington, DC: National Academy Press.

Chataway, C. (1997). An examination of the constraints on mutual inquiry in a participatory action research project. *Journal of Social Issues, 4,* 747–766.

Chávez, V., Israel, B. A., Allen, A. J., III, Lichenstein, R., De Carlo, M., Schulz, A. J., Bayer, R., & McGranaghand, R. (in press). A bridge between communities: Video making and community based participatory research. *Health Promotion Practice.*

Cooper, T. (1989). The rewards of racial prejudice. *Journal of Housing, 46*(3), 105–107.

Cornwall, A., & Jewkes, R. (1995). What is participatory research? *Social Science and Medicine, 41,* 1667–1676.

Duran, B., & Duran, E. (1999). Assessment, program planning, and evaluation in Indian Country: Toward a postcolonial practice. In R. M. Huff & M. V. Kline (Eds.), *Promoting health in multicultural populations: A handbook for practitioners* (pp. 291–311). Thousand Oaks, CA: Sage.

Duran, B., Duran, E., & Brave Heart, M.Y.H. (1998). Native Americans and the trauma of history. In R. Thornton (Ed.), *Studying Native America: Problems and prospects in Native American studies* (pp. 60–78). Madison: University of Wisconsin Press.

Erzinger, S. (1994). Empowerment in Spanish: Words can get in the way. *Health Education Quarterly, 21,* 417–419.

Foucault, M. (1980). *Power/knowledge: Selected interviews and other writings, 1972–1977* (Ed. C. Gordon). New York: Pantheon Books.

Freire, P. (1970). *Pedagogy of the oppressed.* New York: Seabury Press.

Freire, P. (1973). *Education for critical consciousness.* New York: Continuum.

Garrett, L. (2000). *Betrayal of trust: The collapse of global public health.* New York: Hyperion.

Gutierrez, L., & Lewis, E. (1998). Education, participation, and capacity building in community organizing with women of color. In M. Minkler (Ed.), *Community organization and community building for health* (pp. 216–229). New Brunswick, NJ: Rutgers University Press.

Hatch, J., Moss, N., Saran, A., Presley-Cantrell, L., & Mallory, C. (1993). Community research: Partnership in black communities. *American Journal of Preventive Medicine, 9,* 27–31.

Hogue, C.J.R., Hargraves, M. A., & Collins, K. S. (2000). *Minority health in America: Findings and policy implications from the Commonwealth Fund Minority Health Survey.* Baltimore: Johns Hopkins University Press.

Hurtado, A. (1996). *The Color of privilege: Three blasphemies on race and feminism.* Ann Arbor: University of Michigan Press.

Israel, B. A., Schulz, A. J., Parker, E. A., & Becker, A. B. (1998). Review of community-based research: Assessing partnership approaches to improve public health. *Annual Review of Public Health, 19,* 173–202.

James, S. A. (1994). John Henryism and the health of African-Americans. *Cultural Medical Psychiatry, 18,* 163–182.

Jones, C. P. (2000). Levels of racism: A theoretic framework and a gardener's tale. *American Journal of Public Health, 8,* 1212–1215.

Jones, C. P. (2001). Invited commentary: "Race," racism and the practice of epidemiology. *American Journal of Epidemiology, 4,* 299–304.

Kim, J. Y., Irwin, A., Gershman, J., & Millen, J. (Eds.). (1999). *Dying for growth: Global inequality and the health of the poor.* Monroe, ME: Common Courage Press.

Kivel, P. (1996). *Uprooting racism: How white people can work for racial justice.* Gabriola Island, British Columbia, Canada: New Society Press.

Krieger, N., Rowley, D. L., Herman, A. A., Avery, B., & Phillips, M. T. (1993). Racism, sexism, and social class: Implications for studies of health, disease, and well-being. *American Journal of Preventive Medicine, 9*(6), 82–122.

Krieger, N., Williams, D. R., & Zierler, S. (1999). "Whiting out" white privilege will not advance the study of how racism harms health. *American Journal of Public Health, 5,* 782–783; discussion 784–785.

Lin, S. S., & Kelsey, J. L. (2000). Use of race and ethnicity in epidemiologic research: Concepts, methodologic issues, and suggestions for research. *Epidemiology Review, 22,* 187–202.

Marmot, M., & Wilkinson, R. (Eds.). (1999). *Social determinants of health.* Oxford: Oxford University Press.

McIntosh, P. (1998). White privilege: Unpacking the invisible knapsack. In M. McGoldrick (Ed.), *Re-visioning family therapy: Race, culture, and gender in clinical practice* (pp. 147–152). New York: Guilford Press.

McKnight, J. (1995). *The careless society: Community and its counterfeits.* New York: Basic Books.

Mills, C. W. (1998). *Blackness visible: Essays on philosophy and race.* Ithaca, NY: Cornell University Press.

Omi, M. A. (2000). The changing meaning of race. In N. J. Smelser, W. J. Wilson, & F. Mitchell (Eds.), *America becoming: Racial trends and their consequences* (Vol. 1, pp. 243–263). Washington, DC: National Academy Press.

Perkins, D. D., & Wandersman, A. (1990). You'll have to work to overcome our suspicions: The benefits and pitfalls of research with community organizations. *Social Policy, 21*(1), 32–42.

Scott, J. (1985). *Weapons of the weak.* New Haven, CT: Yale University Press.

Sherover-Marcuse, R. (1986). *Emancipation and consciousness: Dogmatic and dialectical perspectives in the early Marx.* New York: Blackwell.

Smelser, N. J., Wilson, W. J., & Mitchell, F. (Eds.). (2000). *America becoming: Racial trends and their consequences* (Vol. 1). Washington, DC: National Academy Press.

Spigner, C. (2000). African Americans, democracy, and biomedical and behavioral research: Contradictions or consensus in community-based participatory research? *International Quarterly of Community Health Education, 3,* 259–284.

Stoller, E. P., & Gibson, R. P. (1999). *Worlds of difference: Inequality in the aging experience* (3rd ed.). Thousand Oaks, CA: Pine Forge Press.

Sullivan, M., Koné, A., Senturia, K., Chrisman, N., Ciske, S., & Krieger, J. W. (2001). Researcher and researched-community perspectives: Toward bridging the gap. *Health Education and Behavior, 2,* 130–149.

Themba, M. N. (1999). *Making policy, making change: How communities are taking law into their own hands.* Berkeley, CA: Chardon Press.

Tilley, C. (1990). Michel Foucault: Towards an archaeology of archaeology. In C. Tilley (Ed.), *Reading material culture: Structuralism, hermeneutics, and post-structuralism* (pp. 281–347). Oxford: Blackwell.

Trinh, T. M. (1989). *Woman, native, other.* Indianapolis: Indiana University Press.

Vasquez, H., Myhand, N., & Creighton, A. (2002). *Celebrating diversity, building alliances: A curriculum for making the peace in middle school.* Alameda, CA: Hunter House.

Walker, A. (Ed.). (1979). *I love myself: A Zora Neale Hurston reader.* New York: Feminist Press.

Wallerstein, N. (1999). Power between evaluator and community: Research relationships within New Mexico's healthier communities. *Social Science and Medicine, 49,* 39–53.

Williams, D. R. (1997). Race and health: Basic questions, emerging directions. *Annals of Epidemiology, 5,* 322–333.

CHAPTER FIVE

Are Academics Irrelevant?

Approaches and Roles for Scholars in Community Based Participatory Research

Randy Stoecker

The word "academic" is a synonym for irrelevant.
—Saul Alinsky (1946/1969, p. ix)

I remember the moment my academic career changed. I was a graduate student, sitting in the Cedar-Riverside Project Area Committee (PAC) office to interview Tim Mungavan about this amazing Minneapolis neighborhood that had instituted a radical grassroots community-controlled redevelopment program. Tim, the group's architect and organizer, leaned back in his chair, put his feet up on his desk, and looked me sternly in the eye. He said "We have students and reporters coming through all the time, asking neighborhood people to give their time and answer their questions. And we don't get so much as a copy of a paper from them. If I agree to talk with you, then I want you to agree that you'll give us a copy of the paper you write" (Stoecker, 1994, p. 25). Tim tells the story of how I then tried to make myself relevant, and he set me to work cleaning the PAC's storeroom, thinking that if I stuck with it after that, I might really be serious. I stuck, at least partly because the storeroom was a treasure trove of neighborhood information. My relationship with the neighborhood continues to this day.

When I got my first academic job at the University of Toledo, I met Dave Beckwith, a community organizer with the Center for Community Change and the University of Toledo Urban Affairs Center. Dave handed me a list of

Note: This chapter was adapted from "Are Academics Irrelevant?" by R. Stoecker, *American Behavioral Scientist*, 42(5), pp. 840–854. Copyright © 1999 by Sage Publications, Inc. Reprinted by permission of Sage Publications, Inc.

community-generated research needs almost the day I arrived. I negotiated with him and other activists to do a resource and needs assessment of Toledo's community based organizations. This project, involving neighborhood activists throughout, built a coalition that brought in over $2 million to support those groups. As time went on, however, I found myself working with bankers, foundation officials, and large nonprofits that did not share my desire to transform all power structures to participatory democracies and community-controlled economies. I consequently became involved in a factional power struggle that destroyed the coalition built by that first project (Stoecker, 1997). Then I was in two very different participatory research projects in 1996. The first project I initiated. It began with academics, never made the transition to community control, and died. The second began with community members, and I became involved as one of many. This project is thriving (Stoecker & Stuber, 1999). Since then, when the original version of this chapter was written, I have worked increasingly closely with a number of community organizers, helping me to clarify my role in CBPR (Stoecker, 1999). I have also been working with the Bonner Foundation's Community Research Project, which is building CBPR programs in more than a dozen universities, and have begun to see the diversity of approaches to CBPR-related approaches out there (Stoecker, 2001). All of this has confirmed what I wrote in the original version of this chapter and reinforces in me the haunting question of how I, as an academic, can become relevant.

APPROACHES TO CBPR AND OPTIONS FOR THE ACADEMIC

I have now made a career of CBPR, and I do finally feel relevant when I am working with community groups. But I still worry. The original goal of participatory research was for the members of the community to do things themselves and become self-sufficient knowledge providers and social change producers (Gaventa, 1991, 1993). Now, with people like me doing CBPR, are we furthering or hindering the long-term goals of community-controlled knowledge production and progressive social change? As Heaney (1993, pp. 43–44) has argued:

> However well-intentioned and zealous the efforts of individual faculty who have brought participatory research into the academic arena, one can only question by what compromises such researchers are likely to survive. . . . Having made our work acceptable in academic terms, we see that work now being incorporated into academic curricula. Our papers have become required readings for professional researchers who are expected to master the theory and methods of participatory research. It is not difficult to imagine the day when Third World governments and community organizations will hire only professional participatory researchers trained and certified by graduate institutions.

Participatory researchers seem to do increasingly well in the university (Cancian, 1993; Gedicks, 1996). But there are often compromises. Graduate students trying to do CBPR are still forced to take control of the research in order to get credit to graduate (Heaney, 1993). The reward system of universities discourages collaboration, and community members have to make time and even money sacrifices to collaborate in research, while academics get rewards (Hall, 1993; see also Appendix D). And in many institutions, community research is still seen as a kind of "community housework" that is not socially valued and hence does not receive much attention (Hubbard, 1996).

So how, as academics, do we keep our eyes on the twin prizes of community-controlled knowledge and progressive social change while still doing relevant work? Today academics seem to adopt three roles when approaching CBPR: the initiator, the consultant, and the collaborator.

The Initiator

One thing that most distinguishes CBPR from more conservative approaches is the belief that the research question should be generated by the community, not the researcher (Brown & Tandon, 1983; Deshler & Ewert, 1995). However, Peter Reason (1994) notes that "paradoxically, many PAR projects would not occur without the initiative of someone with time, skill, and commitment, someone who will almost inevitably be a member of a privileged and educated group" (p. 334). Researchers usually initiate contact with community organizations, even if they do consequently respond to requests coming from the community (Maguire, 1987).

Some also see the researcher as an educator or leader who helps the community overcome its false consciousness. This is tricky, however, because "for the alternative ideology to result from a collective effort throughout the research process, all forms of indoctrination and ideological imposition had to be ruled out" (de Roux, 1991, p. 50). Mohammad Anisur Rahman (1991) accuses some PAR practitioners of placing themselves in a vanguard role. And Stringer (1996) cautions, "When we try to 'get' people to do anything, insist that they 'must' or 'should' do something, or try to 'stop' them from engaging in some activity, we are working from an authoritative position that is likely to generate resistance" (p. 43).

Can an academic adopt an "initiator" approach that is truly empowering? Mary Brydon-Miller (1993) describes how her initial research led to a "community accessibility committee" that began taking action on its own. In this case, the research process strengthened people's awareness of their own skills and resources, requiring the researcher to take on more of a process-facilitating role and less of a product-producing role. Conversely, in a CBPR project I initiated, we were never able to switch control over to the community, as too many of our academic members were not skilled at community organizing and process facilitating (Stoecker & Stuber, 1999).

The Consultant

In the strictest sense, the original participatory research model says that community members should do the research themselves (Gaventa, 1991, 1993). However, in many cases, academics find themselves consulting with community groups (Stoecker, 2001). The community commissions the research, and the academic carries it out while being held accountable to the community. In some cases, the accountability process can be intense, with the researcher getting community input at each stage of the research project. I have used the consultant approach regularly, at the community's request. To ask already overburdened community members to do the research when they could be doing other more important things contradicts the social change goal of CBPR. A community group armed with a PhD-authored study may also be more influential than a group with research authored by someone not regarded as following scientific standards (Beckwith, 1996).

John Gaventa (1993), however, critiques both the initiator and the consultant approaches. Because not just material wealth but also intellectual knowledge is power, we need to change material relations and knowledge relations. Consequently, "to the extent that the research still remains in the hands of the researcher, a real transfer of ownership of knowledge may not have occurred. The dichotomy between those who produce knowledge and those who are most affected by it still exists. Eventually, the researcher may decide to leave, taking the skills, experience, and newly acquired knowledge along with him or her" (pp. 33–34).

The Collaborator

The Policy Research Action Group (PRAG) in Chicago (http://www.luc.edu/depts/curl/prag) pioneered the practice of "collaborative research" (Nyden, Figert, Shibley, & Burrows, 1997). In this approach, "it is recognized that the researcher may have certain technical expertise and the community leader may have knowledge of community needs and perspectives. Rather than either side using these resources to gain control in a research relationship, they need to be combined to provide a more unitary approach to research" (Nyden & Wiewal, 1992, p. 45). In contrast to those who fear that CBPR practitioners might further disempower the community, the PRAG model wonders if CBPR sometimes makes the researcher subservient to the community, and thus less useful than he or she might otherwise be.

But collaboration is hard. Rahman (1991) worries that it is not easy to establish a truly equal relationship at the outset with people who are traditionally victims of a dominating structure. Community members are not used to the "talk" world of academics, and they are often skeptical of it. And real collaboration takes a lot of time—for meetings, for accountability processes, for working through the inevitable conflicts—a commodity that may be in especially short supply for community group members. The collaborative approach may be less efficient than the consultant approach in that it asks community members to participate in ways they aren't interested in or don't have time for. Patricia Maguire (1987) reminds us, "While researchers may be able to invest their total work time in a [CBPR] project, participants continue their regular life activities" (p. 46). But does collaborative participation go far enough in changing existing knowledge relations? If the collaboration generates new knowledge and understanding for both community members and academics, then perhaps so, but if the collaboration is just each doing what they do best, then maybe not.

PARTICIPATORY RESEARCH IN CONTEXT AND RECOMMENDATIONS FOR ACADEMICS

The three CBPR approaches available to academics—as initiator, consultant, and collaborator—seem unsatisfactory and fraught with tensions. The problem, however, is not with the approaches but with a conception that CBPR is a *research project*. It's not. It's a social change project of which the research is only one piece. As such, it has three goals:

- Learning knowledge and skills relevant to the task at hand
- Developing relationships of solidarity
- Engaging in action that wins victories and builds self-sufficiency

"Doing research" is not, in itself, a goal. Research is only a method to achieve these broader goals. And that is where the crux of the issue lies. In real social change, the researcher role is only one of many, and we need to consider the other roles that make for successful CBPR.

Roles in Social Change

Achieving the social change goals of CBPR requires that four roles be fulfilled: leader or "animator," community organizer, popular educator, and participatory researcher.

Part translator, part facilitator, part self-esteem builder, the leader may be the most general and combines parts of the other roles but in essence is an indigenous or adopted community member who helps people develop a sense that they and their issues are important. For Rahman (1991), this "animator" has "a sense of commitment and a desire to live and work in the villages; innovativeness in work and a willingness to experiment with new approaches; communication skills, in particular the ability to dialogue, discuss and listen to the people; flexibility and a readiness to learn from one's own and others' experiences; and intellectual ability and emotional maturity" (p. 96).

The community organizer, a role many associate with Saul Alinsky (1946/1969, 1971; see also Beckwith & Lopez, 1997), is often confused with the researcher's role in CBPR—devaluing the importance of organizer skills and misleading academics as to what the real tasks are. Two important CBPR authors describe "researchers" in ways that better fit the organizer's role. Ernie Stringer (1996) portrays the "researcher" as a catalyst who stimulates people rather than imposes on them, emphasizes process over product, enables people to do things themselves, starts where people are, helps people plan and act and evaluate (rather than advocates for them), and focuses on human development as well as solutions to problems. Peter Park (1993) says that a community's "sense of the problem may not always be externalized as a consensually derived and objectified target of attack in the community, although there may be suffering, a sense of malaise and frustration, and anger. For this reason, the situation characteristically requires outside intervention in the guise of a researcher . . . to help formulate an identifiable problem to be tackled" (p. 8). The tragedy of conflating the organizer and researcher roles, which I have painfully learned, is that only a few academics are good organizers. Those trained in the 1960s social movements have real organizing skills. Those of us not trained in active mobilizations know *how* to do research. But we only know *about* organizing. I am among the latter group—too young to have gotten on-the-job training and too geographically isolated from the good organizing efforts out there today. My most successful CBPR experiences, then, have been working with those who are good organizers (Stoecker, 1999; Stoecker & Beckwith, 1992).

The popular educator, discussed earlier, facilitates the learning process. This is not a teacher who is assumed to have knowledge that he or she gives to people who are assumed to be ignorant. Rather, it is a facilitator who helps people discover for themselves what they already know and create new knowledge (Freire, 1970; Horton & Freire, 1990; Williams, 1996). As a consequence, people develop greater self-confidence along with greater knowledge. Ideally, in such a setting, the expert knowledge of the educator combines with the experiential knowledge of community members, creating entirely new ways of thinking about issues (Fear & Edwards, 1995).

Finally, the participatory researcher knows how to find the references quickly, can construct a survey blindfolded, and can create a research process either with strong guidance from community members or in collaboration with them. The concept of participatory researcher in this context is stripped of the other tasks of the initiator approach and is limited to conducting the research. But this role is also about more than being technically skilled. It is also about being committed to transforming the social relations of knowledge production and to democratic participation in the research process.

One person can occupy multiple roles. For example, a researcher who is a good organizer can be an initiator. Several people can also occupy the same role, especially in the research process, where there might be a variety of people collectively making research decisions.

Guideposts for the Academic

It is important to understand the relationship between the academic approaches to CBPR (initiator, consultant, collaborator) and roles in social change (community leader, community organizer, popular educator, participatory researcher). The academic engages with the community as an initiator, a consultant, or a collaborator. In doing so, he or she may fill one or more social change roles. For example, an academic who engages with the community as an initiator may be filling not just the participatory researcher role but perhaps the others as well. An academic who engages as a consultant may only need to fill the participatory researcher role.

We should ask three questions whenever we enter a CBPR situation to help us determine which of the approaches (initiator, consultant, collaborator) fits the community best. The answers will depend on whether one is working with an organized community or an unorganized community (Maguire, 1993).

What Is This CBPR Project Trying to Do? Some CBPR projects begin in a less well organized community and are actually community organizing projects—using the research to bring people together and build skills and relationships. The Appalachian Alliance conducted a massive eighty-county, six-state study that continues to inform communizing efforts (Horton, 1993). Yellow Creek Concerned Citizens, fighting toxic industrial waste polluting their water, found that doing their own health survey "gave them a reason and an incentive to call at every household along the fourteen-mile length of the creek, and sit down and discuss with them the problems they were experiencing. [It also] broadened and strengthened the leadership within the group. The prime activists in the health survey were women who became better informed and more vocal and confident through their work with the survey. . . . Now, you have to remember that none of us were trained health scientists, and some of the people who were doing this research had not graduated from high school" (Merrifield, 1993, pp. 78, 80).

If you are entering a less organized, low-resource community, members may not have filled the leader, organizer, educator, and researcher roles. If that is the case, see our next discussion, "What Are Your Skills?" Because depending on which social change roles are filled, and which ones *can* be filled by others, you may find yourself occupying the rest. Less organized communities, when they lack members who can fill the roles of leader, educator, organizer, and researcher, need an initiator researcher. These situations are the most difficult for the academic to enter, since they require so many skills beyond simply doing research.

Some projects create special difficulties. A coalition, in its early stages, is no different from any other relatively unorganized community, even if its individual member organizations are stable. Complications also arise with service organizations. If the research project is to "study" the service population but the only people making decisions are service providers, it violates the most fundamental characteristic of CBPR—that the people affected help control the research.

Other CBPR projects may come from already well organized communities that realize they need research to achieve their goals. For instance, I received a call from a neighborhood group concerned about outside landlords' and real estate agents' attempts to transform their neighborhood from homeowners to student renters. The group wanted to document how many rental houses they had. They had done the research themselves and only sought technical advice on their research process. In this situation, the consultant researcher approach fits well, as the group didn't need ongoing assistance.

What Are Your Skills? Researchers with good organizing skills can potentially walk into any community so long as they are aware of the basic issues confronting any organizer such as insider or outsider status, being sponsored or invited, and understanding the preexisting community members' skills and leaders. Researchers with organizer skills can practice an initiator approach in less organized communities, helping people define their needs and organizing action research projects to fill those needs.

If those are not your skills, however, be critically reflective of yourself and the community and ask:

- How organized is this community?
- To what extent are the functional roles of leader, organizer, educator, and researcher filled?
- To what extent can the unfilled social change roles be filled by others?
- Which of the unfilled social change roles can I play?

If you are only comfortable researching, then you are probably limited to a consultant approach and are thus limited to working only with well-organized communities. Be wary of communities with lots of internal conflict or weak organizational structures unless there are others who are effective at filling the other roles (Simonson & Bushaw, 1993). If you are not good at facilitating discussion in the classroom, you won't be good at it on the streets either. Communicating abstract academic ideas so that people think about their practical implications, discussing research in a way that helps people organize action, and helping people build confidence in their own knowledge are special skills indeed.

If you are comfortable with the leader and popular educator roles, then you may use the collaboration approach. Here also, be wary of less well organized groups, since any group needs some degree of organization to collaborate. Interpreting and communicating with a diverse membership is also central to the collaborator approach and can only occur after the academic has been "adopted" into the community. In contrast to traditional research, "going native" is the most desirable condition in CBPR. True collaboration may even mean dramatically altering the character of the research, as tastes for research differ, and you may find yourself doing theater, storytelling, and other forms of creative education (Comstock & Fox, 1993).

There are other skill issues to be aware of. First, are there some kinds of research you are good at and others that you are not? CBPR has a habit of changing midstream, sometimes requiring dramatic shifts in the research process. When I began researching Toledo philanthropic foundations for a neighborhood coalition, I expected to do interviews but found myself copying numbers from poorly microfiched foundation tax returns. Second, how are your writing skills? Academics are often asked to write, both because a PhD author is still seen as having credibility in some quarters and because academics are seen as having time and writing skills. But if your writing looks like a journal article, no one will read it, and no one will use it. In a participatory evaluation project I recently facilitated, I wrote the group's final report using framed sidebars, varied fonts, graphics, and other "magazinelike" qualities. Group members told me it helped them actually read the report.

Third, what are your time constraints? Deadlines in the real world aren't like those in academia. Missing a deadline means missing a grant opportunity, missing a government hearing, missing a legislative vote. You can't make up those kinds of misses, and you can't get extensions. And consistent with Saul Alinsky's (1971) rules of community organizing, a CBPR project that drags on is a drag. Find out ahead of time what the group's deadlines are, and either commit to them or stay out of the project. And remember, there's no spring break in the real world.

How Much Research Participation Does the Community Need and Want? This may be the most contentious issue in CBPR today. Rahman's (1991) and Gaventa's (1993) concern that we change the social relations of both material production and knowledge production must be heeded. At the same time, we must worry that overemphasizing participation can undermine the need to act quickly and forcefully.

For well-organized communities with a sense of empowerment that are moving on an issue, participation in every aspect of the research may not make sense. Often these groups could do their own research but have more important things to do. Having an outside academic facilitate and even do the research does not hinder them from learning new skills and does not maintain knowledge inequality. In these cases, a consultant approach may be perfectly acceptable. In cases where the research will be ongoing, a collaborator approach may be more desirable. An initiator approach will likely *not* work because an outsider academic pushing an agenda will be seen as an attempt to undermine the community.

With less organized communities, the research process is also a community organizing process. In these cases, participation must be organized and maximized. If there are no organizers available and the researcher has organizer skills, the initiator researcher approach may be appropriate. It is extremely important, however, that the initiator researcher strictly follow good organizer practice that builds community control as the project progresses and makes the research serve the community organizing.

There are mixed cases, however, where it is less clear what to do. Those difficult middle cases, where there is some degree of organization and a looming deadline, often require a trade-off between efficiency and democracy, which is no different from the tension between democracy and efficiency that affects any community organizing or development project (Stoecker, 1994). We found this in a CBPR project building a community network in Toledo (Stoecker & Stuber, 1999). As the grant deadline approached, we had to decide whether to fill in some blanks with less participation than we wanted or miss the deadline. We chose to fill in the blanks, building in opportunities for later participation in the event the grant arrived. There is another even more difficult case where the researcher does most of the project when the target population can't participate. This is especially the case with undocumented populations who have no rights of assembly to meet or attend demonstrations and who can't be safely identified in the research process (Hondagneu-Sotelo, 1993).

The most important thing is for communities to consciously choose which decision points to control and which to let a researcher control. These decision points are

- Defining the research question
- Designing the research
- Implementing the research design
- Analyzing the research data
- Reporting the research results
- Acting on the research results

The community must always define the research question. The academic can use an initiator approach to help develop the question, perhaps by surveying the community's information needs, but should not choose the question itself.

The academic can design the research, but community involvement in this step can prevent many a foolish decision. When we developed an eight-page survey for community groups as part of an Internet access study, our community participants pointed out that anything over two pages would be ignored.

Community involvement in implementing the design will serve only two specific objectives—to help individuals build specific skills and to help them build relationships with one another. If the research process will not also be a community organizing process, it may be more effective for the researcher to do the research. Also, as other contributors to this volume make clear, community involvement in implementing the design can significantly lengthen how long it takes to collect data, since the individuals carrying out the research may need extensive training. The only unsuccessful CBPR project I was involved in was one in which community members conducted interviews without any training or preparation for this role. We were working with a neighborhood whose members spoke predominantly Spanish, and neither of us researchers was a strong Spanish speaker, so we used our small grant to pay community members to interview each other. We were unprepared for the social stresses that prevented them from completing the interviews quickly and for the problems created by lack of training. In retrospect, providing training in interviewing techniques and helping these community team members attend to the social stresses they experienced, though adding to the project's timetable, would have increased the quality of data collected while also addressing CBPR's commitment to individual and community capacity building (see Chapter Three).

Analyzing the data, if it cannot be done collaboratively, should at least be done with strict accountability to the community. One method is to present or show rough drafts of the analysis to community members, who can then modify the findings and interject new data. Even in my graduate school research of the Cedar-Riverside neighborhood, I quickly learned that I got more information from people's reactions to my written reports than I did from the original interviews.

Who should take responsibility for reporting the results is another tricky issue. There may be a strategic purpose, as I've noted, for having the "PhD" on the cover of the report. But many communities are also very concerned that academics not use community research to enhance their own careers. Some communities demand ownership of the data and the results, while others have little concern about this. But you should at least talk with the community about issues of authorship in the event that they have not thought about it. Never attempt to publish an article from the research without the community's permission.

Organizing action can be the weakest part of a CBPR project, often because the researcher sees the project as research rather than as community organizing and the roles of leader, educator, and organizer have been neglected. But this phase is also the most important part of the project, and another one where community control is paramount. A researcher who is a good organizer can help the community think about what possible strategies and tactics might be, but the community has to make strategic and tactical choices based on what its members can and are willing to do.

There are cases where the academic is irrelevant and where we can do little or nothing to contribute to a community project. But neither should we sell ourselves short. Even where the academic is not needed, you may be able to help by documenting the struggle so that others may learn from it. As a graduate student academic in Cedar-Riverside, when community members first got me thinking about CBPR, I was of little use to them. I had no expert knowledge in anything that they didn't have more of. I ended up being relevant, however, in documenting the neighborhood's struggle and spreading the word of what happened so that the neighborhood could remember itself and others could adapt its model.

Finally, this chapter is written by an academic speaking mostly to other academics. Dave Beckwith (1996) offers an organizer's perspective on recommendations for academics who want to help:

- Be quick.
- Listen.
- Don't just listen, participate.
- Know the sources.
- Use your priestly power for good.
- Be creative.
- Use people.
- Help us get ahead of the curve.
- Look to all your work for opportunities to help.
- *Pecca tortiter* (sin bravely)!

The last may be the most important. We academics, so concerned with doing the right thing and so trained to evaluate everything from every angle before we act, often end up paralyzed. If we have real respect for the communities we work with, we will understand that they will tell us when we make mistakes, and they won't let us lead them astray. We must learn from our own mistakes and successes, but if we are doing CBPR in the right way, our mistakes and successes will both be shared. And that is the comfort, ultimately, of being relevant.

References

Alinsky, S. D. (1969). *Reveille for radicals*. New York: Vintage Books. (Original work published 1946)

Alinsky, S. D. (1971). *Rules for radicals.* New York: Vintage Books.

Beckwith, D. (1996). Ten ways to work together: An organizer's view. *Sociological Imagination, 33,* 164–172.

Beckwith, D., & Lopez, C. (1997). Community organizing: People power from the grassroots. *COMM-ORG: The On-Line Conference on Community Organizing and Development* [http://comm-org.utoledo.edu/papers97/beckwith.htm].

Brown, L. D, & Tandon, R. (1983). Ideology and political economy in inquiry: Action research and participatory research. *Journal of Applied Behavioral Science, 19,* 277–294.

Brydon-Miller, M. (1993). Accessibility self-advocacy at an independent living center: A participatory research approach. In P. Park, M. Brydon-Miller, B. L. Hall, & T. Jackson (Eds.), *Voices of change: Participatory research in the United States and Canada* (pp. 125–143). Westport, CT: Bergin & Garvey.

Cancian, F. M. (1993). Conflicts between activist research and academic success: Participatory research and alternative strategies. *American Sociologist, 24,* 92–106.

Comstock, D. E., & Fox, R. (1993). Participatory research as critical theory: The North Bonneville, USA, experience. In P. Park, M. Brydon-Miller, B. L. Hall, & T. Jackson (Eds.), *Voices of change: Participatory research in the United States and Canada* (pp. 103–124). Westport, CT: Bergin & Garvey.

de Roux, G. I. (1991). Together against the computer: PAR and the struggle of Afro-Colombians for public service. In O. Fals-Borda & M. A. Rahman (Eds.), *Action and knowledge: Breaking the monopoly with participatory action research* (pp. 37–53). New York: Apex Press.

Deshler, D, & Ewert, M. (1995). *Participatory action research: Traditions and major assumptions.* Ithaca, NY: Cornell Participatory Action Research Network.

Fear, K., & Edwards, P. (1995). Building a democratic learning community within a PDS. *Teaching Education, 7*(2), 12–24.

Freire, P. (1970). *Pedagogy of the oppressed.* New York: Seabury Press.

Gaventa, J. (1991). Toward a knowledge democracy: Viewpoints on participatory research in North America. In O. Fals-Borda & M. A. Rahman (Eds.), *Action and knowledge: Breaking the monopoly with participatory action research* (pp. 121–133). New York: Apex Press.

Gaventa, J. (1993). The powerful, the powerless, and the experts: Knowledge struggles in an information age. In P. Park, M. Brydon-Miller, B. L. Hall, & T. Jackson (Eds.), *Voices of change: Participatory research in the United States and Canada* (pp. 21–40). Westport, CT: Bergin & Garvey.

Gedicks, A. (1996). Activist sociology: Personal reflections. *Sociological Imagination, 33,* 55–72.

Hall, B. L. (1993). Introduction. In P. Park, M. Brydon-Miller, B. L. Hall, & T. Jackson (Eds.), *Voices of change: Participatory research in the United States and Canada* (pp. xiii–xxii). Westport, CT: Bergin & Garvey.

Heaney, T. W. (1993). "If you can't beat 'em, join 'em: The professionalization of participatory research." In P. Park, M. Brydon-Miller, B. L. Hall, & T. Jackson (Eds.),

Voices of change: Participatory research in the United States and Canada (pp. 41–46). Westport, CT: Bergin & Garvey.

Hondagneu-Sotelo, P. (1993). Why advocacy research? Research and activism with immigrant women. *American Sociologist, 24,* 56–68.

Horton, B. D. (1993). The Appalachian Land Ownership Study: Research and citizen action in Appalachia. In P. Park, M. Brydon-Miller, B. L. Hall, & T. Jackson (Eds.), *Voices of change: Participatory research in the United States and Canada* (pp. 85–102).Westport, CT: Bergin & Garvey.

Horton, M., & Freire, P. (1990). *We make the road by walking: Conversations on education and social change* (B. Bell, J. Gaventa, & J. Peters, Eds.). Philadelphia: Temple University Press.

Hubbard, A. (1996). The activist academic and the stigma of "community housework." *Sociological Imagination, 33,* 73–87.

Maguire, P. (1987). *Doing participatory research: A feminist approach.* Amherst: University of Massachusetts, Center for International Education.

Maguire, P. (1993). Challenges, contradictions, and celebrations: Attempting participatory research as a doctoral student. In P. Park, M. Brydon-Miller, B. L. Hall, & T. Jackson (Eds.), *Voices of change: Participatory research in the United States and Canada* (pp. 157–176). Westport, CT: Bergin & Garvey.

Merrifield, J. (1993). Putting scientists in their place: Participatory research in environmental and occupational health. In P. Park, M. Brydon-Miller, B. L. Hall, & T. Jackson (Eds.), *Voices of change: Participatory research in the United States and Canada* (pp. 65–84). Westport, CT: Bergin & Garvey.

Nash, F. (1993). Church-based organizing as participatory research: The Northwest Community Organization and the Pilsen Resurrection Project. *American Sociologist, 24,* 38–55.

Nyden, P., Figert, A., Shibley, M., & Burrows, D. (Eds.). (1997). *Building community: Social science in action.* Thousand Oaks, CA: Pine Forge Press.

Nyden, P., & Wiewel, W. (1992). Collaborative research: Harnessing the tensions between researcher and practitioner. *American Sociologist, 23,* 43–55.

Park, P. (1993). What is participatory research? A theoretical and methodological perspective. In P. Park, M. Brydon-Miller, B. L. Hall, & T. Jackson (Eds.), *Voices of change: Participatory research in the United States and Canada* (pp. 1–20). Westport, CT: Bergin & Garvey.

Rahman, M. A. (1991). The theoretical standpoint of PAR. In O. Fals-Borda & M. A. Rahman (Eds.), *Action and knowledge: Breaking the monopoly with participatory action research* (pp. 13–23). New York: Apex Press.

Reason, P. (1994). Three approaches to participative inquiry. In N. K. Denzin & Y. S. Lincoln (Eds.), *Handbook of qualitative research* (pp. 324–339). Thousand Oaks, CA: Sage.

Simonson, L. J., & Bushaw, V. A. (1993). Participatory action research: Easier said than done. *American Sociologist, 24,* 27–38.

Stoecker, R. (1994). *Defending community: The struggle for alternative redevelopment in Cedar-Riverside.* Philadelphia: Temple University Press.

Stoecker, R. (1997). The imperfect practice of collaborative research: The "Working Group on Neighborhoods" in Toledo, OH. In P. Nyden, A. Figert, M. Shibley, & D. Burrows (Eds.), *Building community: Social science in action* (pp. 219–225). Thousand Oaks, CA: Pine Forge Press.

Stoecker, R. (1999). Making connections: Community organizing, empowerment planning, and participatory research in participatory evaluation. *Sociological Practice, 1,* 209–232.

Stoecker, R. (2001). Community-based research: The next new thing. [http://comm-org.utoledo.edu/drafts/cbrreportb.htm].

Stoecker, R., & Beckwith, D. (1992). "Advancing Toledo's neighborhood movement through participatory action research: Integrating activist and academic approaches. *Clinical Sociology Review, 10,* 198–213.

Stoecker, R., & Stuber, A.C.S. (1999). "Building an information superhighway of one's own: A comparison of two approaches." *Research in Politics and Society, 7,* 291–309.

Stringer, E. T. (1996). *Action research: A handbook for practitioners.* Thousand Oaks, CA: Sage.

Williams, L. (1996). First enliven, then enlighten: Popular education and the pursuit of social justice. *Sociological Imagination, 33,* 94–116.

CHAPTER SIX

Community-Researcher Partnerships

Perspectives from the Field

Marianne Sullivan
Stella S. Chao
Carol A. Allen
Ahoua Koné
Martine Pierre-Louis
James Krieger

Collaborative partnerships between communities and public health researchers are increasingly being promoted to ensure that research and programs are relevant, meaningful to the community, and culturally appropriate (Bruce, 1995; Committee on Community Engagement, 1997). In such partnerships, however, challenging issues are frequently encountered concerning how community is defined, how community representation is achieved, and how to engage community members in meaningful roles. Researchers and communities have employed various approaches to address these concerns, some of which have been characterized as ensuring mutual benefits to both communities and researchers, the development and use of culturally sensitive methodologies, and clarification of the roles and expectations of community members and researchers (Durch, Bailey, & Stoto, 1997; Lillie-Blanton & Hoffman, 1995; Maurana & Goldenberg, 1996; Orlandi, 1992; Sullivan et al., 2001; Vega, 1992).

In this chapter, we draw on the findings of the Community Interview Project, which was conducted by Seattle Partners for Healthy Communities, hereafter called Seattle Partners, to capture the perspectives of urban Seattle communities about challenging issues in community-researcher partnerships and

Note: Portions of this chapter were adapted from "Improving Collaboration Between Researchers and Communities," by A. Koné, M. Sullivan, K. D. Senturia, N. J. Chrisman, S. J. Ciske, and J. W. Krieger, *Public Health Reports, 115*(2–3), pp. 243–248. Copyright © 2000 by Oxford University Press. Adapted with permission of the publisher.

to understand what members of these communities viewed as strengths and weaknesses of such partnerships. By listening to the voices of a diverse group of community residents and professionals from the ethnically diverse neighborhoods of Central and Southeast Seattle, we hoped to uncover attitudes, beliefs, and experiences that could help Seattle Partners in its efforts to further collaborative action-oriented research with these communities.

Following a brief introduction to Seattle Partners and the Community Interview Project, we share the interview participants' perspectives on three major themes that emerged: (1) the definition of community and representation of communities, (2) the role of community members in research collaborations and ensuring community involvement, and (3) the importance of attending to race or ethnicity and culture. For each theme, we provide some examples of how Seattle Partners has used the findings to improve its own effectiveness as a community-researcher partnership committed to collaborative research aimed at eliminating health disparities. We conclude by offering suggestions for other partnerships whose effectiveness, like that of Seattle Partners, will depend in large part on their ability to hear and respond to community concerns in ways that enable communities to be full collaborators in the community based participatory research (CBPR) process.

BACKGROUND

Seattle Partners is a CDC-funded urban research center whose primary goal is to support research and evaluate programs that address the social determinants of health in the urban, low-income, ethnically diverse communities of Central and Southeast Seattle. Housed in the Epidemiology, Planning, and Evaluation Unit of Public Health–Seattle & King County, Seattle Partners is well positioned to make use of the most current assessment data and to bring together concerned community members, public health practitioners, and academic researchers.

Recognizing the challenges it was likely to face, Seattle Partners began in 1995 by establishing a board of community members, groups, agencies, and academic and public health institutions that meets monthly to provide overall direction, priority setting, and budget allocation for Seattle Partners. The board is made up of both community members and institutional partners from diverse racial and ethnic backgrounds and disciplines. Following the adoption of a set of community collaboration principles (Eisinger & Senturia, 2001) and an intensive process of issue selection, the board established two issues for focused efforts: assuring community interests when research is conducted in the community and addressing social determinants of health. Although a full discussion of Seattle Partners projects is beyond the scope of this chapter, they have included participatory interventions in the areas of senior immunization, childhood asthma, lifelong learning, youth leadership development, and domestic violence (see Krieger et al., 2002, for a fuller discussion of these projects).

Prior to establishing the board, Seattle Partners conducted the Community Interview Project (CIP), a qualitative study designed to uncover community members' definitions of community, the communities with which they identified, what individuals or organizations they felt would best represent their communities in working with Seattle Partners, what roles community members should play in research projects, and their recommendations on how community members and researchers could work together more effectively. A diverse group of eighty-five community members participated in the study, sharing their insights through one- to two-hour-long interviews that captured a wide range of thoughts and opinions. Two Health Department researchers conducted the interviews. The community participants in the CIP constituted the community members who were later invited to become part of the Seattle Partners board. The findings of the research were reported to the community participants who attended the first community board meeting. These findings were then used as a basis for developing our structure and collaboration principles. The insights gained from the CIP (Koné et al., 2000) have been referred to over the life of Seattle Partners and continue to inform our work.

Following principles of community collaboration, the authors of this chapter are three members of the community who serve on the Seattle Partners board (including the former chair) and three staff members (including the principal investigator). Through extensive dialogue based on what was learned from participants in the CIP, as well as on our own unique perspectives and experiences, we offer a variety of viewpoints on community attitudes, beliefs, and concerns relevant to collaborative partnerships. The views presented do not necessarily represent those of the entire Seattle Partners board or all of our collaborators but are offered to further discussion and debate in several key areas relevant to CBPR. Following the presentation of each set of key CIP findings, we describe briefly some of the attempts Seattle Partners has made to incorporate and address these concerns in our work.

COMMUNITY INTERVIEW PROJECT FINDINGS: DEFINITION OF COMMUNITY AND COMMUNITY REPRESENTATION

The CIP participants typically defined a community as a group of people with existing relationships who share a common interest. For the majority of the participants, the common interest consisted of living in the same geographic area or sharing a similar ethnic or cultural background. Many also noted the importance of relationships in making community a reality; they felt that the concept of community became meaningless if its members did not relate to and interact with one another. Several participants noted that researchers tend to define communities on the basis of demographic characteristics and recommended that they not overlook the importance of existing relationships, especially when dealing with low-income and minority communities, because doing so could lead to inappropriate definitions and stereotyping. Reflecting on a past research project, one community based research staff member said, "There were some assumptions made about the way people move about in these communities based on a geographic definition of community that in reality didn't play out. So that's important to note, because there were some presumptions made without bothering to ask anybody that actually lived in that community if that were the way [people defined their community]."

Many participants saw the question of who best represents a community as a complex problem that defies easy answers. Participants often mentioned local organizations such as religious institutions, neighborhood groups, women's organizations, and PTAs as important representatives of communities because their memberships come directly from the community. These organizations were recognized for having a broad understanding of the true needs and concerns of their respective communities.

At the same time, however, some participants perceived these organizations as most concerned about their own agendas, which may take precedence over the needs of the community as a whole. A few participants added that in some circumstances, formal community organizations are resistant to new ideas and become unwanted gatekeepers. Some participants noted that people who work in certain job categories, such as outreach workers, tend to be more in touch with community concerns than other organizational employees.

Another source of representation is grassroots people, or activists without organizational links, acknowledged by many participants for their ability to understand the true needs of their communities. Participants felt that unlike organizational representatives, activists were not constrained by organizational agendas. As one respondent put it, "It's absolutely essential to have the grassroots people represented. Often agency people have a certain way of doing business, and they're turf-protecting, whereas the community members really know what they need and want in their community." Several participants added that community activists are often not invited to participate in research projects because in advocating strongly for their communities, they may challenge traditional research practices. Although many participants stressed the importance of including individual activists as community representatives, some expressed concern that activists often lacked the big picture of the community that is necessary for development.

Another suggestion was that representation should be tailored to the specific nature of a project on the theory that different projects may call for different types of representation. For example, one participant said, "As far as representation goes, you really have to make it specific to the need. Representation can increase when there's a specific need in the community that's been identified."

Above all, participants recommended that researchers maintain close ties in the communities with which they hope to work by cultivating diversity among community representatives and by ensuring that the different voices of community members are heard in the collaboration.

ADDRESSING THE FINDINGS

In both the operation of the Seattle Partners board and the implementation of research and evaluation projects, we face continuing challenges that stem from defining and representing community. Seattle Partners uses no single definition of *community*. Different definitions among board members give rise to conflicting perspectives that are revisited numerous times throughout the implementation of specific projects. Defining *community* becomes especially important in the voting structure of the Seattle Partners board, where 60 percent of the votes are from "community" members.

The CIP findings describe definitions of *community* based on demographic groupings and relationships. From an institutional perspective, *community* is frequently defined on the basis of demographic characteristics (geography, ethnicity, income). As a result, the projects implemented by Seattle Partners have defined the community of interest based on geography (the senior immunization intervention focused in a specific neighborhood), ethnicity (the Domestic Violence Project intervention focused on immigrant and refugee communities), or health status and income (the Healthy Homes intervention focuses on low-income asthma patients). However, community members often define *community* on the basis of personal relationships and assess the legitimacy of an individual's claim to represent the community according to the level of interaction between that person and the group he or she is representing.

In board operations, definitions of *community* are rooted in social and professional relationships, as well as involvement in community activities. Demographic and relational definitions are used simultaneously at Seattle Partners, recognizing the value of both institutional and community cultures. However, this also creates confusion and contributes to ongoing conflict in the work of the board—for instance, when deciding on the number of community representatives its membership should include.

We continually struggle with defining "who is community." Definitions of *community* seem more complicated in Seattle, where there is no single predominant ethnic minority, than in urban areas in which a greater proportion of the population consists of people of color and one or two ethnic groups may be predominant. In Seattle, racial and ethnic identity have less to do with community membership than the active social and professional relationships individuals have and their level of participation in community activities. We do not assume that a person of color represents the entire community, any more than we assume that a Caucasian ethnic minority group member (for example, a person of Middle Eastern or eastern European extraction) represents the community of which he or she is a part. An individual's relationships to the "right" people play a strong role in practice. Someone who is affiliated with a particular community group or well-known community activist gains credibility ("community credentials") in the same manner as one's affiliation with a university or a well-known researcher establishes institutional credentials. These definitions of *community* are used when the Seattle Partners board plays a gatekeeper role for diverse, marginalized communities. For instance, such community credentials become important when Seattle Partners selects community projects.

Seattle Partners board members self-define their representation, and some wear multiple hats. This may bring richness in perspectives to discussions and the decision-making process as well as facilitate learning. But such self-definition can also hinder and confuse the process. Although individual board members may define themselves as "community," their roles are often interpreted differently by other members. For example, some board members employed by Public Health or the university see themselves as "community" because they are involved as volunteers or board members of community based organizations (CBOs), or they identify ethnically or geographically with the community. In some cases, board members accept institutional members' self-definition as a community member, and in other cases, they do not. The distinction seems to depend on the relationships that an institutional person has in that particular community. For example, an institutional employee who not only works in the community but is also involved in the community in nonwork settings, such as attending church or social functions, is most likely to be viewed as a community member. University faculty members who are people of color may be viewed as community members by some board members in spite of their affiliation with an institution. Other board members, however, may not see faculty of color as community members but rather as institutional representatives because of their affiliation with the dominant power structure. Their contributions may be interpreted differently by board members, depending on which hat they are seen as wearing.

Power relationships are an important aspect of community representation (Feagin & Feagin, 1994; Robertson & Minkler, 1994; Wallerstein, 1999). In board discussions, some CBO employees self-identified as representatives of the community, only to be challenged by a community member with no agency or institutional affiliation. A few Seattle Partners researchers have also challenged the notion that CBO representatives are true community representatives, as opposed to grassroots community members. Some CBO representatives also share this view, while others do not. The stronger an individual's relationship is with a particular community, the greater his or her acceptance as a representative of that community appears to be. Conversely, the lack of relationship may create distrust.

Representation of "community" and "institution" is seen as a spectrum rather than as an absolute, and its dynamic nature is recognized. In one case, a board member identified as "community" was subsequently hired by the Public Health Department. Her new professional position changed the way she was perceived by other board members at both ends of the spectrum. While she continued to see herself as a community representative, and members of community organizations with which she volunteered also saw her in this role, others on the board relabeled her as an institutional representative.

Such changes in perceived representation present a challenge to CBPR projects whose goal is to hire people from the community. From a community perspective, people working for institutions may be seen as co-opted— "outsiders within"—unless there is a strong focus in their work on actively bringing resources back to the community. Community groups expect these individuals to increase the capacity of institutions to understand community perspectives and to be culturally competent. Since most of the positions occupied by community members are not decision-making or policymaking posts, the ability to meet such an expectation is limited. This creates a greater burden on the individual bridging both ends of the spectrum. If there is commitment from institutions and community to actively support the individual in this sharing of resources the burden is eased and cross-cultural capacity is developed.

While acknowledging that defining and representing community is complex and dynamic, the board recently decided to take the pragmatic approach of deciding on an operational definition of *community* for the purposes of enumerating voting members and determining eligibility for board leadership roles. Each board member is now required to assume a primary role as either a community, academic, or public health representative. If a member receives a salary from an academic or public health institution, then his or her role is determined by the salary source. Otherwise, a member can choose his or her primary role, although the board may question the choice. The board also agreed not to draw distinctions between community members who are affiliated with community based agencies and those who are grass roots community members (that is, unaffiliated with an agency, member of target community, and having an authentic interest in community issues unrelated to financial compensation).

The challenges Seattle Partners has faced around community definition and representation are also the foundations for its potential success. Bringing together people at various points along the spectrum provides a forum for discussion among groups that traditionally have not worked well together. However, the lack of clarity with respect to defining and representing community has impeded board decision making. It remains to be seen whether or not the board's newly adopted approach of making members' roles explicit using the guidelines just described will advance the work of the board.

COMMUNITY INTERVIEW PROJECT FINDINGS: ROLE OF COMMUNITY MEMBERS AND ENSURING COMMUNITY INVOLVEMENT

CIP participants emphasized that contributions from community members are essential to the success of community-research partnerships. A typical remark was, "If you don't include people that you're working with from the get-go, you're likely to end up on the wrong track. You just get disconnected from reality."

All participants agreed that community input in collaborative research is essential, but they differed about the appropriate level of community participation. The majority described the role of community members as advisory—advising researchers on community issues and concerns. Others advocated a stronger role, with community members as decision makers in all research project activities. A smaller group felt that it was possible for community members to assume a dual role in which they advise in some areas and play a decision-making role in others.

Those who suggested an advisory role for community representatives were confident that in such a capacity, community members would be instrumental in identifying priority issues, suggesting appropriate research projects to address community concerns, and providing feedback on ongoing activities. Several proponents of this model also added that when community members play an advisory role, they have the opportunity to formally maintain a voice in the partnership.

Consistent with the views of Labonté (1997) and others (Israel, Schulz, Parker, & Becker, 1998; Schulz, Israel, Selig, & Bayer, 1998; Wallerstein, 1999), participants who suggested a decision-making role for the community stressed that the community must be an *equal* partner in collaborative efforts. They added that when this is the case, a sense of ownership develops that may further enhance community participation and cultivate community trust. Some participants indicated that advocating a decision-making role for community members is a way to avoid tokenism and to promote power sharing among institutions, researchers, and communities. Said one, "If you really want [the partnership] to be useful, then you equalize power. And if you really want to equalize power, then you bring [community] people in on a decision-making peer basis. Giving advisory status without power is tokenism."

CIP participants recommended mechanisms through which community involvement in community-research partnerships could be sustained, including providing direct and concrete benefits to communities and creating tangible roles for community members.

Most participants suggested that community members should be actively involved on research project boards. They visualized such boards as diverse with regard to ethnicity, profession, religion, age, socioeconomic status, and sexual orientation. They particularly favored boards on which technical and grassroots community people work together as co-learners (see Chapter Three) to share expertise and recognize the knowledge and experience all have to offer. Several participants recognized that the process of running such a board can be difficult because it requires members to make a strong commitment to cooperation and patience but added that it is a worthwhile way to promote community participation.

Some participants recommended that communities receive concrete benefits in return for their involvement in research partnerships, noting that without such tangible benefits, the partnership may not be advantageous to the community. Some examples of benefits include the delivery of relevant health and social services; sustainability of worthy, community-initiated programs; and sharing of study results with communities in a culturally appropriate fashion. Specific services mentioned in exchange for community participation were food, child care, and transportation.

The CIP participants saw researchers as the major beneficiaries of most collaborative research projects. Researchers were perceived by some as motivated by opportunities for publications and funding. To help counter this perceived imbalance in the reward system, participants considered it respectful and fair to compensate community people for their time and effort. As previously mentioned, some participants indicated that in past collaborative projects, community involvement had amounted to tokenism, used mainly to fulfill requirements for getting funding. Because of this, they pointed out, many community members are suspicious of researchers' intentions. To reinforce the value of community participation, participants suggested that community members take on tangible roles in these partnerships, assuming positions of responsibility according to their expertise and experience.

ADDRESSING THE FINDINGS

While it sounds straightforward to commit to decision-making power for community members in community based participatory research, we have learned that implementing this is more complex. In its first year, Seattle Partners committed to community members' playing a decision-making role and developed a governance structure to facilitate this. The structure originally included the board (described earlier) and the policy board (made up of seven community members and five researchers, including the two coinvestigators). Originally, the policy board was the decision-making body for Seattle Partners. However, we quickly learned that having a subset of the board making decisions was not a workable structure in a group in which building trust was and is an important ongoing task. For more than four years, we have followed our current structure in which an executive committee sets agendas for board meetings and provides overall guidance while decisions are made by the entire board. For all votes, community members must constitute 60 percent of those voting.

Despite this structure, there are still significant constraints on a decision-making role for community members on the board. First, there are structural factors that set parameters for decision making. The University of Washington and the Public Health Department share fiscal and administrative responsibility for Seattle Partners. Thus they wield institutional control over the funding, with both institutions having policies and procedures with which Seattle Partners must comply. The Public Health Department, however, has taken steps to be flexible in both following Seattle Partners' collaboration principles and meeting system requirements. For example, Seattle Partners has requested and received waivers to recruit external and internal candidates concurrently for positions where internal candidates previously would have been given priority.

A second factor that limits decision making by the board is that it is often difficult for board members to have in-depth knowledge of the issues that they are considering. Staff are often more thoroughly acquainted with the issues because of their involvement with Seattle Partners on a day-to-day basis. Different strategies have been tried (including e-mail, personal phone calls, presentations at board meetings, and retreats for in-depth discussion of particular issues) and have had varying degrees of success in making sure that all board members are fully informed. It takes time to absorb, discuss, and reflect on all of this information, however, and sometimes it has been difficult to build sufficient time into the process for this to occur given external timelines.

While the focus of the findings from the Community Interview Project was on advisory versus decision-making roles, our experience in Seattle Partners has taught us that although this is an important consideration, there are clearly more facets to community members' roles. For example, community members have played important roles in linking researchers to communities, providing input on how to do the work in culturally competent ways, and representing community views and concerns on the board.

The role that community members can play in Seattle Partners also is limited by time constraints. Nearly all have full-time jobs, some directing community based agencies, and some have parenting responsibilities. Therefore, it is difficult for many to participate beyond monthly board meetings and limited committee work, and few board members play a direct role in Seattle Partners projects. Some board members have suggested that the community role might be more meaningful if board members were more engaged in specific Seattle Partners projects, including making site visits and participating in designing and conducting the research. However, although board members may not be involved at this level, other community representatives do participate in research and evaluation projects either as staff members or as collaborative partners.

Seattle Partners has used several strategies to sustain community involvement. Basic logistical measures include holding meetings in a central community location and providing dinner at evening meetings. Staff work to maintain relationships with board members—with a great deal of time devoted to follow-up through e-mail, phone calls, and in-person meetings. Not infrequently, staff consult or provide technical assistance to board members' agencies.

Paying board members for their involvement was raised by CIP participants, but the idea has not been adopted by Seattle Partners. Some board members believe that this is an issue of equity (if staff have the option to be paid for board meetings, so should community members). Others believe that volunteerism is important in community based projects. Early on, the board voted not to compensate its members. However, paying board members for their time may need to be revisited since the process of writing this chapter sparked renewed debate on this issue. Both board members and staff have been financially supported to attend conferences, meetings, and training sessions.

COMMUNITY INTERVIEW PROJECT FINDINGS: RACE, ETHNICITY, AND CULTURE

Although we did not directly ask questions about issues related to race, ethnicity, or culture, these issues emerged in many of the interviews. Specific concerns included racial imbalance among research staff and lack of cultural appropriateness of research projects. The following quote reflects the intersection of race and power experienced by a community member during a research project:

> A significant number of the community people and a significant number of people of color were saying, "This is how we want this done." I don't think they [the researchers] really paid much attention to it. So that's a part of the frustration. They felt really put on the spot. They felt a little out of control. And that is not how they conduct business. Their usual way of working is to sit in a closed room with doors closed to make their decisions and then go out and do things to people. Not have people say, "Wait a minute. We want to figure out what needs to be done here and whether or not this is the most effective thing to be doing."

Many participants said that white people dominate collaborative research projects, particularly those in ethnic minority neighborhoods. Often these researchers do not relate to the communities in which they are working. The need for research projects to recruit and involve minority communities, especially communities of color, was stressed heavily by participants. In the words of one, "In establishing the core center and the network of technical consultants, clearly making sure there are people of color and people who are of the national makeup of the recent [immigrant] populations [represented]" is crucial. Hiring people of color was seen as a particularly important step in increasing the cultural competency of research teams and also as a means of providing training and opportunities for skill building for members of these communities. In the words of one participant, "If we're talking about ethnic communities, then it's imperative that [community members] have to be on staff. This would enhance [researchers'] ability to better serve the population they're supposed to be serving." Participants also mentioned that researchers must understand the cultural context of communities in which collaborative projects are conducted. Participants recommended that researchers cultivate sensitivity to cultural differences in communities and that they conduct themselves in a culturally competent manner.

ADDRESSING THE FINDINGS

Issues of race or ethnicity and culture have played a central role in the Seattle Partners board and in our research and evaluation projects, and they have played out at both institutional and interpersonal levels. All Seattle Partners projects have collaborated predominantly with communities of color, including immigrant and refugee communities. Together, the board and staff represent various racial, ethnic, and cultural groups. In addition, as a community-academic–public health department partnership, we are trying to bridge the cultural differences inherent in these three settings.

All authors agreed that Seattle Partners functions within a larger cultural context of institutionalized racism, discussed in Chapter Four and defined by Camara Jones (2000, p. 1212) as "differential access to the goods, services, and opportunities of society by race. Institutionalized racism is normative, sometimes legalized, and often manifests as inherited disadvantage. It is structural, having been codified in our institutions of custom, practice, and law, so there need not be an identifiable perpetrator. Indeed, institutionalized racism is often evident as inaction in the face of need."

So far, the institutions affiliated with Seattle Partners have not made great strides in diversifying faculty and staff and in working in a more culturally competent way with communities.

One of the issues raised in the CIP was the importance of the involvement of principal investigators (PIs) of color in community based participatory research. This continues to be an issue for Seattle Partners. The PI and the codirector are European American. Of the four other PhD-level investigators who play a leadership role in Seattle Partners or one of its research projects, only one is a person of color. While it is clear that diversity among investigators is just as important as among staff and board members, this has been harder to achieve, in part because of the limited number of faculty of color at the University of Washington's School of Public Health.

With respect to hiring staff of color and staff from the communities with which we work, Seattle Partners has had some success. Board members have taken an active role in recruitment and hiring decisions. In the Healthy Homes intervention, for example, Vietnamese, Latina, and African American staff play a key role in making the research more culturally appropriate. A Vietnamese staff member, for instance, was able to effectively address the practice of burning incense in homes as part of Buddhist practice, which can trigger asthma. He suggested that Buddhist clients switch to electric candles, which they did, and parents noticed less coughing among their children with asthma as a result.

From an institutional perspective, the participation of staff of color in Seattle Partners has been central to its success. However, as discussed in more detail in Chapter Fourteen, community health workers (CHWs) are in the position of bridging two very different cultures, the culture of their community and the institutional culture, which can present unique difficulties. For example, the concept of research may be difficult to explain to some community members, and research protocols may be difficult to follow when CHWs have personal relationships or community connections to participants. An example from the Healthy Homes asthma intervention is that it employed a crossover design. The group receiving the full intervention was compared to a group receiving a lower-intensity intervention rather than the typical control group, which receives only usual care. Members of the low-intensity group received the full intervention after one year of enrollment. It was difficult for some CHWs to explain to community members why some participants were receiving immediate benefits while others were not, since CHWs are often looked to by community members as providers of immediate help.

An approach that has worked in some Seattle Partners projects has been to closely partner with community based agencies led and staffed by members of the communities with which we're working. Our partner, a refugee and immigrant service organization, is taking the lead role in developing a culturally appropriate domestic violence social support intervention for refugee and immigrant domestic violence survivors. Seattle Partners is conducting a participatory evaluation of this intervention.

Within Seattle Partners, racial tensions have at times contributed to conflict among board members. Some authors believe that this is the result of institutionalized racism playing out at the board level. The primary example discussed among the authors is the institution (in this case, Seattle Partners) controlling the funding and our community based partner agencies contracting with us. The power differential inherent in this relationship was seen by some as an example of institutionalized racism.

Others argued that board conflict may not be a result of racism but rather that conflict within the group gets framed in racial terms. None of the authors thought that racial tensions within the group are a result of interpersonal racism and as such amenable to interventions such as sensitivity training. However, after a number of conflicts among board members centering around race, the board did take the important step of hiring an outside facilitator to address race and power issues and assist us in understanding ways that we can address institutionalized racism within our group.

DISCUSSION

The themes originally identified through the CIP in 1995 have proved to be important and continuing challenges for Seattle Partners and have implications for those contemplating community based participatory research. In our case, Seattle Partners has taken steps toward more inclusive definitions of community, including diverse perspectives on the board, sharing decision-making power, diversifying staff, and hiring community members. Though these are important steps toward effective collaboration and power sharing, the themes that frame this chapter are long-term issues that will continue to be revisited in CBPR, since many projects are situated within a larger context of social inequality (Israel et al., 1998; see also Chapter Three).

As others have noted, an important consideration for anyone embarking on a CBPR project is the complexity of defining and representing community (Labonté, 1997; Walter, 1997). This will likely vary by geographic region, based on local demographics and relationships among groups. We have tried to represent a range of examples in which Seattle Partners has struggled with the issue of community definition. This issue has been part of a challenging learning process for the board. In Seattle Partners, although we have found that issues of geography and race are important, the individuals who seem to have the most legitimacy in representing community on the board are those with strong relationships with community members and institutions.

Structural issues in CBPR projects must be acknowledged and addressed. It is important to recognize up front the constraints imposed by funding sources and institutional affiliations (Minkler & Pies, 1997). It is also important to be able to differentiate between short-term goals of conducting effective community based research projects and long-term goals of changing institutions to be more effective at doing CBPR (increasing faculty of color, improving the cultural competency of the institution, providing incentives to faculty) (Fawcett, 1991; Sullivan et al., 2001). Such issues are critical, and it is important to prioritize concrete actions in relation to them.

It is also important to recognize that CBPR takes place in a social context deeply influenced by institutionalized racism. Along with addressing institutionalized racism, there must be open discussion about other isms that may impede collaboration, including interpersonal racism, sexism, and homophobia.

Developing a governance structure for CBPR projects that ensures meaningful community participation and representation is a critical step in doing this work. Others have described in detail governance structures used in other research centers and projects and their benefits and shortcomings (Eisinger & Senturia, 2001; Lantz, Viruell-Fuentes, Israel, Softley, & Guzman, 2001; Plough & Olafson, 1994; see also Chapter Three). Projects may start with one structure and change it over the course of the project if it is not meeting participants' needs. It is important to include participatory evaluation from the beginning (Fawcett et al., 1996) as a way to assess how well the governance structure of the project is working and to be flexible if midcourse correction appears warranted.

Another important consideration is that the costs of participating in CBPR projects for community representatives may be more significant than the costs for researchers. If CBPR projects "go wrong," individual community representatives and community based agencies may be held responsible by the community. This may damage personal and professional relationships that have taken years to develop.

For all participants in CBPR projects, it is important to be thick-skinned. It is essential to understand that you may not always be seen as an individual but rather as a representative of a particular community or institution. For example, if you are a white male researcher, you may be viewed as representing mainstream, white, male institutional culture, regardless of how you view yourself. Similarly, if you are an African American community member, you may be viewed as representing the "African American community," regardless of how you personally define your community membership. Over time, the development of trusting relationships helps participants move beyond these stereotypical representations of individuals.

Seattle Partners has learned that the more time we spend in developing and maintaining relationships with communities and among all of the players in the collaboration, the more effectively we are able to facilitate CBPR projects. Honest and open communication is essential, and that can be achieved only if time is spent developing relationships among participants. The more we work across cultures, the clearer it becomes that we are all heavily shaped by our multiple cultural influences, as these play out both where we live and where we work. Part of the process of learning how to work together is developing a greater understanding of our cultural differences (Gutierrez & Lewis, 1994; Jones, 2000; National Institute of Environmental Health Sciences, 1997). Since the dominant culture is often in a position to establish cultural norms and ways of working collaboratively, institutional partners must be particularly aware of the need to respect and be open to alternative norms and ways of working together. It may be a cliché to say there are no easy answers, but in our experience, there really aren't any. There is only commitment to the process, to the goals, to relationships with each other, and to improving the health of the community.

References

Bruce, T. A. (1995). Community health science: A discipline whose time has already come. *American Journal of Preventive Medicine, 11*(suppl.), 7.

Committee on Community Engagement. (1997). *Principles of community engagement.* Atlanta: Centers for Disease Control and Prevention/Agency for Toxic Substances and Disease Registry.

Durch, J. S., Bailey, L. A., & Stoto, M. A. (Eds.). (1997). *Improving health in the community: A role for performance monitoring.* Washington, CD: Institute of Medicine/National Academy Press.

Eisinger, A., & Senturia, K. D. (2001). Doing community-driven research: An evaluative description of Seattle Partners for Healthy Communities. *Journal of Urban Health, 78,* 519–534.

Fawcett, S. B. (1991). Some values guiding community research and actions. *Journal of Applied Behavior Analysis, 24,* 621–636.

Fawcett, S. B., Paine-Andrews, A,. Francisco, V. T., Schultz, J. A., Richter, K. P., Lewis, R. K., et al. (1996). Empowering community health initiatives through evaluation. In D. M. Fetterman, S. J. Kaftarian, & A. Wandersman (Eds.), *Empowerment evaluation: Knowledge and tools for self-assessment and accountability* (pp. 161–187). Thousand Oaks, CA: Sage.

Feagin, J. R., & Feagin, C. B. (1994). *Social problems: A critical power-conflict perspective* (4th ed.). Upper Saddle River, NJ: Prentice Hall.

Gutierrez, L., & Lewis, E. (1994). Community organizing with women of color: A feminist approach. *Journal of Community Practice, 1*(2), 23–43.

Israel, B. A., Schulz, A. J., Parker, E. A., & Becker, A. B. (1998). Review of community-based research: Assessing partnership approaches to improve public health. *Annual Review of Public Health, 19,* 173–202.

Jones, C. P. (2000). Levels of racism: A theoretic framework and a gardener's tale. *American Journal of Public Health, 90,* 1212–1214.

Koné, A., Sullivan, M., Senturia, K. D., Chrisman, N. J., Ciske, S. J., & Krieger, J. W. (2000). Improving collaboration between researchers and communities. *Public Health Reports, 115,* 243–248.

Krieger, J. W., Allen, C. A., Cheadle, A., Ciske, S. J., Schier, J. K., Senturia, K. D., & Sullivan, M. (2002). Using community-based participatory research to address social determinants of health: Lessons learned from Seattle Partners for Healthy Communities. *Health Education and Behavior, 29,* 361–382.

Labonté, R. (1997). Community development and the forming of authentic partnerships: Some critical reflections. In M. Minkler (Ed.), *Community organizing and community building for health* (pp. 88–102). New Brunswick, NJ: Rutgers University Press.

Lantz, P. M., Viruell-Fuentes, E., Israel, B. A., Softley, D., & Guzman, J. R. (2001). Can communities and academia work together on public health research? Evaluation results from a community-based participatory research partnership in Detroit. *Journal of Urban Health, 78,* 495–507.

Lillie-Blanton, M., & Hoffman, S. (1995). Conducting an assessment of health needs and resources in racial/ethnic minority communities. *Health Services Research, 30,* 225–236.

Maurana, C. A., & Goldenberg, K. (1996). A successful academic-community partnership to improve the public's health. *Academic Medicine, 71,* 425–431.

Minkler, M., & Pies, C. (1997). Ethical issues in community organization and community participation. In M. Minkler (Ed.), *Community organizing and community building for health* (pp. 120–138). New Brunswick, NJ: Rutgers University Press.

National Institute of Environmental Health Sciences. (1997, October 27–29). *Advancing the community-driven research agenda.* Symposium held at the Environmental Justice and Community-Based Prevention/Intervention Research Grantee meeting, Washington, DC.

Orlandi, M. A. (1992). *Cultural competence for evaluators: A guide for alcohol and other drug abuse practitioners working with ethnic/racial communities.* Rockville, MD: U.S. Department of Health and Human Services, Office for Substance Abuse and Prevention, Division of Community Prevention and Training.

Plough, A., & Olafson, F. (1994). Implementing the Boston Healthy Start Initiative: A case study of community empowerment and public health. *Health Education Quarterly, 21,* 221–234.

Robertson, A., & Minkler, M. (1994). New health promotion movement: A critical examination. *Health Education Quarterly, 21,* 295–312.

Schulz, A. J., Israel, B. A., Selig, S., & Bayer, I. (1998). Development and implementation of principles for community-based research in public health. *Journal of Community Practice,* Suppl. 1, 83–110.

Sullivan, M., Koné, A., Senturia, K. D., Chrisman, N. J., Ciske, S. J., & Krieger, J. W. (2001). Researcher and researched community perspectives: Toward bridging the gap. *Health Education and Behavior, 28*(2), 130–149.

Vega, W. A. (1992). Theoretical and pragmatic implications of cultural diversity for community research. *American Journal of Community Psychology, 20,* 375–390.

Wallerstein, N. (1999). Power between evaluator and community: Research relationships within New Mexico's healthier communities. *Social Science and Medicine, 49,* 39–53.

Walter, C. L. (1997). Community building practice: A conceptual framework. In M. Minkler (Ed.), *Community organizing and community building for health* (pp. 68–87). New Brunswick, NJ: Rutgers University Press.

PART THREE

IDENTIFYING STRENGTHS AND SELECTING ISSUES WITH COMMUNITIES

As community organizer Mike Miller (1985) has argued, one of the biggest challenges in community work is differentiating between problems and issues. A *problem,* he notes, is what an outsider looking in would identify as something "wrong" with a community and in need of fixing. An *issue,* in contrast, is something the community identifies and feels strong enough about that it is willing to work on to bring about change.

One of the hallmarks of community based participatory research is, of course, its commitment to starting with an issue that the community, rather than the "outside expert," identifies. In the ideal case, community members will have identified such an issue on their own and will have approached the outsider about working collaboratively with them. Often, however, as suggested in Part Two, it is the outside researcher who has the time and resources to play the role of initiator in a potential CBPR project. In such cases, the outsider may use a variety of methods to help community members identify an issue about which they care deeply and around which a CBPR effort might take place.

In the first chapter in Part Three, Meredith Minkler and Trevor Hancock describe and illustrate a host of such techniques and methods, ranging from risk mapping and walking or "windshield" (driving) tours to Delphi techniques and the development of community health indicators. Yet such issue selection efforts must be accompanied by equal attention to helping communities identify their strengths and resources—the "building blocks" (McKnight & Kretzmann, 1988) that can help them in collaboratively studying shared issues and engaging in subsequent community problem solving. Many of the issue selection techniques and methods explored in this chapter (such as windshield tours, interviews with local residents, town hall meetings, and the development of community indicators) are equally useful as a means of helping communities identify their strengths.

Chapter Eight introduces another set of tools that can similarly be used both for issue selection and for helping communities take stock of their assets and resources. In this chapter, community psychologist Steve Fawcett and colleagues at the University of Kansas explore how Internet based tools can be used in the context of CBPR and other community health and development work in pursuit of community-determined goals. A five-component framework for building capacity for this shared work ranges from understanding the context in which the work occurs to planning for sustainability. Core competencies related to CBPR are presented, along with examples of Internet based tools that can make these activities both more rewarding and easier to accomplish. The chapter then takes a detailed look at one such tool, the Community Work Station of the Community Tool Box and its utility for CBPR partners as they work together in identifying community assets and issues, as well as in other stages of the CBPR process. The chapter concludes with a discussion of the challenges and benefits of using Internet based tools to enhance CBPR and other efforts to improve community health and development.

As Hilary Bradbury and Peter Reason point out in Chapter Eleven, "Conversation and paper writing are valuable tools, but the worlds of theater, dance, video, poetry, and photography invite us to be inspired in the service of better theory and practice." In Chapter Nine, the final chapter in Part Three, Caroline Wang, developer of the widely used "photovoice" method, offers a fascinating case study of this potent tool in a community based participatory research project with the homeless in Ann Arbor, Michigan. Drawing on documentary photography, the dialogical methods of Paulo Freire, and feminist theory, photovoice involves the provision of inexpensive cameras and training to often marginalized groups, who capture their own images of what matters in their world. Through this process, community members are also aided in developing a collective new voice for sharing their issues and strengths with diverse audiences. Wang discusses the multiple ways in which photovoice can facilitate issue selection and community assessment and in doing so facilitate individual and community capacity building. Considering the many ethical and practical challenges, particularly with already stigmatized and devalued populations, Wang concludes with a frank discussion of the advantages and limitations of this approach to issue selection and its potentials for use in diverse settings.

References

McKnight, J. L., & Kretzmann, J. P. (1988). *Mapping community capacity.* Evanston, IL: Northwestern University, Center for Urban Affairs and Policy Research.

Miller, M. (1985). *Turning problems into actionable issues.* Unpublished manuscript.

CHAPTER SEVEN

Community-Driven Asset Identification and Issue Selection

Meredith Minkler
Trevor Hancock

When residents of Tillery, North Carolina, began to suspect that the chronic sore throats, itchy eyes, and other health problems besetting their community were tied to the open lagoons and other practices of the hog production industry, they began their own "barefoot epidemiology" to document what was taking place. Impressed by their efforts, a journalist connected their organization, Concerned Citizens of Tillery (CCT), with researchers at the University of North Carolina's School of Public Health, and an exemplary CBPR project got under way (Wing, Grant, Green, & Stewart, 1996).

The Tillery case study, which is presented in Chapter Eleven, is in many ways an ideal case. The issue around which CBPR took place came directly from the community, which subsequently began its own study and then partnered with both a university and the local health department to conduct the more detailed research needed and advocate for change. Yet in many cases, it is outside researchers or practitioners, rather than communities themselves, who wish to embark on a CBPR project. As Randy Stoecker suggests in Chapter Five, in such cases, the outsider frequently plays the role of initiator, approaching community organizations about the possibility of a collaboration and setting the process in motion. In other instances, typified by the Healthy Communities approach, a neighborhood or community may decide that it wishes to create a better and healthier environment for its citizens and embark on a process of identifying its assets and studying and addressing the things it hopes to change.

In this chapter, we examine the processes of community-driven issue selection, giving particular attention to the roles that outside researchers or practitioners may play in facilitating this process. In keeping with the emphasis in CBPR on recognizing and building on community capacity, however, the chapter is equally concerned with the often similar processes through which communities may be helped to identify and build on their resources. We begin with a brief review of the core principles guiding a participatory and strengths-based approach to community asset identification and issue selection. Next we present a variety of methods and approaches for assisting communities in identifying their assets and resources as well as their concerns and issues. We then review some key criteria, adapted from the field of community organizing, that may usefully guide community issue selection in CBPR. Finally, we highlight the challenge that arises when categorical funding and other factors constrain issue selection in a participatory research effort. Using as an example the federal Healthy Start program to reduce infant mortality, we illustrate how even within such constraints, a commitment to community participation and empowerment can lead to high-level community involvement in deciding on the issues on which collective research and action will take place.

CORE PRINCIPLES AND CONSIDERATIONS

The approaches to community identification of assets and issues described in this chapter are grounded in a conceptual framework that builds on three core principles. First, and central to the other two, is the principle that reminds us to "start where the people are." Articulated by health education leader Dorothy Nyswander (1956) nearly fifty years ago, starting where the people are is critical not only for demonstrating to communities our faith in them but also in ensuring that the issues we jointly address are the ones that really matter. As sociologist John McKinlay is fond of saying, professionals frequently suffer from an unfortunate malady known as "terminal hardening of the categories." We get the kinds of answers we are comfortable dealing with because we ask the kinds of questions that will give us those answers. In community health research, for example, residents may be told that HIV/AIDS or heart disease is a major health problem in their community and asked their opinions about various preventive health approaches. Although this may yield some valuable information, it may miss the fact that different issues, such as drugs, violence, or unemployment, may be of far greater concern to the community. Starting where the people are would have us shelve more traditional approaches, in which the researcher enters the community with his or her research topic and methods predetermined. Instead, and consistent with the principles of CBPR, it would have us foster a dialogical process though which the community's felt concerns heavily shape and determine the topic chosen, how it is explored, and to what ends (Hall, 1992).

As suggested in Chapter Four, starting where the people are also means listening for and honoring what James Scott (1990) has called the "hidden transcripts," or private discourse of an oppressed community. The hidden transcripts may include stories, jokes, dreams, and fantasies and the kind of "plain talk" that cannot safely be expressed within earshot of the dominant class. Although much of the content of hidden transcripts is, by definition, not for public consumption by researchers and others outside the group, methodic listening and a willingness to take seriously the messages conveyed can be an important avenue for improving one's understanding of an oppressed group. Makani Themba (1999) points to rap music as "one of very few venues for expressing rage at the status quo as well as holding a candid discussion of social issues" (p. 22). Despite the commodification of and contradictions within some rap music, its ability to "chronicle the lived experience" of a sizable group of African American and other youth in America make it a powerful medium for CBPR participants committed to better understanding an oppressed group. Methodic listening to rap music and keen attention to other cultural expressions can form the basis for the dialogue that lies at the heart of CBPR.

Another dimension of "starting where the people are" involves a second core principle, which reminds us to recognize and begin with community strengths and assets, rather than problems. In their classic indictment of traditional "needs based" approaches to health and human welfare, Kretzmann and McKnight (1993) argue that well-meaning professionals and bureaucracies frequently hurt communities by characterizing them as "bundles of pathologies" or problems to be solved. Although such characterizations may be useful in attracting outside funding, they may do substantial damage by reinforcing a deficit mentality in which both community members and outsiders view the community in terms of its problems—needs and deficiencies to be "fixed" by outside experts (McKnight & Kretzmann, 1992).

The past two decades have witnessed a growing appreciation of the importance of a more balanced perspective, which begins by helping communities identify and build on their strengths. Community asset identification is used here as a broad concept to capture a variety of different processes through which communities themselves, often with the assistance of outside professionals, engage in the collection of such information. As Sharpe, Greany, Lee, and Royce (2000) have argued, "An assets orientation does not imply ignoring needs and problems or throwing out rational, strategic planning." But "by involving community members in visual, intuitive, and nonlinear processes of self-assessment and discovery, assets-oriented approaches invite more creativity in assessment and planning than collection and perusal of statistical data alone can engender" (p. 206).

The third and final principle embedded in community-driven approaches to asset identification and issue selection involves the heavy accent placed in CBPR on authentic dialogue. As discussed in Chapter Two, dialogue as described by Paulo Freire (1970, 1973) helps people "look at the 'whys' of their lives, inviting them to critically examine the sources and implications of their own knowledge" (Sohng, 1996, p. 86). In so doing, it facilitates co-learning by community members and researchers, and, as Sohng points out, avoids presupposing a frame of reference that is in fact the researcher's rather than the community's. Dialogical approaches thus lead to a far richer and deeper understanding of both community strengths and locally identified problems and issues than traditional researcher-as-interviewer-and-interrogator methods alone are likely to achieve.

In this discussion, we draw on each of these principles—starting where the people are, emphasizing and building on community strengths and assets, and using the power of dialogue—as they help inform community, rather than researcher-driven identification of community assets and selection of issues for community based participatory research.

IDENTIFYING COMMUNITY RESOURCES AND ISSUES: TOOLS AND APPROACHES

A host of tools and approaches that can be used to help communities identify their strengths and assets, as well as the problems or issues they wish to address, have been developed and refined over the past three decades. Although a full discussion of each of these is beyond the scope of this chapter, we attempt to provide an overview of several of the most promising approaches, as well as resources for finding more detailed information on each.

Walking and Windshield Tours

Crucial to identifying both community assets and potential issues or problems is being able to see one's community "through fresh eyes." One effective way of beginning this process is by walking, wheeling, or driving slowly through the community on weekends and weekdays, at different times of the day, observing and recording one's observations (Eng & Blanchard, 1990; Sharpe et al., 2000). In CBPR, both community residents and outside researchers may take part in this process, working individually or as teams and later sharing their impressions and observations. Although tape recorders, cameras, and even videotapes have been employed, windshield and walking tours typically involve simply handwritten notes or maps that highlight key observations. Such tours can provide valuable impressionistic data about things like the condition and types of local housing, the extent and nature of social interactions, the presence of vacant lots and commercial and recreational facilities, and the general maintenance of buildings, yards, and common grounds (Eng, Briscoe, & Cunningham, 1990; Sharpe et al., 2000). Looking at the content of bulletins boards in community centers, libraries, houses of worship, and local stores or the public notices stapled to utility poles or fences can provide clues to local "hot" issues in the community.

Interviews with Formal and Informal Leaders and "Regular Folks"

As Sung Sil Lee Sohng (1996) has cautioned, the frequent reliance in community assessment on interviews with "key informants" necessarily limits the frame of reference of an interaction to that of the interviewer and further misses the co-learning that can come with more dialogical inquiry approaches. Yet there is clearly a place for thoughtful interviewing in community assessment, particularly if questions are formulated in ways that invite participants to share their pride and vision for their community, as well as their concerns and felt needs.

Interviews may be conducted with both formal leaders and informal ones— those "natural helpers" to whom people go for advice or help and who are often key behind-the-scenes players in helping neighborhoods function effectively. To identify such informal leaders, Israel (1985), Eng et al. (1990), Sharpe et al. (2000), and others have suggested that residents be asked questions like these:

- Whom do people in this neighborhood go to for help or advice?
- Whom do children go to?
- When this community has had a problem in the past, who has been involved in working to solve it?
- Who gets things done in the community?

Interviews with "regular folks," and particularly longtime residents are clearly key to identifying a core group of informal leaders who then should also be interviewed and ideally would be valuable participants in a CBPR project. Interviewers may also ask residents a variety of other questions, such as these:

- What do you like best about living in this neighborhood?
- What would you most like to see changed?
- What are some of the things other people are proud of in the community?
- Is this a good neighborhood in which to raise kids? (Why or why not?)
- When challenges or problems arose in the past, did the community come together to meet them? If so, can you give an example? How well did this collaboration work?

- Where in the community do kids go for fun or just to hang out?
- If youth get into a fight in this community, are adult residents likely to intervene?
- Do people in the neighborhood socialize with one another often? Do you socialize with others here?
- How would you characterize the relationships between members of different racial or ethnic groups in the neighborhood?

These and additional questions may be found in Duhl and Hancock (1988); Eng and Blanchard (1990); Hancock and Minkler (1997); Healthy Cities Network (http://www.healthycommunities.org); Israel (1985); and Sharpe et al. (2000). See also Appendix I.

The answers to questions like these can provide a wealth of initial data and stories about a community and may be compiled in narrative form or in the form of charts summarizing the key findings (Sharpe et al., 2000). As epidemiologist Chuck McKetney and his colleagues found in the Healthy Neighborhoods Project in Contra Costa County, California, however, the richest answers—and the best understanding of those answers—came when the interviews were conducted by local residents and then analyzed with their help (Minkler, 2000).

The Modified Delphi Process

The Delphi survey is a method for getting an opinion from a large group without needing to meet, while allowing for feedback and interaction. Trevor Hancock used a modified version of this in Toronto in the early 1980s to identify key health issues in the community. In each of two health areas, a panel of approximately one hundred community leaders from all walks of life were identified. In the first round of the survey, they were asked to identify what they saw as the three to five most important issues perceived as a threat to the health of the community. The results of this open-ended survey were collated, resulting in a list of around eighty issues. In the second round, the participants were sent this list (arranged in alphabetical order) and asked to score each item on a scale of 1 to 10 in terms of the item's importance as a determinant of the health of the community. These results were then compiled to generate a list ranked in order of priority. This list was then sent to participants, who were given a chance to reconsider their previous scoring on the basis of the collective opinion. (This resulted in little or no change in the rank ordering.) It should be noted that the issues identified through this process were not strictly within the mandate of public health. Nonetheless, the public health system had to respond and did so, thus ensuring that the community's identified issues were taken seriously.

The advantage of this process is that it enabled a wide variety of individuals to participate in a way that was not too time-consuming, with both the list of issues and the rank ordering of those issues determined by the participants themselves. Although it is true that the participants were "community leaders," having approximately one hundred of them allowed for a wide range of perspectives. Given that this was the early 1980s, when a recession was under way, it is perhaps not surprising that the group identified unemployment, poverty, and similar issues as the major threats to the health of their community at that time. This had interesting implications for the health department, as discussed later.

Community Capacity Inventories

As we have suggested, an important alternative to the "community needs assessments" traditionally relied on in fields like public health and social welfare are capacity-focused efforts, which form a critical part of CBPR. The simplest such approaches often involve creating a capacity inventory, typically by developing a written list of the skills and talents of individual community members as well as the associations and other resources of the neighborhood as a whole. Although a simple survey can be used to help create this list, the information gleaned from windshield and walking tours, interviews, and other assessment methods described in this chapter can be used as well. Similarly, community newspapers or directories may contain references to dozens of individual and neighborhood-level resources while also themselves constituting important community assets. For a detailed guide to undertaking a comprehensive community capacity inventory, see Kretzmann and McKnight's *Building Communities from the Inside Out* (1993).

As McKnight and Kretzmann (1992) have pointed out, conducting a capacity inventory can be an important way of drawing attention to the gifts of "labeled" or stigmatized people as well as members of such often forgotten groups as elders and children. The earlier mentioned Healthy Neighborhoods project provided an excellent case in point. Project facilitators taped to the wall of a community center large pieces of butcher paper on which they listed headings such as "child care provision," "artistic abilities," "cooking for large groups" (as at wedding or funeral gatherings), and "non-English-speaking ability." Residents who previously had seen themselves as lacking any talents and special skills soon were signing their names under several skill categories (El-Askari et al., 1998; Minkler, 2000). Of particular importance in the aftermath of several anti-immigrant proposals and initiatives on the state level, moreover, was turning "speaking a language other than English" from a liability into a strength through the capacity inventory process.

Community Asset Maps

Closely related to community capacity inventories is the process through which community members themselves "map" local resources, abilities, and other building blocks for community growth and change (McKnight &

Kretzmann, 1992). A community asset map represents a means of laying out in a visual format the physical assets of a community—library, playgrounds, schools, parks, houses of worship—that may constitute important physical and social support structures for achieving community goals. Asset maps are often first drawn by individuals or teams who walk or ride through their neighborhood and indicate the assets they observe on their own hand-drawn maps. Using push pins on a large street map or land use map or through a collectively drawn asset map, they then share their individual perceptions and develop a map that represents the collective views of the group about community strengths or building blocks.

Although asset mapping is sometimes conducted by outsiders with minimal contact with residents, it becomes a potent tool in CBPR when community members play an active role in the process. Sharpe and her colleagues (2000) thus describe how the visual mapping of a South Carolina neighborhood by outsiders at first suggested that a local church was an important community meeting place. Through dialogue with residents, however, it became apparent that nearly all of the church's members lived outside the neighborhood, leaving local residents with little sense of identification with the institution. Asset mapping efforts that are driven by local residents are better able to accurately map community-perceived strengths and resources and can be a potent tool in CBPR.

Risk Mapping

The technique known as risk mapping was first developed by workers in an auto plant in Italy in the 1960s. Using a blueprint of the factory's production line and drawing on it circles of varying sizes and colors to indicate different workplace hazards, the workers then had their findings verified by a group of scientists (Labor Occupational Safety and Health Program, 1996). The risk mapping method was adapted and used by Mexico City health and safety activists in the 1970s and by the 1980s had achieved popularity in the United States as well. Health departments, university based occupational health centers, community based organizations concerned with environmental health issues, and unions are among the entities that have effectively used this approach (see Appendix G; Labor Occupational Safety and Health Program, 1996), which is now widely employed in the field of occupational health in the United States.

Risk mapping need not involve a shared work setting to be an effective tool in CBPR. Residents of a housing complex (such as an apartment building or a single-room-occupancy hotel) or pupils in a school can focus on shared spaces such as multipurpose rooms, hallways, and elevators to collectively identify hazards to which they are exposed. Typically under the guidance of a trained leader, community members sharing such a space are given a large piece of butcher paper and asked to draw a floor plan of the site, indicating boundaries, doorways, windows, and other key features. Colored markers then are used to identify different types of hazards (physical, chemical, and so on) as described in Appendix G. Community members then discuss the various risks identified on their map, decide on those they most wish to address, and develop plans for further studying and taking action to address the chief hazards of concern to the group. Whether with workers, apartment dwellers, or others who share a geographic space, however, risk mapping can be a potent method for issue selection (see Appendix G).

A variant of the risk map is the community safety audit conducted by groups of women who examine potential threats to safety in their neighborhood by walking through it in a group at night, identifying poorly lit areas and other safety hazards (Wekerle & Whitzman, 1995). The problem areas thus identified can then be used as a basis for study and action to bring about change.

Community Dialogues or Guided Discussions

Engaging community members in dialogues or guided discussions about their communities has become an increasingly popular means of community assessment and issue selection. Within this broad category of approaches, focus groups are among the most popular, typically involving six to twelve diverse community members under the direction of a trained moderator. In a confidential and nonthreatening discussion, members address a series of questions about their communities, which are designed to elicit their beliefs about the strengths of their neighborhoods and the changes they'd like to see. Whether tape-recorded and transcribed or summarized through detailed handwritten notes, the output of focus groups can provide a wealth of information for thematic analysis and use in subsequent community-driven asset assessment and issue selection (Krueger & Casey, 2000).

Nominal group process (Delbecq, Van de Ven, & Gustafson, 1975) is a second small group method with considerable appeal for community assessment and issue selection. A structured process designed to foster creativity, encourage conflicting opinions, and prevent domination by a few vocal individuals, nominal group process is especially helpful in encouraging the participation of marginal group members (Hancock & Minkler, 1997; Siegel, Attkisson, & Cohn, 1977).

The Healthy Communities "community dialogues" (http://www.healthy-communities. org) represent a method that can involve either small groups or literally hundreds of individuals in diverse settings in a process of discussing their hopes and dreams for their communities and the issues about which they are concerned. Sample dialogue questions include the following:

- What do you believe are the two or three most important characteristics of a healthy community?
- What makes you most proud of our community?

- What are some specific examples of people or groups working together to improve the health and quality of life of our community?

- What do you believe is keeping our community from doing what needs to be done to improve health and quality of life?

- What would excite you enough to become involved (or more involved) in improving our community?

(See Appendix I for a full listing of the Healthy Communities dialogue questions and prompts or subquestions intended to deepen the dialogue in each of these issue areas.)

Finally, community dialogues also can be facilitated through town hall meetings and neighborhood forums. In Pasadena, California, some 150 residents participated in a daylong forum in which they decided on ten areas of concern, including housing, local employment, and alcohol and drugs. They then worked together in small groups to determine the "critical issues" in each of these ten areas for which indicators could be developed (Lasker, Abramson, & Freedman, 1998) as a prelude to community action for change.

Voting with Your Feet

An interesting and simple way to assist a group in identifying its priorities involves having members list their priorities and then asking people to move into groups for the priorities that have been identified. Since people cannot be in more than one place at a time, the level of commitment to the priority issues becomes apparent very quickly. An issue that is deemed very important (such as poverty) may in fact fail to attract any people to a work group forming to deal with it, perhaps because the issue is too big and people feel helpless in the face of it. Conversely, if most of the people in the room were to move into one particular group, this would indicate that a lot of time and energy should be committed to that issue, and in fact those people could form the core of a work group. (The fact that an issue receives no support from the participants on that day does not mean it is not an important issue but rather that the people in the room that day are not the right ones to deal with it.)

Developing Community Indicators

In recent years, much attention has been focused on the development and use of community health indicators (CHIs) that characterize a neighborhood or community as a whole, rather than simply the individuals or subgroups of which it is comprised (Cheadle, Wagner, Koepsell, Kristal, & Patrick, 1992; Hancock, Labonté, & Edwards, 1999). As Patrick and Wickizer (1995) suggest, such indicators take several forms and may be thought of as "a community analogue to health-risk appraisal for individuals" (p. 72). The number, type, and visibility of No Smoking signs in workplaces, the proportion of space in grocery stores devoted to low-fat foods (Patrick & Wickizer, 1995), and the proportion of a community's children under age two with up-to-date immunizations are all examples of potent community health indicators.

Although such indicators are often created and employed by outside professionals, the very process of developing CHIs can be an important part of CBPR. Constituting as they do a limited set of quantitative and qualitative measures that reflect the current health status of the complex system that a community represents, CHIs can also suggest how the community's health status, broadly defined, is changing over time (Bauer, 1997). Ideally, as Hancock and his colleagues (1999) have pointed out, good community indicators should reflect six key determinants of health: environmental quality, economic activity, social cohesion and "civicness," equity (including power), sustainability, and livability. They should further capture four process dimensions—education, participation, empowerment and civil rights, and government performance—as well as the outcome of health status. Finally, Hancock et al. suggest that to be relevant to both policymakers and the general public, community indicators should have several key qualities:

- Face validity—they make sense to people
- Theoretical and empirical validity—they measure an important health determinant or dimension
- Social value—they measure things people care about
- Valency—they are powerful and carry social and political punch

Based on earlier work by Norris and Hancock, these investigators further propose the development of a CD-ROM based indicator selection tutorial that communities could use to choose indicators while learning about what indicators are and how to use them. Such a tutorial could be linked to web based data sets that would enable users to develop indicator reports.

As Georg Bauer has noted, "Because community health indicators draw attention to selected aspects of community health, they are crucial in setting the action agenda for our communities" (1997, p. 4). Consistent with this philosophy, an ambitious effort was undertaken in the late 1990s to develop community health indicators on the neighborhood level for and with the Fruitvale and San Antonio areas of Oakland, California, as a prototype for use in other neighborhoods. Coordinated by Bauer, a doctoral student at the School of Public Health, University of California, Berkeley, who was also a member of Oakland's Community Health Academy, the project was conducted through a partnership involving residents of the Fruitvale and San Antonio neighborhoods in Oakland; the Alameda County Department of Public Health; and the University of California, Berkeley, School of Public Health (see Appendix F). The Community Health Academy, a community based organization that grew out of the

W. K. Kellogg Foundation–funded Oakland Community Based Public Health Initiative (OCBPHI), was integral to the development and implementation of the community indicators project. Carrying forward the OCBPHI's original mission of moving away from "the domination and control of the health system by professionals through greater community involvement in local networks, cooperative planning, and collaborative partnerships" (Oakland Community Based Public Health Initiative, 1996), the Academy placed a heavy accent on local community development, capacity building, and advocacy for policy-level changes that can improve community health (see Appendix A).

The Fruitvale–San Antonio community health indicators project was committed to the notion of information as a vehicle for both change and community empowerment (Hancock & Minkler, 1997). As such, the small working group that met monthly to develop an initial list of indicators was guided by theoretical frameworks from community organizing, ecological perspectives on community health and sustainability, and the accent of the "new public health" on community partnerships, participation, and empowerment. Broad indicator categories included the following:

- Community capacity building and empowerment
- Community relations
- Community attraction (satisfaction with neighborhood, intention to stay, and so on)
- Cultural affirmation
- Youth development
- Community health and safety
- Physical environment
- Ecological sustainability
- Population health

For each of the issues identified in the working group meetings, local residents were asked about both their level of concern and their level of interest in taking action (Bauer, 1997). An area such as street violence (under "community health and safety"), to which almost three quarters of residents assigned "high importance" and over half reported "high interest in action," helped point the way for subsequent issue selection and community mobilization.

Visioning Processes

Community dialogues and the creation of healthy community indicators are often part of a larger visioning process through which a group of community members "collectively define a shared dream of what their community can become" (Sharpe et al., 2000, p. 209). Varying in length and format from a daylong retreat to a yearlong process with multiple phases, visioning typically involves both small group work and large group convenings under the leadership of trained facilitators (see Appendix I).

The vision workshop process has been extensively used in healthy community projects. Groups as large as one hundred or more participants are taken through a process of guided imagery in which they see their community at some point in the future when it is as healthy as it could be. Then in small groups of six to eight, they are asked to draw a shared group picture of what they saw in their mind's eye. These pictures are then shared with the group as a whole, and common themes can be identified that are evident in most of the pictures. These common themes can then be the basis for issue development, since they reflect the most important factors that the participants recognize as being fundamental to the health of their community (Hancock, 1993).

In Clark County Community Voices 2010, in Vancouver, Washington, teen mothers, members of a Russian church group, and participants in a local senior organization were among a wide variety of community members who took part in a yearlong visioning process. Through focus groups, they addressed such questions as "What do you most like about your community?" "What are your hopes for your community's children twenty years from now?" and "Where would you put your energy to make the community a better place?" (Lasker et al., 1998).

As in the other community dialogue approaches described in this chapter, the processes involved in this activity can constitute a critical phase of CBPR, while the findings concerning community perceived strengths and issues in need of redress can form an important basis for subsequent research and praxis.

Creative Arts

Growing appreciation of the role that a variety of creative arts can play in helping communities identify their strengths and assets, as well as their shared problems and concerns (McDonald, Antuñez, & Gottemoeller, 1998), is grounded in part in the philosophy and methods of Paulo Freire. As he asked rhetorically, "How is it possible for us to work in a community without feeling the spirit of the culture that has been there for many years, without trying to understand the soul of the culture?" (Horton & Freire, 1990, p. 131).

A variety of techniques have been used to capture visual and oral expressions of the history, sources of pride, and shared concerns of a people. Key among these are community murals, vision workshop drawings, poetry and arts workshops, community plays about the history and present issues faced by the community, and videotapes capturing a wealth of perspectives on community life. As Marian McDonald and colleagues (1998) observed, "While art and literature are often solitary activities in the creation stage, the act of sharing art and literature is profoundly social and collective. By creating common reference points through culture, communities begin to break down isolation, share their common experience, and build collective vision" (p. 273).

Illustrating this message, the photovoice process described in Chapter Nine provides a powerful means of helping community members document, through their own photographs, community assets and problems that in turn form the basis of dialogue, collective analysis, and action for social change. The process has been successfully used by such diverse groups as rural women in China (Wang & Burris, 1994), residents of low-income multicultural neighborhoods (Spears, 1999), homeless people (Wang, Cash, & Powers, 2000), and people with active tuberculosis (Butler & Xet-Mull, 2001) and has demonstrated considerable promise with each of these diverse populations (see Chapter Nine).

FROM ASSET AND PROBLEM IDENTIFICATION TO ISSUE SELECTION IN CBPR

The approaches we have described can provide a wealth of stories and data by and about a community and its resources, strengths, perceived problems or needs, and dreams for the future. The outside researcher or professional can often play a valuable role in helping community members learn about and use one or more of these methods and then critically reflect on what they have learned about their community as a basis for next steps in the CBPR process.

Because the methods described in this chapter are likely to reveal a wide range of problems of concern to the community, however, a critical step in CBPR involves helping community members "turn problems into issues" or identify those concerns they feel deeply enough about to systematically study and take action. In this process, the outsider can play a valuable role in asking the kinds of questions that can help community members decide on a specific issue or concern that can in turn form the basis of collective study and action for social change.

Community organizers provide a variety of guidelines and criteria for issue selection that can be adapted in CBPR. Borrowing from organizer Lee Staples (1997, p. 177), for example, and using *community* rather than *community organization* as the frame of reference, residents engaged in CBPR may evaluate the pros and cons of an issue they are considering by dialoguing about the following questions:

- Is the issue consistent with the long-range goals or agenda of the community (as identified, for example, through a visioning process)?
- Will the issue be unifying or divisive?
- Will the issue contribute to community capacity building?

- Will the process of CBPR on this issue provide a good educational experience for leaders and community members, developing their consciousness, independence, and skills?
- Will the community receive credit for a victory?
- Will working on this issue result in new partnerships or alliances?
- Will CBPR on this issue result in concrete action for change and produce new issues for subsequent CBPR efforts?
- Will CBPR on this issue lead to an improved health or social outcome for the community?
- Is the issue important enough to people that they are willing to work on it?

As suggested by this list, a good issue for a CBPR effort will be consistent with the community's overall vision of itself as a healthy community and help it move toward that vision. Similarly, and while recognizing that communities are not homogeneous in their goals and values (Labonté, 1997), a good issue will be selected through a democratic process that helps avoid the kind of divisiveness that can weaken rather than strengthen the community (Staples, 1997). A good issue will not only appeal to a broad range of community members but also lend itself to the provision of multiple opportunities for participation in the CBPR process. Similarly, a good issue will attract new leaders and provide both leaders and members of the community with opportunities for developing a variety of skills and abilities that contribute to capacity building on the individual, organization, and community levels. Ideally as well, the issue chosen will attract external funding and other outside supports that can further help expand the community's resource base (Staples, 1997). In a related way, an issue may attract other potential community or institutional partners whose participation may further enhance aspects of the CBPR process while contributing to local capacity building.

Like community organizing, CBPR for health is ultimately concerned with bringing about social change that will promote the health and well-being of the community. The process of issue selection should therefore also involve dialogue about whether and how CBPR on the issue under consideration could ultimately help bring about conditions in which the community can be a better and healthier place in which to live. An issue that excites people but has little or no prospect of leading to actions that could ultimately help improve community health would not meet this important criterion as a "good issue" for CBPR.

In sum, many factors need to be considered by communities as they decide on the issue or issues that will drive a CBPR effort. By fostering a dialogue using the types of questions and guiding considerations discussed here, the outside researcher or professional can play an important role in helping community members with this critical stage in the CBPR process.

WHEN PREEXISTING (EXTERNAL) GOALS CONSTRAIN ISSUE SELECTION: A FINAL NOTE

This chapter has been written from the perspective that communities can and should have a major role in determining the problem or issue to be studied and addressed through a CBPR process. Yet as earlier chapters have made clear, achieving true community-driven issue selection is often difficult in practice. Public health researchers thus frequently approach a community concerned about its high rates of HIV/AIDS or substance abuse and wishing to collaborate in studying the problem and developing a community based intervention. Similarly, funding mandates may sharply circumscribe the areas within which issue selection may take place.

The federal government's initiative to eliminate disparities in health represents a good case in point. When the Centers for Disease Control and Prevention (CDC) made substantial funds available for eliminating health disparities, it earmarked six "areas of focus" within which such efforts must take place: cancer screening and management, cardiovascular disease, child and adult immunizations, diabetes, HIV/AIDS, and infant mortality (U.S. Department of Health and Human Services, 1998). All six of these represent areas where serious disparities in both health access and health outcomes continue to exist by race and ethnicity. Yet for communities upset over drugs in their children's playgrounds, violence, or high unemployment rates, none of these six may represent an issue of central concern.

The federal campaign to eliminate health disparities represents a classic dilemma for communities and the outside professionals with whom they collaborate in CBPR. On the one hand, the availability of funds to conduct CBPR can be a boon to communities, providing resources and stimulating partnerships that can help them tackle major health problems. On the other hand, however, limiting funding to the six specified areas may violate the basic principle of community-driven issue selection.

For communities and their professional allies engaged in CBPR within the constraints imposed by initiatives like the federal effort to eliminate health disparities, some useful lessons may be learned from such related efforts as the National Healthy Start Program (NHSP) to reduce infant mortality. When the NHSP commenced in 1991, the U.S. ranked twenty-second in the world in infant mortality, and the black infant death rate was more than twice that of the white rate (Public Health Service, 1996). The program's goal was to reduce infant mortality by half over a five-year period in fifteen demonstration sites, plus an additional eighty sites added by the late 1990s. Although specifically targeting infant mortality, however, program guidelines also emphasized the need for "substantive and informed" community participation through consortia and other means designed to foster community-driven approaches at every stage of the process (Health Resources and Services Administration, 1991, p. 4). As a consequence, community consortia often engaged participants in studying and addressing issues *they* identified. In Cleveland, for example, residents successfully took on a local hospital's use of an incinerator that was creating an environmental hazard, while in Chicago, participants, through their consortia, studied the new welfare reform time limits and work requirements and worked to get waivers in place for mothers with special needs children (Minkler, Thompson, Bell, & Rose, 2001; Thompson et al., 2000).

Taking a cue from such examples, CBPR projects that begin in response to problem-specific community based health initiatives can, with creativity and attention to the interconnections between many health and social issues, often "broaden the net" so that issues of primary concern to the community become a driving force for the collaborative research and action undertaken.

This chapter has provided a broad overview of the core principles underlying community-driven asset identification and issue selection and their relevance for CBPR. We also have described and illustrated by example a number of different tools and approaches that may be useful in helping communities recognize and build on their strengths and collectively identify issues about which they feel strongly enough to engage in systematic inquiry and action. Our overview of tools and methods has intentionally omitted an important and growing category of approaches, those that involve the use of computer technology in assessing community resources and potential issues for CBPR. It is to these increasingly potent tools for assessment and issue selection that we turn in the next chapter.

References

Bauer, G. F. (1997). *Community health indicators on the neighborhood level: A prototype for the Fruitvale/San Antonio area in Oakland.* Oakland, CA: Oakland Community Based Public Health Initiative/Community Health Academy.

Butler, L. M., & Xet-Mull, A. M. (2001, November 8). *Through our eyes: Understanding the experience of tuberculosis with photovoice.* Paper presented at the Human Rights Summer Fellowship Conference, University of California, Berkeley.

Cheadle, A., Wagner, E. A., Koepsell, T. D., Kristal, A., and Patrick, D. (1992). Environmental indicators: A tool for evaluating community-based health promotion programs. *American Journal of Preventive Medicine, 8,* 345–350.

Delbecq, A., Van de Ven, A. H., & Gustafson, D. H. (1975). *Group techniques for program planning: A guide to nominal group and Delphi processes.* Glenview, IL: Scott, Foresman.

Duhl, L., & Hancock, T. (1988). *A guide to assessing healthy cities.* Copenhagen, Denmark: FADL.

El-Askari, G., Freestone, J., Irizarry, C., Kraut, K. L., Mashiyama, S. T., Morgan, M. A., & Walton, S. (1998). The Healthy Neighborhoods Project: A local health department's role in catalyzing community development. *Health Education and Behavior, 25,* 146–159.

Eng, E., & Blanchard, L. (1990). Action-oriented community diagnosis: A health education tool. *International Journal of Community Health Education, 11*(2), 93–110.

Eng, E., Briscoe, J., & Cunningham, A. (1990). The effect of participation in water projects on immunization. *Social Science and Medicine, 30,* 1349–1358.

Freire, P. (1970). *Pedagogy of the oppressed.* New York: Seabury Press.

Freire, P. (1973). *Education for critical consciousness.* New York: Continuum.

Hall, B. L. (1992). From margins to center: The development and purpose of participatory action research. *American Sociologist, 23,* 15–28.

Hancock, T. (1993). Seeing the vision, defining your role" *Healthcare Forum Journal, 36*(3), 30–36.

Hancock, T., Labonté, R., & Edwards, R. (1999). Indicators that count: Measuring population health at the community level. *Canadian Journal of Public Health, 90*(Suppl. 1), 22–26.

Hancock, T., & Minkler, M. (1997). Community health assessment or healthy community assessment: Whose community? Whose health? Whose assessment? In M. Minkler (Ed.), *Community organizing and community building for health* (pp. 139–156). New Brunswick, NJ: Rutgers University Press.

Health Resources and Services Administration. (1991). *Guidance for the Healthy Start program.* Washington, DC: Author.

Horton, M., & Freire, P. (1990). *We make the road by walking: Conversations on education and social change* (B. Bell, J. Gaventa, & J. Peters, Eds.). Philadelphia: Temple University Press.

Israel, B. A. (1985). Social networks and social support: Implications for natural helper and community-level interventions. *Health Education Quarterly, 12,* 66–80.

Kretzmann, J. P., & McKnight, J. L. (1993). *Building communities from the inside out: A path toward finding and mobilizing a community's assets.* Chicago: ACTA.

Krueger, R. A., & Casey, M. A. (2000). *Focus groups: A practical guide for applied research* (3rd ed.). Thousand Oaks, CA: Sage.

Labonté, R. (1997). Community, community development, and forming of authentic partnerships: Some critical reflections. In M. Minkler (Ed.), *Community organizing and community building for health* (pp. 88–102). New Brunswick, NJ: Rutgers University Press.

Labor Occupational Safety and Health Program. (1996). *A group method for improving risk mapping: Workplace health and safety.* Los Angeles: University of California, Labor Occupational Safety and Health Program.

Lasker, R. D., Abramson, D. M., & Freedman, G. R. (1998). *Pocket guide to cases of medicine and public health collaboration.* New York: Center for the Advancement of Collaborative Strategies in Health/New York Academy of Medicine.

McDonald, M., Antuñez, G., & Gottemoeller, M. (1998). Using the arts and literature in health education. *International Quarterly of Community Health Education, 18,* 269–282.

McKnight, J. L., & Kretzmann, J. P. (1992). *Mapping community capacity.* Evanston, IL: Center for Urban Affairs and Policy Research, Northwestern University.

Minkler, M. (2000). Participatory action research and healthy communities. *Public Health Reports, 115,* 191–197.

Minkler, M., Thompson, M., Bell, J., & Rose, K. (2001). Contributions of community involvement to organizational-level empowerment: The federal Healthy Start experience. *Health Education and Behavior, 28,* 783–807.

Nyswander, D. (1956). Education for health: Some principles and their application. *Health Education Monographs, 14,* 56–70.

Oakland Community Based Public Health Initiative (OCBPHI). (1996). *Annual report to the W. K. Kellogg Foundation.* Oakland, CA: Community Health Academy.

Patrick, D. L., & Wickizer, T. M. (1995). Community and health. In B. C. Amick, S. Levine, A. R. Tarlov, & D. C. Walsh (Eds.), *Society and health* (pp. 46–92). New York: Oxford University Press.

Public Health Service. (1996). *Health: United States, 1995.* DHHS Publication No. (PHS)96-1232. Hyattsville, MD: U.S. Department of Health and Human Services.

Scott, J. (1990). *Domination and the arts of resistance: Hidden transcripts.* New Haven, CT: Yale University Press.

Sharpe, P. A., Greany, M. L., Lee, P. R., & Royce, S. W. (2000). Assets-oriented community assessment. *Public Health Reports, 113,* 205–211.

Siegel, L. M., Attkisson, C. C., & Cohn, I. H. (1977). Mental health needs assessment: Strategies and techniques. In W. A. Hargreaves & C. C. Attkisson (Eds.), *Resource materials for community mental health program evaluation* (2nd ed., pp. 46–65). Washington, DC: U.S. Government Printing Office.

Sohng, S.S.L. (1996). Participatory research and community organizing. *Journal of Sociology and Social Welfare, 23*(4), 77–97.

Spears, L. (1999, April 11). Picturing concerns: The idea is to take the messages to policy makers and to produce change. *Contra Costa Times,* pp. A27, A32.

Staples, L. (1997). Selecting and cutting the issue. In M. Minkler (Ed.), *Community organizing and community building for health* (pp. 175–194). New Brunswick, NJ: Rutgers University Press.

Themba, M. N. (1999). *Making policy, making change: How communities are taking law into their own hands.* San Francisco: Jossey-Bass.

Thompson, M., Minkler, M., Allen, Z., Bell, J. D., Bell, J. K., Blackwell, A. G., et al. (2000). *Community involvement in the federal Healthy Start program.* Oakland, CA: PolicyLink.

U.S. Department of Health and Human Services. (1998). *Call to action: Eliminating racial and ethnic disparities in health.* Washington, DC: Author/Grantmakers in Health.

Wang, C. C., & Burris, M. A. (1994). Empowerment through photo novella: Portraits of participation. *Health Education Quarterly, 21,* 171–186.

Wang, C. C., Cash, J. L., & Powers, L. S. (2000). Who knows the streets as well as the homeless? Promoting personal and community action through photovoice. *Health Promotion Practice, 1,* 81–89.

Wekerle, G., & Whitzman, C. (1995). *Safe cities: Guidelines for planning, design, and management.* New York: Van Nostrand Reinhold.

Wing, S., Grant, G., Green, M., & Stewart, C. (1996). Community based environmental justice: Southeast Halifax environmental awakening. *Environment and Urbanization, 8,* 129–140.

CHAPTER EIGHT

Using Internet Based Tools to Build Capacity for Community Based Participatory Research and Other Efforts to Promote Community Health and Development

Stephen B. Fawcett
Jerry A. Schultz
Valorie Lynn Carson
Valerie A. Renault
Vincent T. Francisco

A Vision of Internet-based Supports for the Work

Some years ago, our community established All Our Children, an action group with the mission of improving outcomes for all our children and youth through public education, advocacy, and caring connections among children and adults. The Internet has transformed how we do our work. For example, our group's members used tools available on the Internet to guide social marketing efforts to encourage parents to get their children immunized. Our members stay connected through an Internet based forum in which any one of us can post a question or offer guidance about how to solve a problem or dilemma. To document and analyze our accomplishments, we use an on-line system that provides reports and graphs whenever we need them. We use this information to learn, adjust, and be accountable to those who support our work. Although no substitute for face-to-face contact, using the Internet makes our work easier and more rewarding. How could we achieve our big goals without it?

Note: We deeply appreciate the contributions of our many colleagues in community initiatives, university based organizations, and grantmaking institutions who have taught us about building capacity for community work. These include our colleagues at the KU Work Group, including Renee Boothroyd, Rod Bremby, Jenette Nagy Del Rosario, Paul Evensen, and Rachel Oliverius; our technology partners at Athenix, Inc.; and those on the broader Community Tool Box team, especially Tom Wolff, Bill Berkowitz, and Phil Rabinowitz. This ongoing work was funded in part by grants from the Robert Wood Johnson Foundation, the Kansas Health Foundation, the Office of Prevention of the Kansas Department of Social and Rehabilitative Services, the John D. and Catherine T. MacArthur Foundation, and the Ewing Marion Kauffman Foundation.

Why is this vision of integrated, Internet based supports relevant to community based participatory research and action?

Community based participatory research can be used to enhance the process and outcomes of efforts to understand and improve community health and development (Fawcett, Francisco, Hyra, et al., 2000; Green & Kreuter, 1991; Minkler, 1997, 2000; Wallerstein, 1999, 2000). Consider the interrelated tasks in this complex, dynamic, and unfolding work: community members, and those who support them, must understand the context and situation in which an identified problem or goal exists. Together, they must be able to define a common purpose such as assuring clean drinking water or neighborhood safety, eliminating health or education disparities, or promoting child development or independent living for older adults. They must also have the tools or know-how to take action, design, and adapt effective interventions to fit the local context. Using a variety of strategies, they can bring about and document changes in the community or broader system, such as a new public education campaign or a policy to promote access to basic needs and services. The aim is to effect widespread behavior change, such as increases in caring engagements or reduced use of tobacco products, and improvement in population-level outcomes (such as community-level measures of well-being or rates of smoking and associated chronic diseases). Finally, to be successful, they must maintain the effort long enough to affect and engage all those who can benefit and contribute.

Since 1975, our work group at the University of Kansas has been collaborating with community based organizations to try to understand and improve conditions affecting community health and development. Since 1990, we have used a common measurement system (Francisco, Paine, & Fawcett, 1993) in multiple case studies with more than thirty different community and state partnerships (in such areas as substance abuse, adolescent pregnancy, immunization, cardiovascular diseases, systems change for public health improvement, and neighborhood development). This participatory research has focused on two overarching questions (Roussos & Fawcett, 2000): (1) what factors affect a community's capacity to bring about community and systems change? and (2) under what conditions are community and systems changes associated with improvements in population-level outcomes? Emerging answers to these questions helped identify core competencies (for example, formulating a clear vision and mission; action planning; leadership) and broader conditions (such as resources for community organizers or making outcome matter) that appear to contribute to sufficient rates and distributions of community and systems change. Using this information and the work of others, in 1995 we began developing an on-line resource, known as the Community Tool Box (http://ctb.ku.edu) (Fawcett, Francisco, Schultz, et al., 2000), for enhancing core competencies and enabling the work of those doing, supporting, and evaluating community based efforts for change and improvement.

Following a brief review of community based participatory research and related traditions, along with their underlying principles and values, we describe Internet resources that can play an important role in supporting such work. We outline a five-component framework for building capacity for this shared work: (1) understanding context and collaborative planning, (2) community action and intervention, (3) community and systems change, (4) widespread behavior change and improvement in population-level outcomes, and (5) sustaining the effort. The focus is on sixteen core competencies related to this work (for example, assessing community needs and resources and evaluating the initiative) and how a variety of Internet based resources can make these activities easier and more rewarding. We illustrate with a variety of Internet based tools, featuring a case example of integrated supports through the Community Tool Box. The concluding discussion outlines challenges and prospects of using Internet based tools to enhance the shared work of understanding and improving community based participatory research for health and development. (All Web addresses were working at the time of publication, though some may have changed since.)

SOME TRADITIONS AND VALUES GUIDING THE WORK

Multiple and interrelated traditions help inform community based inquiry and action. These include methods and values from the fields of community organization and development (for example, Dunham, 1963; Fawcett, 1999; Rothman, 1999; Rothman, Erlich, & Tropman, 1995), action research (Lewin, 1946), applied anthropology (Stull & Schensul, 1987; Tax, 1958), community psychology (Chavis, Stucky, & Wandersman, 1983; Fawcett, 1990; Tolan, Keys, Chertok, & Jason, 1990), behavioral community psychology (Fawcett, 1991), action science (Argyris, Putnam, & Smith, 1985; Schön, 1983), empowerment evaluation (Fetterman, Kaftarian, & Wandersman, 1996), and education for social change (Freire, 1973; Horton & Freire, 1990).

The sister tradition of participatory action research (George, Green, & Daniel, 1996; Green et al., 1995; Israel, Schurman, & Hugentobler, 1992; Whyte, 1991) has several common values and attributes: *participation* of both community members with experiential knowledge of local issues and context and (often) outside researchers and supporters with specialized knowledge of methods of inquiry and intervention; *co-learning* for community members and outside supporters and researchers; *capacity-building* for doing, supporting, and evaluating the work; and *empowerment* or enhanced influence over the research and action among those local people doing the work (Israel et al., 1992; Minkler, 2000).

As noted in earlier chapters, in CBPR, control of the research agenda and intervention methods shift from sole determination by outside experts (the "professional researchers") to shared determination with community members who have experiential knowledge of the local issues and context. The results of CBPR—new knowledge and methods—are used to inform practice and support the work of understanding and bringing about change in communities and systems. These related approaches emphasize action and learning, self-determination and support, and recognition of the value of both local and outside knowledge. These traditions acknowledge that community members, with their experiential knowledge, can contribute to the definition of the problem or goal, the methods of research and intervention, interpretation of results, and shared learning and adjustments among all those doing and supporting the work. The common objective is enhancing "community capacity" (Goodman et al., 1998): local people and organizations equipped with the knowledge and skills to effectively address the issues that matter most to them.

Community based work often involves a broad collaboration among three parties: local people who work together to address a problem or goal, such as decent jobs or housing; those (often outside) professionals who provide technical assistance and evaluation; and grantmakers who offer financial assistance and other resources (Fawcett, Francisco, Paine-Andrews, et al., 1993). Through the emerging social and technical relationships (Schwab & Syme, 1997), each party is respected for the knowledge and experience he or she brings to this shared work. In a spirit of humility, all recognize the need for additional information and competency and may use enabling or support systems to assist with this complex work (see, for example, Fawcett, Paine-Andrews, Francisco, et al., 1995).

Yet those working on community based efforts to improve health and development often find it difficult to gain access to the support they need, when they need it, at an affordable cost. Support organizations and research teams, who may provide technical assistance and evaluation, are similarly challenged to provide what is needed at a scale that matches the abundance of community work that is being done at local, state, and national levels. Although technical assistance often requires direct personal contact, new communications technologies, such as the Internet, offer additional forms of support for cross-learning among generations of diverse and geographically distributed people doing this work.

Internet technology can help communities become more capable of understanding and effecting community-determined improvements in community health and development (Fawcett, Francisco, Schultz, et al., 2000; Milio, 1996; Schultz, Fawcett, Francisco, & Berkowitz, in press). It can deliver information of enormous breadth and depth, with the potential to provide support for a widespread (and growing) network of people and places. It can provide access to relevant and just-in-time information while reducing barriers of location, eligibility, or cost. Ironically, communication over the Internet can be community-enhancing; instantly connecting those working together on a common issue, either within a community or across communities in a state or nation or globally.

This chapter presents some prospects for achieving the opening vision—community members, and those supporting them, using Internet based resources to inform and amplify their community work.

A FRAMEWORK, CORE COMPETENCIES, AND INTERNET BASED RESOURCES FOR THE WORK

Here we will set out a framework for the process of understanding and improving community based (and community-determined) efforts to improve community health and development. It is based on prior research and experience of our KU work group (see Fawcett, Francisco, Hyra, et al., 2000) and many others (for example, Green & Kreuter, 1991; Wallerstein, 2000). The framework has five basic components: understanding context and collaborative planning, community action and intervention, community and systems change, widespread behavior change and improvement in population-level outcomes, and sustaining the effort. Its components are *interactive* or mutually influencing; for instance, documenting the process of community and systems change may affect (and be affected by) our understanding of the context of the effort. The process is also *iterative* or repeating; consider, for example, how successful and sustained efforts to improve original outcomes may yield to subsequent collaborative planning and action to address other community-determined goals.

Exhibit 8.1 presents sixteen core competencies (and the related framework) for the shared work of understanding and improving efforts to promote community health and development. The core competencies are often related to one or more aspects of the framework (for example, leadership may apply to both taking action and sustaining the effort). The Internet provides access to a vast (and potentially overwhelming) array of resources related to these core competencies. Although particular Web sites may come and go on the Internet, we highlight current resources to illustrate the Internet based supports available for the core competencies. For each aspect of this framework, key questions may help guide the user's exploration of Web sites to find support, resources, and tools for CBPR and other efforts to promote community health and development.

Understanding Context and Collaborative Planning

What do we know about the local people, situation, needs, and assets? How do people define the problem (goal) and see its causes (contributing factors)? What is the community's vision for success, and how do community members plan to get from here to there? An appreciation of people, problems, goals, and places—of past history, current conditions, and future dreams—is the critical basis for community work. For example, a community initiative to reduce the

Exhibit 8.1. A Conceptual Map of the Community WorkStation Aspect of the Community Tool Box.

Community Tool Box
Framework for Promoting Community Health and Development

Understanding Context and Collaborative Planning	*Community Action and Intervention*	*Community and Systems Change*	*Widespread Behavior Change and Improvement in Population-Level Outcomes*	*Sustaining the Effort*

Sixteen Core Competencies Supported by the Community WorkStation
What kind of community work do you want to do today?

1. Create and maintain coalitions and partnerships
2. Assess community needs and resources
3. Analyze problems and goals
4. Develop a framework or model of change
5. Develop a strategic or action plan
6. Build leadership
7. Develop an intervention
8. Increase participation and membership
9. Enhance cultural competency
10. Advocate for change
11. Influence policy development
12. Evaluate the initiative
13. Implement a social marketing effort
14. Write a grant application for funding
15. Improve organizational management and development
16. Sustain the work or initiative

CONNECTING WITH SUPPORT
What kinds of support do I need?

Building Capacity	**Learning and Adjustments**	**Documentation and Evaluation**
• Help in planning the work • Solve a common problem • Quick tips and tools for how to do the work • See a story or example • Learn a specific skill • Training curriculum	• Link to other on-line resources • Connect with others about this work • Ask a question of an adviser • Knowledge base from collective experience • See how this work fits together	• Document community and systems change • Enter or see community-level indicators • Display trends and discontinuities • Analyze the contribution • Sense making and adjustments • Capture success stories • On-line and print reporting

Source: Courtesy of Community Tool Box.

spread of HIV/AIDS should be grounded in an understanding of the concerns of those most affected, the incidence and prevalence of HIV/AIDS among local people, traditional barriers to healthy behaviors and exposures to risks, and community assets to support improvement. In addition, such efforts are well served by strategic plans that communicate the community's vision for success (for example, "Health for All") and a concrete action plan for getting there.

Core Competencies for the Work. Six core competencies, or fundamental abilities, contribute to the work of understanding context and collaborative planning. First, *creating and maintaining coalitions* and collaborative partnerships is a common strategy for engaging the variety of sectors, such as government agencies or faith communities, in a common purpose (Berkowitz & Wolff, 2000; Brown, 1984; Kaye & Wolff, 1997). Second, *assessing community needs and resources* (Berkowitz, 1982; Kretzmann & McKnight, 1993; McKnight, 1992; Neuber & Associates, 1980), such as the need for more accessible health services or the presence of grassroots advocacy groups, grounds the work in what is locally important and available. Third, working with community partners in *analyzing community-identified problems and goals* helps pinpoint the personal and group factors (such as knowledge and skills or history of care or discrimination) and environmental factors (access and barriers, support and resources, broader policies, and the like) that may affect the current problem and future prospects for goal attainment (Cox, 1995; Quinlivan-Hall & Renner, 1994).

Fourth, *developing a framework or model of change* (Milstein & Wetherhall, 1999; Wong-Reiger & David, 1995) helps define how the community intends to go from the current situation, such as low rates of childhood immunization, to sustained improvements in population-level health outcomes. Fifth, *developing strategic and action plans* sets the blueprint for getting from a community's vision, such as the Healthy Youth program, to improvements in population-level outcomes (for example, changes in estimated pregnancy rates or prevalence of drug and alcohol use) (Berkowitz, 1982; Bryson, 1982). Sixth, *building leadership* helps ensure that the community has a team of people to develop and sustain relationships and transform conditions necessary for community health improvement (Chrislip & Larson, 1994; Gardner, 1990).

Illustrative Internet Based Supports. The Internet, or World Wide Web, can help link people and resources for nearly all aspects of the shared work of understanding and improving community based efforts to promote community health and development. For example, some Web sites offer tips from experienced practitioners on creating and maintaining community partnerships and coalitions such as the national Healthier Communities initiative (http://www.healthycommunities.org) and the National Civic League (http://www.ncl.org). From the AHEC/Community Partners Web site (http://www.ahecpartners.org), for instance, a coalition director could download or print a tip sheet titled "Coalition Barriers and How to Overcome Them" to use in a board meeting or in a training session to facilitate discussion of problems the group may be encountering.

Other sites support the work of assessing community needs by offering on-line data on the incidence and prevalence of community outcomes. For example, at the U.S. government's Healthy People 2010 Web site (http://www.health.gov/healthypeople/state/toolkit/progress.htm), a community leader could learn how to develop baseline information about a community health issue. Similarly, at the U.S. Health Resources and Services Administration (HRSA) Web site (http://www.communityhealth.hrsa.gov), a member of a partnership for maternal and child health could find the infant mortality rate for his or her particular county. Other Web sites supported development and use of community indicators, including the Sustainable Communities Network (http://www.sustainable.org), Redefining Progress (http://www.rprogress.org), the Aspen Institute Roundtable (http://www.aspenroundtable.org), the Public Health Foundation (http://www.phf.org), and the Urban Quality Indicators Newsletter (http://people.mw.mediaone.net/cyoakam/index.html). A Geographic Information Systems site (http://www.mapcruzin.com/learn_to_map) provides on-line training in creating and using maps to display the distribution of community problems or assets.

For those interested in developing a framework or logic model to guide the work, the U.S. Centers for Disease Control and Prevention's Evaluation Working Group collected an extensive set of resources on creating frameworks or logic models (http://www.cdc.gov/eval/resources.htm#logic%20model). On-line forums and chat rooms, an additional form of Internet based support, permit access to peers and experts for advice on common tasks such as building leadership. For example, in the on-line forum of the Leadership Challenge (http://www.theleadershipchallenge.com/index.html), contributors commented on and replied to each other about the core functions and challenges of leadership.

Community Action and Intervention

What will we do to address the identified problems or goals? How can we develop the most appropriate and effective interventions? A community's dreams, such as for safe places or social connections for elders, and related population-level outcomes, such as rates of crime or caring engagements, communicate the vision and measures for success. But to move forward, community members must convert a clear and shared vision and framework into community action and intervention. The more specific components of the intervention should reflect an analysis of contributing factors and available assets. To be successful, community efforts must mobilize and engage all those who can benefit and contribute, including those representing diverse cultures and experiences.

Core Competencies for the Work. Three additional core competencies appear to affect success with community action and intervention. Seventh, *developing an intervention* involves selecting and using intervention components and elements based on an analysis of contributing factors and available resources (Fawcett et al., 1994; Green & Kreuter, 1991; Homan, 1994). For example, a comprehensive intervention to increase childhood immunization might include multiple components such as providing information and enhancing skills (for example, a new computerized tracking and notifying system), modifying access, barriers, and opportunities (expanded outreach programs), and modifying policies (offering immunizations as part of other clinic visits). Eighth, *increasing participation and membership* promotes voice and influence from those with deep experience, such as youth or ethnic minorities, but limited engagement (Fisher & Cole, 1993; Kaye & Wolff, 1997). Ninth, *enhancing cultural competency* helps build cross-cultural relationships and create more inclusive and just organizations and communities (McCoy, 1997; Rivera & Erlich, 1992). An understanding of cultural beliefs and practices, for example, the Hmong belief that illness is largely a spiritual matter (Fadimon, 1997), can aid community based efforts to improve health. In addition, several fundamental abilities identified here have a continuing influence on the intervention (for example, building stronger leadership and developing strategic and action plans).

Illustrative Internet Based Supports. Selected Internet sites, such as those of government agencies and national associations, can help support intervention aspects of the work. Forums and chat rooms provide opportunities to communicate with others about key considerations in designing an intervention. For instance, the Office of the Assistant Secretary of Planning and Evaluation in the U.S. Department of Health and Human Services supports a listserv for exchanges among those working on issues of disability, aging, and long-term care (http://aspe.hhs.gov/daltcp/group.htm). There are many useful Web sites that provide tools and supports for taking action in a local community. For example, the U.S. Environmental Protection Agency's site (http://www.epa.gov/iaq/schools/tools4s2.html) offers downloadable checklists, coordinators' guides, manuals, and other materials to support a community intervention to improve indoor air quality. Those interested in enhancing cultural competency might consult available Web sites, such as the U.S. Administration on Aging's on-line guide (http://www.aoa.gov/minorityaccess/guidbook2001/default.htm), to find recommendations that could be adapted to better engage underserved or underrepresented groups such as African Americans, youth, or people with special needs.

Community and Systems Change

How are we using different strategies to bring about change? How will we know if the initiative is a catalyst for community and systems change? Many CBPR and other community efforts to promote health and development act as catalysts for change: they help launch the changes in the environment, such as new programs or policies, that can contribute to improvement in more distant population-level outcomes (Roussos & Fawcett, 2000). For example, a school-community effort to reduce risks for adolescent pregnancy may help bring about new or modified programs (for example, supervised after-school activities), policies (required sexuality education curricula), and practices (enhanced access to contraceptives through school-linked clinics) (Paine-Andrews et al., 1999). Multiple strategies are often needed to have the intended effect. For instance, as part of a community building and CBPR effort to study and promote a safer community in a low-income area in Contra Costa County, California, residents worked with the housing authority, the police, the mass media, the health department, and other partners to successfully advocate for speed bumps, improved lighting, and youth activities. Some residents became active in affecting city and county policies, serving on a Partners for Health initiative and participating in county planning on transportation and welfare reform (El-Askari et al., 1998; Minkler, 2000).

Core Competencies for the Work. Several additional core abilities are associated with bringing about community and systems change. Tenth, *advocating for change* involves overcoming resistance and barriers to bring about new programs and policies related to the mission of a CBPR or other community effort (Altman, Balcazar, Fawcett, Seekins, & Young, 1994; Bobo, Kendall, & Max, 1991; Wallack, Dorfman, Jernigan, & Themba, 1993; see also Chapter Eighteen). For example, a statewide effort to reduce use of alcohol, tobacco, and other drugs might need to anticipate and counteract different forms of opposition, such as denying there is a problem or discounting the potential effectiveness of prevention efforts. Eleventh, *influencing policy development* requires being able to affect the policy agenda and the array of policy options presented to decision makers for consideration (Dearing & Rogers, 1996; Seekins, Maynard-Moody, & Fawcett, 1987). As described in Chapter Nineteen, for instance, a CBPR effort to promote public policies that support the community reintegration of prisoners with substance abuse problems involved the collection of information on factors contributing to this problem on the individual, family, service provider, neighborhood, and broader policy levels. This included policy-relevant information about treatment resources (for example, at the individual and family levels), correctional policies (releasing inmates in the middle of the night without adequate discharge plans), and employment policies (permitting discrimination against former inmates). Twelfth, *evaluating the initiative* includes being able to document the unfolding of community and systems changes over time and their potential impact on more distant population-level indicators of success (Fawcett, Sterling, et al., 1995; Milstein & Wetherhall, 1999; Rootman et al., 2001). For example, a participatory evaluation of a community initiative to reduce risk for (and protect against) adolescent substance abuse documented the onset of new programs (such as after-school programs) and policies (police crackdowns on drinking and driving) and analyzed their contribution to more distant population-level outcomes (rates of single nighttime vehicle crashes) (Fawcett et al., 1997).

Illustrative Internet Based Supports. Some Web sites, such as the Network for Good (http://www.networkforgood.org/npo/advocacy), offer informational tips about how to advocate for change as well as newsletters or forums for connecting with peers or experts doing this work. Similarly, the American Library Association's on-line advocacy handbook (http://www.ala.org/pio/advocacy/libraryadvocateshandbook.pdf) provides tools and worksheets that can be adapted by a community leader interested in advocating for a cause (such as environmental protection or health care access for the uninsured). Some Web sites provide guidance on policy development (one is Service Leader, http://www.serviceleader.org/manage/lobby.html) and access to related exchange networks. For example, Citizen Works (http://www.citizenworks.org), a social justice site, offers links and tools for organizing and lobbying . Other Internet sites provide help with evaluation of community based initiatives (including the American Evaluation Association's "topical interest groups" in participatory evaluation, http://www.eval.org) and chat rooms and electronic discussion lists for dialogue among community evaluators (see the American Evaluation Association's discussion list, available at evaltalk-request@bama.ua.edu or http://ua1vm.ua.edu/cgi-bin/wa?SUBED1 = evaltalk&A = 1).

Widespread Behavior Change and Improvement in Population-Level Outcomes

How do we affect the behavior of enough people in enough places to improve overall outcomes? To effect population-level outcomes, such as the incidence of civic engagement, requires changing the behaviors (for example, voting or making proposals for change) of large numbers of people (such as all adults and youth). To affect the behavior of large numbers of people, states and communities may use social marketing efforts that include promotional messages (touting, say, the beneficial consequences of civic engagement) and environmental changes that make the desired behaviors easier (enhanced access to polling places) and more rewarding (actual influence on the policy agenda).

Core Competencies for the Work. An additional core competence, the thirteenth, is *implementing a social marketing effort*—using promotional techniques to effect widespread behavior change related to socially important goals (Andreasen, 1995; Kotler & Roberto, 1989). For example, our colleague Jim Caccamo and the Kansas City Partnership for Children developed media messages and billboards to promote use of the "Number One Question: Is it good for the children?" in all local decision making. Those who used the Number One Question were honored for their accomplishments in changing programs (for example, immunization tracking) and policies (school revenue bonds) to benefit children (see Community Tool Box, http://ctb.ku.edu). Other previously noted abilities, such as building leadership and evaluating the initiative, also have relevance to this aspect of the work.

Illustrative Internet Based Supports. Some Internet sites provide access to social marketing information for specific goals—for instance, preventing drug abuse (National Council on Alcoholism and Drug Dependence, http://www.ncadd.org), promoting immunizations (PATH, http://www.path.org/about/program_goals.htm), advocating for children's' issues (Children's Defense Fund, http://www.childrensdefense.org), or promoting community support for children and youth (America's Promise, http://www.americaspromise.org). In addition, on-line forums permit exchanges among individuals doing the work of social marketing (Social Marketing Institute, http://www.social-marketing.org/sm.html).

Sustaining the Effort

How well, and in what ways, are valued aspects of the community's work sustained? How do we tell others of our accomplishments? It usually takes time—perhaps ten years or more—to change the environment and behavior sufficiently to improve population-level outcomes. To be successful, communities will need to sustain both the overall change effort and the particularly effective programs and policies that they launch, as well as promote their organizations.

Core Competencies for the Work. Several of the sixteen core competencies are particularly important to this final aspect. Fourteenth, *writing a grant application for funding* can help gain access to resources needed for the work (Robinson, 1996; see also the *Chronicle of Philanthropy* at http://www.philanthropy.com). Virtually all government agencies and private foundations that might support a CBPR project or other community based effort require a clear statement of the community problem or goal, the plan for addressing it, the resources needed, and a plan for evaluation. Fifteenth, *improving organizational management and development* can generate and enhance the needed institutional supports (Herman & Associates, 1994; Unterman & Davis, 1984). For example, having clear lines for decision making and open channels for communication help ensure coordination and collaboration among all aspects of the effort. Finally, sixteenth, *sustaining the work or initiative* helps ensure that human and financial resources are available long enough to make a difference (Brice, 1987; Lefebvre, 1990; Steckler & Goodman, 1989). For example, a CBPR or other community effort to improve positive outcomes for children and youth might use a variety of strategies for keeping the effort going (Paine-Andrews, Fisher, Campuzano, Fawcett, & Berkley-Patton, 2000), such as sharing positions for child health between agencies (as in schools and public health organizations) or embedding the costs for after-school programs as a line item in an existing budget (as in the police or parks and recreation department).

Illustrative Internet Based Supports. Some Internet sites provide information about possible sources for grants and funding in the United States (Council on Foundations, http://www.cof.org). Others offer access to information or guidance about organizational development (http://www.mapnp.org/library, a free management library, or the California Management Assistance Partnership's Nonprofit Genie site, http://www.genie.org). Some sites provide help in planning for how to sustain the effort (the Philanthropy Journal on-line forum for exchange, http://gort.ucsd.edu/newjour/p/msg02367.html).

A CASE EXAMPLE: INTEGRATED SUPPORTS THROUGH THE COMMUNITY TOOL BOX

We now offer a case example to show how a comprehensive set of Internet based resources might be *integrated* in support of community based participatory research for health and development. We describe a feature of the Community Tool Box (http://ctb.ku.edu) known as the Community WorkStation. The mission of the Community Tool Box (CTB) is to promote community health and development by connecting people, ideas, and resources. Established in 1995 and undergoing continuous development, the CTB has over six thousand pages of how-to information relevant to the sixteen core competencies. In a related effort, the KU Work Group has developed an Internet based system for documenting and evaluating community initiatives known as the CTB Online Documentation and Support System.

The Community WorkStation Feature of the Community Tool Box

What kind of community work do you want to do today? What kind of support do you need to do it? The aim of the Community WorkStation (CWS) feature of the CTB is to make the work of community health and development—whatever people need to do—easier and more rewarding. It focuses support, such as an outline for a grant application and real-life examples, on the sixteen core competencies for the work. It enables CBPR partners and other users to connect to different forms of support, such as help planning the work, learning a specific skill, or exchanging information with others doing the work.

Audiences and Attributes of the Community WorkStation

The CTB's Community WorkStation feature was designed to meet the needs and interests of individuals doing and supporting the work of promoting community health and development. The primary audiences (and their related interests) include *leaders and members of community initiatives* (at the local, state, and national level) who are doing this work, *staff of support organizations* who are providing helpful and timely technical assistance and evaluation services, *learners and teachers* from educational institutions who include novices and those with deep experience, and *grantmakers* and funders who are ensuring accountability and brokering connections to other needed resources. Working together in a broad collaborative partnership, these parties all need the ability to build capacity for how to do this work, learn and make adjustments, and document, evaluate, and make sense of the effort's contributions to more distant outcomes.

Consistent with the audiences' needs and interests, the CWS has several attributes. First, the resources are *integrated* in a one-stop "workstation" of multiple supports for what needs to be done to promote community health and development. Second, its content is *comprehensive,* addressing all sixteen core competencies; from creating and maintaining community partnerships to sustaining the initiative. Third, the information is *easily available on demand,* providing a just-in-time response with the tools and links to resources a few clicks away on one Web site. Fourth, the supports are *useful,* providing help in building capacity for doing this work, learning and making adjustments, and evaluating and making sense of the effort's contributions. Fifth, the resources are *appropriate for diverse users and contexts,* including for different types of users (both novices and those with extensive experience), issues (community and public health; child and youth development; community development), and contexts (urban, rural, statewide, global). Sixth, it *promotes equity* by ensuring equal access to guidance for all who have access to the Internet in their organizations or communities. Finally, carrying out the recommended activity results in a *tangible product with benefits* to the community initiative or organization (for example, a functional plan of action or a grant application with prospects for funding).

Technical Features and Capabilities of the Community WorkStation

Use of the Community WorkStation is made possible by advances in Internet technology. This includes development of the Java programming language by Sun Microsystems (http://www.sun.com). Development platforms, such as

SilverStream (http://ww.silverstream.com), help integrate functions offered by Java with preexisting technologies for managing databases such as Microsoft SQL (http://www.microsoft.com). These tools permit the development of a reusable programming infrastructure, such as a Work Flow System, that provides for up to 70 percent of the code needed for navigating and performing routine tasks with the various on-line tools. This also provides for consistency in appearance so that end users can navigate through the Web site without getting lost.

In its most comprehensive form, the CTB's Community WorkStation offers three basic capabilities in support of this work: building capacity for the work; learning and adjustments; and documentation, evaluation, and analysis of the initiative's contribution. The first two aspects are available through the free, public version of the Community Tool Box (http://ctb.ku.edu). Customized and interactive forms of all three aspects are available for those who purchase tailored on-line capabilities for their own community work or for community, state, and national initiatives.

Building Capacity for Doing the Work. For each core competency (such as developing a strategic plan or writing a grant application), the Community WorkStation offers multiple forms of support. First, it provides *help planning the work.* For example, tools for "evaluating the initiative" include a detailed outline for an evaluation plan with links to how-to sections in the Community Tool Box relevant to each task. For instance, for the task "identify stakeholders," there is a link to a CTB section titled "Understanding Community Leadership, Evaluators, and Funders: What Are Their Interests?" Second, the CWS provides help in *solving commonly occurring problems.* The CTB's Troubleshooting Guide lists common problems and dilemmas in doing this work (for example, "We don't have enough members" or "We haven't brought about enough community and systems change"), questions to help clarify the issue (for example, for bringing about change, one question asks, "Do you have a clear, agreed upon action plan in place?"), and links to appropriate sections in the CTB to provide support (for example, "Developing an Action Plan"). Third, the WorkStation offers access to a growing database of *quick tips and tools for how to do the work.* For example, checklists and exercises are offered to guide different aspects of the work. Fourth, it features illustrative *stories and examples* of success doing this work. For example, the CWS unit on social marketing features a description of the Number One Question campaign, a social marketing effort to promote the well-being of children in the Kansas City metropolitan area. Fifth, the CWS provides access to relevant how-to sections for *learning a specific skill.* For each competency (such as strategic planning), there are links to relevant sections from the CTB ("Developing Vision and Mission Statements," "Creating Objectives"). Finally, access to a *training curriculum* is available to those who pay for this service. The CTB training curriculum includes different modules for each core competency (for example, "Evaluating the Initiative"), each with related lessons that include experiential learning activities, assessment ("Developing an Evaluation Plan"), and integrated links with how-to sections in the Community Tool Box.

Learning and Adjustments. The Community WorkStation facilitates co-learning and adjustments in community practice. First, it helps in *linking to other on-line resources.* This includes access to information and materials from the vast array of potentially relevant Web resources for the sixteen core competencies (see our earlier discussion of Internet based supports). Second, it aids in *connecting with others* to learn about this work and make adjustments. It uses a forum or chat room (with e-mail and file transfer capabilities) to create a "learning community" among those doing this work. Forum users may post a puzzle or dilemma (for example, how to constructively involve those traditionally opposed to the group's efforts) or offer guidance to another colleague ("Have you tried . . . ?"). Third, those in particular community efforts for which this is available can gain expert guidance by *asking a question of an adviser.* For example, in a statewide effort to improve child and youth development, experienced community members and national experts might respond on-line to questions from practitioners about particular issues (such as best practices for improving school success). Fourth, the on-line system can offer an evolving *knowledge base from collective experience.* Since the system can code and retrieve emerging knowledge about the work (from the documentation system, success stories, and on-line forums involving peers and outside advisers), we can capture the emerging wisdom across generations of people in distributed communities of research and action. Finally, as illustrated in Exhibit 8.1, the CWS provides a framework showing *how this work fits together.* The sixteen core competencies—what kind of community work to do today—are integrated in a robust framework or road map for organizing this work.

Documentation, Evaluation, and Analysis of the Initiative's Contribution. This final component, the CTB Online Documentation and Evaluation System is based on a common and widely field-tested measurement system for detecting the unfolding of community and systems change (see, for example, Fawcett, Sterling, et al., 1995; Francisco et al., 1993). Since the documentation system is more labor-intensive, it is available only for sponsored community initiatives. First, it supports the on-line *documentation of community and systems change* and other important events. This includes the capacity to provide narrative information about accomplishments (for example, important events such as a new program or policy facilitated by the initiative) and code the events (as a community or system change, service provided, or resource generated). Second, the system supports *entering or seeing community-level indicators.* For instance, a statewide initiative for youth health and development might make available on-line data on estimated pregnancy rates or high school graduation rates for participating cities and counties. Third, it can *display trends and discontinuities* in coded events. On-line graphs of the rate of community and systems changes, for instance, allow for a real-time review of trends and for an exploration of critical events that may be associated with increases or decreases in the pace of change such as new grant funding or a change in leadership.

Fourth, the on-line system permits an *analysis of contribution* of how the initiative is aiding population-level improvement. On-line pie charts can show the distribution of community and systems changes by key aspects of contribution (for example, amount by goal area, duration, and concentration by sector or place). Similarly, on-line time-series graphs can display the relationship between levels of community and systems change, such as facilitated by a teen pregnancy prevention effort, and improvements in community-level indicators (for example, estimated pregnancy rates for adolescent girls). Fifth, it supports *sense making and adjustments.* Users can go from a graph that shows a decrease in the rate of change, for example, to on-line guidance (through the CTB Troubleshooting Guide) on how to accelerate the pace of change. Sixth, the system also *captures success stories* about the initiative. Members of a national initiative to ensure access to health care for all, for example, can communicate stories of accomplishments they are particularly proud of, why their project mattered, and its meaning for the people involved in the effort. Finally, the on-line documentation system supports *on-line and print reporting* about the initiative. Lists of accomplishments, graphs, success stories, and analyses of contributions are available on demand for all those doing and supporting the work, and print capabilities help make the work of reporting easier and more rewarding.

This case example of the Community Tool Box's Community WorkStation highlights the potential power of Internet based supports for building capacity for the work; learning and adjustments; and documentation, evaluation, and analysis of the community's contribution. We anticipate further progress toward a comprehensive and integrated system that enables a diverse and distributed community of doers, supporters, and grantmakers to each add value to the common effort.

The Internet offers unprecedented opportunities to build capacity for CBPR and other community efforts to promote community health and development. But to optimize its contribution, a number of issues must be further addressed. First, access to the Internet itself presents the most obvious barrier to use. Some grassroots organizations do not have access to the Internet, which precludes their use of *any* Internet based tools. Although studies suggest that Internet use is increasing rapidly (reaching well over half of U.S. households), we must ensure a more equitable distribution of computers and networks to reduce the great disparities between the haves and the have-nots nationally and globally (Hoffman & Novak, 1998). Academic partners in CBPR may have an important role to play in writing into research grants computers or Internet access for their community partners to help address this problem.

Second, a community organization may have access to the Internet but be unaware that a particular resource such as the Community Tool Box or the Healthy Communities Web site exists or be unable to find the most appropriate tools for its particular work. In response to the keyword *community*, for instance, search engines such as Google or Yahoo will typically provide tens of thousands of Web sites. So the community member has to become quite skilled in using advanced search techniques to find to the best material. Outside researchers, having greater familiarity with such tools, may contribute by arranging informal educational sessions designed to help bridge the digital divide. In the spirit of co-learning, such forums might be structured so that community partners help outsiders learn the kinds of informational goals and needs most relevant for their community and with outside partners offering more technical information about how these issues might best be addressed with Internet based resources.

Third, sometimes community members and outside experts may not know what would be helpful in a particular situation. For example, an inexperienced or overwhelmed community leader or outside researcher may not know to plan for sustaining the community effort from its earliest days. When members of CBPR and other community efforts are unsure of what is needed or possible, more advanced Internet based supports, such as expert systems that offer a knowledge base derived from experience, could provide valuable guidance based on the whole group's emerging wisdom. Finally, as we have already suggested, community and outside members of the CBPR team may not have the complete skills necessary for this work, even when useful informational resources are available on-line. More intensive supports, such as training workshops or certification through on-line learning, might aid in developing core competencies to increase individual and community capacity and to further work toward enhanced participation of community members and outside researchers in community-determined efforts.

Future research and development can help ensure that Internet based tools, like any shovel or hoe, amplify the efforts of people to address what matters in communities. First, with input from end users, Internet based systems can help provide more tailored support and guidance. Second, as smart systems learn about users' interests, they can become more responsive to the particular needs of those doing and supporting community work. Third, with advances in technology and language translation, people doing community work throughout the world can have rapid connections with a diverse and global community of peers and professional experts. Fourth, refinements in on-line graphing, sense making, and adjustments will permit even fuller integration of the work of understanding and improvement.

Finally, the available Internet based resources must ultimately be useful to those doing and supporting the work of CBPR and other efforts to promote community health and development. To have utility for already overburdened community partners, these tools must make the core tasks easier and more rewarding. The vision of integrated, functional, Internet based supports for community work is becoming a reality in some communities. Its promise is enhanced capacity among generations of change agents in thousands of geographically dispersed communities. Together, we doers, learners, and supporters can be joined—both locally and globally—in this meaningful work of creating just, caring, and healthy communities.

References

Altman, D. G., Balcazar, F. E., Fawcett, S. B., Seekins, T., & Young, J. Q. (1994). *Public health advocacy: Creating community change to improve health.* Palo Alto, CA: Stanford Center for Research in Disease Prevention.

Andreasen, A. R. (1995). *Marketing change: Changing behavior to promote healthy social development and the environment.* San Francisco: Jossey-Bass.

Argyris, C., Putnam, R., & Smith, D. M. (1985). *Action science: Concepts, methods, and skills for research and intervention.* San Francisco: Jossey-Bass.

Berkowitz, B., & Wolff, T. J. (2000). *The spirit of the coalition.* Washington, DC: American Public Health Association.

Berkowitz, W. R. (1982). *Community impact: Creating grassroots change in hard times.* Rochester, VT: Schenkman Books.

Bobo, K., Kendall, J., & Max, S. (1991). *Organizing for social change: A manual for activists in the 1990s.* Chicago: Midwest Academy.

Brice, H. J. (1987). *Financial and strategic management of nonprofit organizations.* Englewood Cliffs, NJ: Prentice Hall.

Brown, C. R.(1984). *The art of coalition building: A guide for community leaders.* New York: American Jewish Committee.

Bryson, J. M. (1982). *Strategic planning for public and nonprofit organizations: A guide to strengthening and sustaining organizational achievement.* San Francisco: Jossey-Bass.

Chavis, D. M., Stucky, P., & Wandersman, A. (1983). Returning basic research to the community: A relationship between scientist and citizen. *American Psychologist, 38,* 424–434.

Chrislip, D. D., & Larson, C. E. (1994). *Collaborative leadership: How citizens and civic leaders can make a difference.* San Francisco: Jossey-Bass.

Cox, F. M. (1995). Community problem solving: A guide to practice with comments. In J. Rothman, J. L., Ehrlich, & J. E. Tropman (Eds.), *Strategies of community organization* (5th ed., pp. 146–162). Itasca, IL: Peacock.

Dearing, J. W., & Rogers, E. M. (1996). *Agenda-setting.* Thousand Oaks, CA.: Sage.

Dunham, A. (1963). Some principles of community development. *International Review of Community Development, 11,* 141–151.

El-Askari, G., Freestone, J., Irizarry, C., Kraut, K., Mashiyama, S. T., Morgan, M. A., & Walton, S. (1998). The Healthy Neighborhoods project: A local health department's role in catalyzing community development. *Health Education and Behavior, 25,* 146–159.

Fadimon, A. (1997). *The spirit catches you and you fall down: A Hmong child, her American doctors, and the collision of two cultures.* New York: Farrar, Straus & Giroux.

Fawcett, S. B. (1990). Some emerging standards for community research and action: Aid from a behavioral perspective. In P. Tolan, C. Keys, F. Chertok, & L. E. Jason (Eds.), *Researching community psychology: Integrating theories and methodologies* (pp. 64–75). Washington, DC: American Psychological Association.

Fawcett, S. B. (1991). Some values guiding community research and action. *Journal of Applied Behavior Analysis, 24,* 621–636.

Fawcett, S. B. (1999). Some lessons on community organization and change. In J. Rothman (Ed.), *Reflections on community organization: Enduring themes and critical issues* (pp. 314–334). Itasca, IL: Peacock.

Fawcett, S. B., Francisco, V. T., Hyra, D., Paine-Andrews, A., Schultz, J. A., Roussos, S. T., et al. (2000). Building healthy communities. In A. Tarlov & R. St. Peters (Eds.), *Society and population health: A state perspective* (pp. 75–93). New York: New Press.

Fawcett, S. B., Francisco, V. T., Paine-Andrews, A., Lewis, R. K., Richter, K. P., Harris, K. J., et al. (1993). *Work Group evaluation handbook: Evaluating and supporting community initiatives for health and development.* Lawrence, KS: Work Group on Health Promotion and Community Development, University of Kansas.

Fawcett, S. B., Francisco, V. T., Schultz, J. A., Berkowitz, B., Wolff, T. J., & Nagy, G. (2000). The Community Tool Box: A Web-based resource for building healthier communities. *Public Health Reports, 115,* 274–278.

Fawcett, S. B., Lewis, R. K., Paine-Andrews, A., Francisco, V. T., Richter, K. P., Williams, E. L., & Copple, B. (1997). Evaluating community coalitions for prevention of substance abuse: The case of Project Freedom. *Health Education and Behavior, 24,* 812–828.

Fawcett, S. B., Paine-Andrews, A., Francisco, V. T., Schultz, J. A., Richter, K. P., Lewis, R. K., et al. (1995). Using empowerment theory in collaborative partnerships for community health and development. *American Journal of Community Psychology, 23*, 677–697.

Fawcett, S. B., Sterling, T. D., Paine-Andrews, A., Harris, K. J., Francisco, V. T., Richter, K. P., et al. (1995). *Evaluating community efforts to prevent cardiovascular disease.* Atlanta: Centers for Disease Control and Prevention/National Center for Chronic Disease Prevention and Health Promotion.

Fawcett, S. B., Suarez-Balcazar, Y., Balcazar, F. E., White, G. W., Paine, A. L., Blanchard, K. A., & Embree, M. G. (1994). Conducting intervention research: The design and development process. In J. Rothman & E. J. Thomas (Eds.), *Intervention research: Design and development for human service* (pp. 25–54). New York: Haworth Press.

Fetterman, D. M., Kaftarian, S. J., & Wandersman, A. (Eds.). (1996). *Empowerment evaluation: Knowledge and tools for self-assessment and accountability.* Thousand Oaks, CA: Sage.

Fisher, J. C., & Cole, K. M. (1993). *Leadership and management of volunteer programs: A guide for volunteer administrators.* San Francisco: Jossey-Bass.

Francisco, V. T., Paine, A. L., & Fawcett, S. B. (1993). A methodology for monitoring and evaluating community health coalitions. *Health Education Research: Theory and Practice, 8*, 403–416.

Freire, P. (1973). *Education for critical consciousness.* New York: Continuum.

Gardner, J. (1990). *On leadership.* New York: Free Press.

George, M. A., Green, L. W., & Daniel, M. (1996). Evolution and implications of PAR for public health. *Health Promotion Education, 3*, 6–10.

Goodman, R. M., Speers, M. A., McLeroy, K., Fawcett, S. B., Kegler, M., Parker, E. A., et al. (1998). Identifying and defining the dimensions of community capacity to provide a basis for measurement. *Health Education and Behavior, 25*, 258–278.

Green, L. W., George, M. A., Daniel, M., Frankish, C. J., Herbert, C. P., Bowie, W. R., & O'Neill, M. (1995). *Study of participatory research in health promotion: Review and recommendations for the development of participatory research in health promotion in Canada.* Vancouver, British Columbia: Royal Society of Canada.

Green, L. W., & Kreuter, M. W. (1991). *Health promotion planning: An educational and environmental approach.* Toronto: Mansfield.

Herman, R. D., & Associates. (1994). *The Jossey-Bass handbook of nonprofit leadership and management.* San Francisco: Jossey-Bass.

Hoffman, D. L., & Novak, T. P. (1998). Bridging the racial divide on the Internet. *Science, 280*, 390–391.

Homan, M. (1994). *Promoting community change: Making it happen in the real world.* Pacific Grove, CA: Brooks/Cole.

Horton, M., & Freire, P. (1990). *We make the road by walking: Conversations on education and social change* (B. Bell, J. Gaventa, & J. Peters, Eds.). Philadelphia: Temple University Press.

Israel, B. A., Schurman, S. J., & Hugentobler, M. K. (1992). Conducting action research: Relationships between organization members and communities. *Journal of Applied Behavioral Science, 28,* 74–101.

Kaye, G., & Wolff, T. J. (Eds.). (1997). *From the ground up: A workbook on coalition building and community development.* Amherst, MA: AHEC/Community Partners.

Kotler, P., & Roberto, W. (1989). *Social marketing: Strategies for changing public behavior.* New York: Free Press.

Kretzmann, J. P., & McKnight, J. L. (1993). *Building communities from the inside out: A path toward finding and mobilizing a community's assets.* Chicago: ACTA.

Lefebvre, R. C. (1990). Strategies to maintain and institutionalize successful programs: A marketing framework. In N. Bracht (Ed.), *Health promotion at the community level* (pp. 209–228). Newbury Park, CA: Sage.

Lewin, K. (1946). Action research and minority problems. *Journal of Social Issues, 2*(4), 34–46.

McCoy, M. (1997). *Toward a more perfect union in an age of diversity: A guide for building stronger communities through public dialogue.* Pomfret, CT: Topsfield Foundation.

McKnight, J. L. (1992). *Mapping community capacity.* Chicago: Center for Urban Affairs and Policy Research, Northwestern University.

Milio, N. (1996). *Engines of empowerment: Using technology to create healthy communities and challenge public policy.* Chicago: Health Administration Press.

Milstein, B., & Wetherhall, S. (1999). Framework for program evaluation in public health. *Morbidity and Mortality Weekly Report, 48*(RR-11), 1–40.

Minkler, M. (Ed.). (1997). *Community organizing and community building for health.* New Brunswick, NJ: Rutgers University Press.

Minkler, M. (2000). Using participatory action research to build healthy communities. *Public Health Reports, 115,* 191–197.

Neuber, K. A., & Associates. (1980). *Needs assessment: A model for community planning.* Beverly Hills, CA: Sage.

Paine-Andrews, A., Fisher, J. L., Campuzano, M. K., Fawcett, S. B., & Berkley-Patton, J. (2000). Promoting sustainability of community health initiatives: An empirical case study. *Health Promotion Practice, 1,* 248–258.

Paine-Andrews, A., Harris, K. J., Fisher, J. L., Lewis, R. K., Williams, E. L., Fawcett, S. B., & Vincent, M. L. (1999). Effects of a replication of a school/community model for preventing adolescent pregnancy in three Kansas communities. *Family Planning Perspectives, 31,* 182–189.

Quinlivan-Hall, D., & Renner, P. (1994). *In search of solutions: 60 ways to guide your problem-solving group.* San Diego, CA: Pfeiffer.

Rivera, F. G., & Erlich, J. L. (1992). *Community organizing in a diverse society.* Needham Heights, MA: Allyn & Bacon.

Robinson, A. (1996). *Grassroots grants: An activist's guide to proposal writing.* Berkeley, CA: Chardon Press.

Rothman, J. (Ed.). (1999). *Reflections on community organization: Enduring themes and critical issues.* Itasca, IL: Peacock.

Rothman, J., Ehrlich, J. L., & Tropman, J. E. (Eds.). (1995). *Strategies of community organization* (5th ed.). Itasca, IL: Peacock.

Rootman, I., Goodstadt, M., Hyndman, B., McQueen, D. V., Potvin, L., Springett, J., & Ziglio, E. (Eds.). (2001). *Evaluation in health promotion: Principles and perspectives.* Copenhagen, Denmark: World Health Organization.

Roussos, S. T., & Fawcett, S. B. (2000). A review of collaborative partnerships as a strategy for improving community health. *Annual Review of Public Health, 21,* 369–402.

Schön, D. A. (1983). *The reflective practitioner: How professionals think in action.* New York: Basic Books.

Schultz, J. A., Fawcett, S. B., Francisco, V. T., & Berkowitz, B. (in press). Using information systems to build capacity: The Public Health Improvement Tool Box. In P. O'Carroll, W. A. Yasnoff, M. E. Ward, R. Rubin, & L.Ripp (Eds.), *Public health informatics and information systems: A contributed work.* New York: Springer-Verlag.

Schwab, M., & Syme, S. L. (1997). On paradigms, community participation, and the future of public health. *American Journal of Public Health, 87,* 2049–2051.

Seekins, T., Maynard-Moody, S., & Fawcett, S. B. (1987). Understanding the policy process: Preventing and coping with community problems. *Prevention in Human Services, 5*(2), 65–89.

Steckler, A., & Goodman, R. M. (1989). How to institutionalize health promotion programs. *American Journal of Health Promotion, 3*(4), 34–44.

Stull, D., & Schensul, J. (1987). *Collaborative research and social change: Applied anthropology in action.* Boulder, CO: Westview Press.

Tax, S. (1958). The Fox project. *Human Organization, 17,* 17–19.

Tolan, P., Keys, C., Chertok, F., & Jason, L. E. (Eds.). (1990). *Researching community psychology: Integrating theories and methodologies.* Washington, DC: American Psychological Association.

Unterman, I., & Davis, R. H. (1984). *Strategic management of not-for-profit organizations: From survival to success.* New York: Praeger.

Wallack, L., Dorfman, L., Jernigan, D., & Themba, M. N. (1993). *Media advocacy and public health: Power for prevention.* Newbury Park, CA: Sage.

Wallerstein, N. (1999). Power dynamics between evaluator and community: research relationships within New Mexico's healthier communities. *Social Science and Medicine, 49*, 39–53.

Wallerstein, N. (2000). A participatory evaluation model for healthier communities: Developing indicators for New Mexico. *Public Health Reports, 115*, 199–204.

Whyte, W. F. (Ed.). (1991). *Participatory action research.* Newbury Park, CA: Sage.

Wong-Reiger, D., & David, L. (1995). Using program logic models to plan and evaluate education and prevention programs. In A. J. Love (Ed.), *Evaluation methods sourcebook II.* Ottawa: Canadian Evaluation Society.

CHAPTER NINE

Using Photovoice as a Participatory Assessment and Issue Selection Tool

A Case Study with the Homeless in Ann Arbor

Caroline C. Wang

Photovoice is an innovative participatory tool based on health promotion principles and the theoretical literature on education for critical consciousness, feminist theory, and a community based approach to documentary photography. Defined as "a process by which people can identify, represent, and enhance their community through a specific photographic technique"(Wang & Burris, 1997, p. 369), it involves providing community people with cameras so that they can photograph their everyday health and work realities. Photovoice has three main goals: (1) to enable people to record and reflect their community's strengths and concerns, (2) to promote critical dialogue and knowledge about important community issues through large and small group discussion of photographs, and (3) to reach policymakers and others who can be mobilized for change. It codifies the goals of involving community members in taking

Note: Portions of this chapter were adapted from "Who Knows the Streets as Well as the Homeless? Promoting Personal and Community Action Through Photovoice," by C. C. Wang, J. L. Cash, and L. S. Powers, *Health Promotion Practice, 1*(1), pp. 81–89. Copyright © 2000 by Sage Publications, Inc. Adapted by permission of Sage Publications, Inc.

The Washtenaw Council for the Arts provided valuable financial support for Language of Light Photovoice. The Shelter Association of Washtenaw County made the project possible with logistic support. Lisa Powers initiated the opportunity for the project to occur and offered her skillful leadership and teaching. Jennifer Cash, Adrian Wylie, and Linda Wan provided important technical support. I am deeply grateful to Lisa Butler and Meredith Minkler for their generous editorial work on this chapter. I thank especially the project participants for their time and insight.

pictures, telling stories, and informing policymakers about issues of concern at the grassroots level (Wang & Burris, 1994).

This chapter focuses primarily on the use of photovoice as a participatory assessment tool that enables people to identify community strengths or assets and their shared concerns as a basis for issue selection and action. Following an overview of the background and conceptual framework of photovoice, the advantages of this approach to community assessment are explained. The chapter then describes the Language of Light Photovoice project, which was designed to create opportunities for men and women living at a shelter in Ann Arbor, Michigan, to conduct their own community assessment as a first step in an ongoing community based participatory research (CBPR) process (Wang, Cash, & Powers, 2000).

As in many other communities, the homeless people in Washtenaw County are a highly stigmatized group with minimal access to the media or to the policymakers whose decisions influence their lives. As this case study suggests, by photographing their everyday health, work, and life conditions, homeless participants were able to document their struggles and strengths and to promote critical dialogue through group discussion about their photographs. This participatory assessment and issue selection process in turn helped position them to reach policymakers and the broader public about their concerns.

PHOTOVOICE BACKGROUND AND CONCEPTUAL FRAMEWORK

The photovoice concept, method, and use for community based participatory research were first developed and applied by Wang and colleagues in the Ford Foundation–supported Women's Reproductive Health and Development Program in Yunnan, China (Wu et al., 1995). Photovoice adheres to basic health promotion principles by involving people at the grassroots level in community action as stated in the *Ottawa Charter for Health Promotion* (World Health Organization, 1986).

Theoretical underpinnings of photovoice and its application as an effective technique for conducting community assessment and participatory evaluation, reaching policymakers, and carrying out participatory health promotion have been described in a series of research articles (Wang, 1999; Wang & Burris, 1994, 1997; Wang, Burris, & Xiang, 1996; Wang, Wu, Zhan, & Carovano, 1998; Wang, Yuan, & Feng, 1996). Photovoice has been used in a variety of settings and with diverse populations, including neighborhood groups in Contra Costa County, California (Spears, 1999); community residents in Flint, Michigan (Vanucci, 1999; Vaughn, 1998; Wang, Morrel-Samuels, Bell, Hutchison, & Powers, 2000); people with mental illness in New Haven, Connecticut (Bowers, 1999); Planned

Parenthood youth peer educators in Cape Town, South Africa (Moss, 1999a, 1999b); young, homeless women and older, marginally housed women in Detroit (Killion & Wang, 2000); teenage "town criers" on AIDS in the San Francisco Bay Area (May, 2001); and a "community of identity" comprised of tuberculosis patients, community health advisers, and health care professionals (Butler & Xet-Mull, 2001). An overview of the approach and its uses may be found on the Web at http://www.photovoice.com.

Photovoice integrates Paulo Freire's (1970) approach to critical education, feminist theory, and a participatory approach to documentary photography. As discussed in Chapter Two, Freire's educational praxis stresses the importance of people's sharing and speaking from their own experience. It further emphasizes people identifying historical and social patterns binding their individual lives, creating an analytical perspective from which to relate their situations to root causes, and developing solutions and strategies for change (Freire, 1970; Wallerstein & Bernstein, 1988). Freire placed great emphasis on the power of the visual image as a means to helping individuals think critically about the forces and factors influencing their lives (Freire, 1970). Photovoice builds on a commitment to social and intellectual change through community members' critical production and analysis of the visual image. Feminist theory suggests that power accrues to those who have voice, set language, make history, and participate in decisions (Smith, 1987). One application of feminist theory to photovoice practice is that participants may wield this approach to influence how their public presence is defined. As a methodology, photovoice represents one attempt to enable participants to help disrupt and ultimately revise depictions that contribute to gender, class, ethnic, and other kinds of oppression. Finally, participatory approaches to documentary photography developed by Wendy Ewald (1985), Jim Hubbard (1991), Jo Spence (1995), and other activist photographers suggest a grassroots approach to representation and demonstrate ways in which women, children, homeless youth, and others can effectively use photography as a personal voice. The photovoice methodology attempts to blend the principle of photography as personal voice with the politics of photography as community voice in order to reach policymakers.

The photovoice concept is designed to enable people to produce and discuss photographs as a means of catalyzing personal and community change. Using cameras, participants document the reality of their lives. By sharing and talking about their photographs, they use the power of the visual image to communicate their life experiences and perceptions. As they engage in a group process of critical reflection, participants may discuss individual change, community quality of life, and policy issues (Wallerstein, 1987). The immediacy of the visual image creates evidence and promotes a vivid participatory means of sharing expertise and knowledge.

CONTRIBUTIONS OF PHOTOVOICE
TO COMMUNITY ASSESSMENT

Chapters Seven and Eight reviewed various community assessment tools and techniques that may be useful in community based participatory research (see also Green & Kreuter, 1991; Israel, Cummings, Dignan, Heaney, & Perales, 1995; Minkler, 1997; Sharpe, Greany, Lee, & Royce, 2000). Several advantages of the photovoice method illustrate how it is distinct from other community assessment and evaluation methods (such as community inventory, community assessment, or formative or process evaluation) (Wang & Burris, 1997). These advantages are summarized here in terms of their contribution to program implementation and sustainability, the assessment process, and equity and community building.

Photovoice offers new approaches for programs, providing a Freirian perspective of "problem-posing education" that allows participants to help define issues and frame the most relevant social actions. Beyond the conventional role of needs assessment, photovoice enables participants to become advocates for their own well-being and that of their community. More than a method of assessment, this is a tool to reach, inform, and organize community members, enabling them to prioritize their concerns and discuss problems and solutions. The method can also sustain community participation during the period between needs assessment and program implementation. The camera is an unusually motivating and appealing device for many people, and photovoice provides a source of community pride and ownership. Furthermore, photovoice provides a way to reaffirm or redefine program goals during the periods when community needs are being assessed. Wang and Burris (1997) noted that in Yunnan, the village women were often asked by friends and neighbors why they were taking pictures. Their explanations served to focus attention on women's status and health, to teach the community about the goals of the project, and to solicit people's feedback about the process.

Photovoice provides powerful assessment opportunities for health researchers and practitioners engaged in community based participatory research. As John Gaventa (1993) has noted, the participatory process assumes the legitimacy of popular knowledge produced outside a formal scientific structure. Photovoice prioritizes the knowledge put forth by people as a vital source of expertise, giving participants "the possibility of perceiving their world from the viewpoint of the people who live lives that are different from those traditionally in control of the means for imaging the world" (Ruby, 1991, p. 50). As an approach to participatory needs assessment or participatory appraisal, this method confronts a fundamental disparity between what researchers think is important and what the community thinks is important. With its powerful use of visual images to capture and reflect a community context, photovoice satisfies the "descriptive mandate" of needs assessment (Wang & Burris, 1997). Photovoice also contributes to assessment by the sampling of different social and behavioral settings. People with cameras can record settings or interactions not available to health professionals or researchers. Photovoice enables participants to bring the explanations, ideas, or stories of other community members to the assessment process. In this way, it affords a flexible, accessible means of incorporating a wide array of perspectives.

Photovoice offers a community- and equity-building component when used as a program or assessment methodology. By focusing on long-term community relationships, it provides tangible and immediate benefits to people and their networks. Returning photographs to neighbors and friends enables participants to express their appreciation, build ties, and pass along something of value created by themselves. This process can affirm the ingenuity and perspective of society's most vulnerable populations. Wang and Burris (1997) describe the success of photovoice with low-income women from Yunnan villages where education for females lacked parental and broader support. Photovoice is accessible to anyone who can learn to use an autofocus camera, whether or not he or she is able to read and write. Photographs collected using this method may serve to capture the full context of a community, its assets as well as its needs. Kretzmann and McKnight (1993) note that the range of community experience includes capacities, collective efforts, informality, stories, celebration, and tragedy. In Yunnan, the village women photographed moments of loss and grief as well as those of celebration and strength, and they elicited stories about the community's imagination, resources, and capabilities (Wang & Burris, 1997). In contrast, conventional methods of needs assessment, such as interviews or questionnaires, may inadvertently reinforce a sense of impotence, inferiority, and resentment. The breadth and depth of public health problems suggests that photovoice can provide a creative approach to enables participants to identify, define, and enhance their community according to their own priorities.

The next section presents a case study illustrating the use of photovoice as a method of participatory community assessment as well as participatory evaluation (Wang, Yuan, & Feng, 1996).

The Language of Light Photovoice project was initiated in Ann Arbor, Michigan, by Lisa Powers, at the time a board member of the Shelter Association of Washtenaw County, Michigan. A professional photographer, she felt she knew relatively little about the people whom she was representing and contacted me to collaborate on a photovoice project. Men and women living at the shelter in Washtenaw County used photovoice as a tool for participatory assessment and to depict issues concerning homeless people. Their photographs and explanations would also be used in a structured evaluation of the effectiveness of the project.

PHOTOVOICE AND THE LANGUAGE OF LIGHT PROJECT

Public understanding of the plight of homelessness is important because public opinion can influence policies affecting homeless persons (Toro & McDonell, 1992). The Language of Light project was established to enable participants to counteract stereotypes about homeless people and to help shape public perceptions about important issues affecting them.

Several projects involving homeless people and self-expression served as forerunners to this effort. In New York City, Hope Sandrow founded the Artist and Homeless Collaborative, a place where artists create artwork with, rather than about, the women, teens, and children living in the city's homeless shelters. Together, they use art to speak out about the personal, social, and political issues that affect homeless people. Such projects have included the creation of an AIDS education poster; a poster addressing rape, abuse, and homelessness; and a writing project yielding a visual collage and exhibit of shelter residents' résumés (Wolper, 1995).

The Artist and Homeless Collaborative has promoted community health by seeking to practice art as an "operating theater in which the often polarized segments of a community come together to create something not seen before" (Wolper, 1995, p. 252). Sandrow also notes that their approach enables people in the shelter to regain what the shelter system and their life circumstances remove: "a sense of individual identity and confidence in human interaction" (p. 253).

Jim Hubbard, founder of Shooting Back, a project with offices in Washington, D.C., and Minneapolis, has taught photography and writing to homeless and Native American youth and engaged them in the process of "creating their own images of themselves and their realities" (Hubbard, 1991, 1994). At an urban drop-in center in Cambridge, Massachusetts, the Women Speak writing project explored the use of writing by homeless women to enhance their self-expression and self-esteem; clinicians reported its value in helping them rethink their relationships with community people (Wolf, Goldfader, & Lehan, 1997).

Finally, the celebrated photographer-educator Wendy Ewald, collaborating with the Self-Employed Women's Association, worked with village children in Vichya, India, to use photography and writing to document their lives (Ewald, 1996). All of these projects focus on the creative process of using photography to help promote a sense of well-being in marginalized communities.

Language of Light built on these successful projects with a firm commitment to the photovoice method of assessment and evaluation. The project had three primary goals: first, to enable people to record and reflect their community's strengths and concerns; second, to promote critical dialogue and knowledge about important community issues through large and small group discussion of photographs; and third, to enable participants to reach policymakers. Major project phases included training the trainers, recruiting participants, conducting workshops, and sharing information with policymakers, journalists, and the broader community.

Training the Trainers and Facilitators

Training of my cofacilitators Lisa Powers and then–public health graduate student Jennifer Cash included providing a full description of the program goals, the theoretical underpinnings of the project, ethical concerns, and photovoice methodology. In addition, they were familiarized with the basics of group process and camera instruction. Although our team did not have prior experience working directly with homeless people, we each had community organizing and advocacy experience.

Participant Recruitment

Participants were recruited at the city's shelters through contact with project facilitators and distribution of flyers. Facilitators welcomed all shelter residents to participate. Eight men and three women volunteered, for which they received a stipend of $20 per session. The men ranged in age from twenty-four to fifty-five years, the women from eighteen to sixty-one. The eleven participants included six white Americans, three African Americans, one Asian American, and one Hispanic American.

Design of the Workshops

Over a one-month period, participants attended three four-hour workshops at one of the city's day shelters, with separate workshops held for men and women. This time frame facilitated maintaining contact with and generating enthusiasm among participants who lead itinerant lives.

The first workshop began with a discussion of cameras, ethics, and power; an introduction to the photovoice concept, method, and goals; careful review of a written informed consent form; camera instruction and self-portraits; a guided photo shoot around the downtown area; and wrap-up and evaluation. Our discussion focused on participants' safety, the camera as a tool conferring authority as well as responsibility, ways to approach people when taking their picture, and giving photographs back to people to express appreciation and build ties. Questions included "What is an acceptable way to approach someone to take his or her picture?" "Should someone take pictures of other people without their knowledge?" "What kind of responsibility does carrying a camera confer?" and "What would you *not* want to be photographed doing?" We also explained that for each roll of film taken by participants, we would provide them with an "acknowledgment and release" form. This form asked participants to obtain the signed permission of each identifiable person photographed, to allow that such images be shared publicly at a future time (see Wang & Redwood-Jones, 2001, for a more detailed discussion of these and other ethical issues and applications).

Procedure

During the introduction to the photovoice concept and method, participants looked at images of downtown Ann Arbor taken by facilitator Powers. In each photograph, participants were able to identify every landmark, alley, and building; provide historical information about each location; and recount recent events that had taken place there. Both facilitators and participants noted the depth and breadth of participants' knowledge of the community.

Participants learned to load reusable Holga cameras. We selected the Holga camera for its simple design and operation, its affordability ($20 per camera), and its appealing and creative format. In this way, participants were provided with something of value that could also be replaced if lost or stolen. One distinguishing feature of the Holga camera is that it permits double and multiple exposures of images, thus allowing the photographer to literally layer meanings. Participants used black-and-white film, which is particularly well suited to the Holga's softer focus and its multiple-exposure feature.

After learning how to load and advance film, participants walked around town together in a guided photo shoot. Facilitators encouraged participants to experiment with angles, reflections, and shadows. At their first session, each participant exposed a full roll of film, learned how to load and unload the film, and discussed the experience of using the camera. This first guided photo shoot enabled participants to see and discuss their first pictures at the very next session.

In the second and subsequent sessions, participants took several more rolls of photographs individually or in small groups formed on their own initiative. They examined photographic contact sheets of each of their images from previous sessions. They also received enlarged prints of images that they felt were most significant or attractive. Some participants performed writing exercises about their photos, following a method that is captured by the mnemonic SHOwED (Shaffer, 1983):

What do you *See* here?

What's really *Happening* here?

How does this relate to *Our* lives?

Why does this problem, concern, or strength *Exist*?

What can we *Do* about it?

Regardless of what they wrote, we invited participants to discuss their photographs in an audiotaped interview. During these discussions, held in a group format, participants described and analyzed the content and context of their photographs. They gave affirming feedback to one another about their images. These discussions helped prepare participants for subsequent public display of their work at a theater. Each participant was provided with a three-ring binder with clear plastic sleeves in which to store their negatives, contact sheets, and enlarged photographs for safekeeping.

Sharing Information with Policymakers, Journalists, and the Broader Community

With participants' approval, and with the understanding that their participation was voluntary, we arranged public forums in which participants could convey their perspectives to community leaders and the public. Participants selected the photographs that they felt were most interesting or attractive and wrote descriptive captions for a series of articles that appeared in local newspapers, in a gallery exhibition, and in a major public forum.

Facilitator Powers, an established local resident, gained a central gallery's invitation to hold an exhibition, as well as free use of the city's largest theater and pro bono union labor for the public forum. She drew on her longtime networks to arrange these local venues and garner community support. We found policymakers, such as city council members, notably responsive to letters and follow-up postcards inviting them to the public events. To gain media coverage, we contacted print and electronic media by mail and by phone. We especially sought out journalists who covered community and local interest beats, as these media representatives were likely to be particularly sensitive to the project outcomes.

Evaluation

The multimethod evaluation included carrying out ongoing formative evaluation throughout the project; surveying participants before and after each workshop; garnering feedback from participants using an open-ended, audiotaped interview; monitoring the extent and quality of media coverage of the project; and assessing audience attendance and feedback. The sample size of participants was too small for the pre- and postworkshop surveys to lend themselves to statistical analyses. Informed by the other evaluation approaches, however, the following discussion is framed by analyzing the extent to which the Language of Light photovoice project met its goals.

The first goal, to enable people to record and reflect their community's strengths and concerns, was achieved by participants, as evidenced by the range of photographs taken and stories told. A fifty-five-year-old man titled one image "Good Times but We're Not Feeling It." He took a picture of a clock and digital display on Main Street. He said, "Not only does it tell the time, but it also shows the Dow Jones as high as it has ever been. Why is the Dow Jones so high? Everyone's making a bundle of money on the stock market—but even though many of us at the shelter have jobs, we can barely find a hamburger to eat sometimes." This participant later taught policymakers and others something that many did not know: it was not uncommon for a person living in the shelter to hold two or three jobs. People also photographed what gave them hope. A fifty-three-year-old man titled a photograph of a canoe in the water "Tranquility." He said, "I was trying to get the peacefulness of it. Water's always interested me, and I have a lot of respect for Mother Nature and the enjoyment of it. The appeal of water and the freedom to go into areas where I control the outcome."

The second goal was to promote critical dialogue and knowledge about important community issues through large and small group discussion of photographs. This goal was achieved as participants shared survival skills necessary for living at the shelter and critiqued stereotypes that they felt attached to themselves and other homeless people. Photovoice facilitators had anticipated that participants might focus attention on the major homeless policy issue being debated, that of moving the shelter out of the city to a remote area near the city dump, and perhaps even wish to mobilize around it. Unexpectedly, they gave minimal attention in their photographs and discussions to this topic. An important aspect of how participants defined this second goal was their ability to increase project facilitators' knowledge about the difficulties of their everyday lives on their own terms.

Discussion

In keeping with the goal of CBPR to balance research with action (Israel, Schulz, Parker, & Becker, 1998), the Language of Light project sought to reach policymakers and other influential audiences. Barrow, Herman, Cordova, and Struening (1999) note that interventions should address not only the health conditions of the homeless but also the general phenomenon of homelessness itself and the societal problem of discrimination that influences it. Participants conveyed their perspectives to a broader audience in three ways. First, they snapped photographs and wrote descriptive text for newspaper articles. Second, their photographs and captions were exhibited locally at a downtown gallery, whose staff reported that it was the best-attended exhibit in the gallery's history. Finally, several hundred people, including policymakers, journalists, researchers, public health graduate students, and the public, attended an exhibit at the city's largest theater where photovoice participants showed their slides with accompanying narrations and spoke to an audience of present and future community leaders. Three newspapers and cable television covered the event.

This photovoice project was conducted at a time when homeless advocates observed that constructing a new 120-bed shelter on the outskirts of the city was "designed to placate downtown merchants" at the expense of homeless people (Hall, 1997). At that particular moment, the city was considering an investment of $3 million in the proposed new facility, which would have made it extremely difficult for shelter users to travel on foot or by bus to their workplaces or other sites of health care, education, and social services. Although the Language of Light project did not substantively alter these plans, it enabled board members, planners, community residents, and community leaders to rethink issues from the perspective of the homeless.

An unstated goal of the project was to help participants adhere to the shelter's sixty-day limit and find permanent shelter without having to ask for an extension. Such extensions had been requested by approximately 75 percent of shelter users. However, within three months of initiating this project, ten of the eleven participants had left the shelter and moved into their own housing. While it is difficult to determine whether the participants represented a skewed sample, in the sense of being more likely to succeed in finding new housing, their success in meeting this unspoken goal was striking. Shelter residents who volunteered for the photovoice workshop may have been especially motivated to explore new strategies to improve their lives or find a way to leave the shelter as quickly as possible. For example, one eighteen-year-old participant had just arrived at the shelter from another state the previous day; despite her personal suffering, she displayed a relentlessly positive attitude and the ability to encourage others.

Participants appear to have benefited from their photovoice involvement in a number of ways. Women and men alike noted that their participation enhanced their self-esteem, peer status, and quality of life by providing an opportunity to creatively express their perspectives and define their concerns in a manner that garnered the attention of media, policymakers, researchers, and the broader society of which they are a part. For example, one fifty-year-old man stated that had he not participated in photovoice, he would have "just been laying around the shelter watching television." He noted that many shelter users were intelligent people seeking to be engaged and stimulated by training such as that provided by Language of Light Photovoice. The eighteen-year-old woman described the project as "awesome" because her participation made her feel important and useful: "I was busy, and that was such a wonderful feeling, and my feeling of esteem went way up." One sixty-one-year-old woman held up her camera and said, "This is history!" She felt that photovoice gave her the opportunity to define her life as she, not outsiders, understood it. Several participants noted that the photovoice project enabled them to view their surroundings in a deliberate fashion, to observe their environment with new curiosity, and to imagine the world from another person's point of view. One participant also said that the process of keeping track of his camera, his unexposed and exposed rolls of film, and his photographs helped him think in a parallel way about how he organized other aspects of his life.

Despite their own extraordinary hardships, the people who participated in the photovoice project had the drive and strength to come to regular sessions.

No one dropped out during the course of the project. One member who found a new job was unable to attend some scheduled sessions; in his place he sent a friend recruited from the shelter. During group discussions, people sometimes described painful experiences, of which they had had more than their share. Facilitators and participants conveyed empathy and support. For both groups, women's and men's, the extent to which the individual's sharing of a difficult life story served as a traumatic or a therapeutic experience—for the individual and for the group—depended on the group's listening skills as well as compassion. Participants tended to close ranks in support of one another if someone shared a debilitating or sad experience.

Outside the photovoice sessions, participants could be seen walking around town together in groups of two to four people. Participating in this project itself enabled participants to get to know one another, build ties and friendships, and therefore bond as a peer support group for problem solving and teamwork. It enabled homeless people to speak from their experience and talk about what mattered to them so that they could help one another survive. The project gave people the opportunity to find solutions together—sometimes simple but important ones—getting to trust one another and then being able to literally borrow the shirt off another person's back for a job interview. Such occurrences appear to illustrate Thoits's finding (1986) that the most effective social support is not likely to be given by professionals but by people who socially resemble the support recipient and who can empathize with stressors based on personal experience.

An unexpected observation was that having a camera around one's neck suggested the luxury of expendable income. Facilitators and participants found that wearing the Holga enabled participants to "pass" as middle-class adults rather than homeless ones. They found that people were more likely to approach them, express curiosity about what they were doing ("Are you in a photography class?"), and strike up conversations ("Are you a photographer?" "Take our picture!"). Given the stigma and shame conferred on homeless people by our society, many participants found this experience more evocative and affirming than they expected and expressed this during each workshop.

Limitations

As illustrated in the Language of Light project, the photovoice approach has its weaknesses. First, we are not able to say whether the housing solutions found by participants have been long-lasting. William Breakey (1997) notes that for some people who lack housing, homelessness may be episodic, and their health profiles are similar to those of others living in poverty. Other people may move into and out of permanent housing in a cyclical pattern. We know that one participant who found an apartment still on occasion uses daytime shelter support services such as the lunch program; we do not know the remaining project participants' long-term housing outcomes. Like other researchers in this domain, we are challenged to follow up with people who may lead essentially nomadic lives (Comover et al., 1997).

Second, the initial workshop stressed participants' safety, but any potential risks to participants in a photovoice project are magnified when the project involves society's most vulnerable members. During the course of the project, a shelter user with a serious mental illness hit one of the project participants in the face with a metal chair in what the latter described as a gay-bashing. We strove to minimize risks as much as possible and view the safety of participants as paramount but could not prevent every serious danger they may have faced daily.

Third, as indicated earlier, we did not ascertain the extent to which participants were representative of other homeless people in initiative, motivation, and resilience. One participant would say, "She has a bad attitude," to describe someone else in the shelter, a nonparticipant, whom she perceived as complaining, negative, and self-pitying. As participation in this photovoice project was voluntary, it may be that people who have the most difficult lives find the method impractical, unappealing, or inaccessible.

Fourth, as a general concern, a photovoice project might enable providers to achieve good public relations at the expense of other substantive approaches to prevent and solve homelessness. Paul Toro and his colleagues support examining how the introduction of a new service for homeless people may affect the ongoing pattern of existing or future services (Toro, Trickett, Wall, & Salem, 1991). Photovoice facilitators ought to appreciate the broader "principle of interdependence" that "alerts researchers, interventionists, and policy makers to attend to the full range of possible positive and negative consequences of their activities" (p. 1212).

Finally, the focus on participants' contribution to representing and enhancing their lives may be seen to be casting homelessness strictly in terms of personal responsibility, rather than broader community or social responsibility (Minkler, 1999). How personal and collective responsibility for homelessness, or any other public health issue, will be understood by the public through photovoice images and narratives ought to be critically discussed by project facilitators and participants.

IMPLICATIONS FOR USE OF PHOTOVOICE WITH VULNERABLE POPULATIONS

Based on the Language of Light Photovoice project, two recommendations are offered to community based participatory researchers considering a photovoice project with people belonging to any of society's most vulnerable groups.

The first recommendation is to recruit at the very outset the policymakers and community leaders who can be mobilized to help implement the change recommended by photovoice participants (Wang, 1999). Participants' photographs and stories can reach policymakers and the broader society, perhaps even influencing healthful public policy, but how? The potential for practitioners' and participants' use of photovoice as a tool for community based health promotion dwells in the conversations and negotiations among participants, health workers, policymakers, journalists, and community leaders over the images of interest. Not by happenstance do these interactions occur. From the start of the Language of Light project, the team facilitators involved, wrote, and informed the mayor, city council members, journalists, and other community leaders. These people were chosen because they might serve as an influential audience for participants' images and stories and could help amplify the participants' insights.

The second recommendation is to be aware of, and find ways to minimize, participants' risks, including physical harm and loss of privacy to themselves or their community. Although researchers and practitioners engaged in CBPR cannot fully prevent all dangers to participants—particularly homeless people or other groups of society's most vulnerable members—they can minimize potential dangers to participants. Among the ways of doing so are (1) underscoring during group discussions the participants' responsibilities when carrying a camera to respect the privacy and rights of others, (2) facilitating critical dialogue that yields specific suggestions and ways to respect others' privacy and rights, and (3) emphasizing that no picture is worth taking if it brings the photographer or subject harm or ill will. As noted earlier, written consent was obtained from participants, and participants were asked to obtain written consent from any people they photographed. This requirement sometimes yielded stiff, less spontaneous pictures but prevented misunderstandings. It also built trust by giving participants an opportunity to describe the project and solicit the subjects' own insights about a community issue. Furthermore, it established the possibility of a long-term relationship that may allow for future photographs and exchange of knowledge, as well as the possibility of acquiring written consent to use the photographs for health promotion aims. Flint Photovoice, a large-scale project subsequent to Language of Light Photovoice, yielded further important ethical lessons and is elaborated upon by Wang and Redwood-Jones (2001).

The Language of Light project suggested that photovoice could make several important contributions to health promotion practice. These contributions synthesize the methodology's theoretical underpinnings: the critical production of knowledge and expertise that influence personal and community action, the accrual of power to those who participate in promoting their own and their community's health, and the analytical use of a community based approach to photography as personal voice.

Contributions to health promotion practice include, first, that health professionals can use photovoice as a tool to learn more about the people with whom they work, to build rapport and trust, and to create productive settings for group discussion and problem solving. The importance of these advantages is substantial; many health professionals learn the hard way that people in the community view them with skepticism, if not outright suspicion. Regardless of the community based participatory researcher's experience, skills, or commitment, he or she may initially be perceived as part of the problem—elitist; ignorant of people's everyday realities, priorities, and survival needs; and motivated by careerism (see Chapters Four, Five, and Six).

Second, important variations in the health needs of homeless people are often overlooked in health planning (Ensign & Santelli, 1997). Photovoice offers a vehicle for gaining needed contextual information for understanding the health status, behavior, needs, strengths, and concerns of homeless people.

Third, community based participatory researchers can use photovoice as a tool to map personal and community assets that can in turn facilitate issue selection and action (Kretzmann & McKnight, 1993). Participants may find photovoice an ideal methodology for creatively documenting their environment and its resources. In doing so, they demonstrate their own ingenuity and imagination.

Fourth, participants may benefit from enhanced self-esteem and peer status as they are listened to—not talked at—and gain a sense of political efficacy (Zimmerman, 1989).

Fifth, sheltered homeless mothers had few social supports to buffer stress and improve well-being (Bassuk et al., 1996), suggesting the positive implications of social networks. Health promotion practitioners may find photovoice a creative and effective tool for fostering social support among participants.

Sixth, photovoice can bring willing, powerful members of a community together with highly stigmatized people and enable the former to assist the latter by first learning from them.

The women and men involved in the Language of Light project are similar to thousands of people who are homeless and looking for means to find adequate shelter, food, health care, education, employment, and dignity. Photovoice may create an opportunity for society's most vulnerable members to speak from their own experience and can change the quality of discussion among themselves and those who advocate their well-being.

References

Barrow, S. M., Herman, D. B., Cordova, P., & Struening, E. L. (1999). Mortality among homeless shelter residents in New York City. *American Journal of Public Health, 89,* 529–534.

Bassuk, E. L., Weinreb, L. F., Buckner, J. C., Browne, A., Salomon, A., & Bassuk, S. S. (1996). The characteristics and needs of sheltered homeless and low-income housed mothers. *Journal of the American Medical Association, 276,* 640–646.

Bowers, A. A. (1999, November). *People with serious mental illnesses using photovoice: Implications for participatory research and community education.* Paper presented at the American Public Health Association annual meeting, Chicago.

Breakey, W. R. (1997). Editorial: It's time for the public health community to declare war on homelessness. *American Journal of Public Health, 87,* 153–155.

Butler, L. M., & Xet-Mull, A. M. (2001, November 8). *Through our eyes: Understanding the experience of tuberculosis with photovoice.* Paper presented at the Human Rights Summer Fellowship Conference, University of California, Berkeley.

Comover, S., Berkman, A., Gheith, A., Jahiel. R., Stanley, D., Geller, P. A., et al. (1997). Methods for successful follow-up of elusive urban populations: An ethnographic approach with homeless men. *Bulletin of the New York Academy of Medicine, 74,* 90–108.

Ensign, J., & Santelli, J. (1997). Shelter-based homeless youth: Health and access to care. *Archives of Pediatrics and Adolescent Medicine, 151,* 817–823.

Ewald, W. (1985). *Portraits and dreams: Photographs and stories by children of the Appalachians.* New York Writers & Readers.

Ewald, W. (1996). *I dreamed I had a girl in my pocket.* Durham, NC: DoubleTake Books/Center for Documentary Studies.

Freire, P. (1970). *Pedagogy of the oppressed.* New York: Seabury Press.

Gaventa, J. (1993). The powerful, the powerless, and the experts: Knowledge struggles in an information age. In P. Park, M. Brydon-Miller, B. L. Hall, & T. Jackson (Eds.), *Voices of change: Participatory research in the United States and Canada* (pp. 21–40). Westport, CT: Bergin & Garvey.

Green, L. W., & Kreuter, M. W. (1991). *Health promotion planning: An educational and environmental approach.* Toronto: Mansfield.

Hall, J. (1997). $3 million homeless shelter opposed: Funding generous but misguided. *Agenda, 129,* 5–6.

Hubbard, J. (1991). *Shooting back: A photographic view of life by homeless children.* San Francisco: Chronicle Books.

Hubbard, J. (1994). *Shooting back from the reservation: A photographic view of life by Native American youth.* New York: New Press.

Israel, B. A., Cummings, M., Dignan, M. B., Heaney, K., & Perales, D. P. (1995). Evaluation of health education programs: Current assessment and future directions. *Health Education Quarterly, 22,* 364–368.

Israel, B. A., Schulz, A. J., Parker, E. A., & Becker, A. B. (1998). Review of community-based research: Assessing partnership approaches to improve public health. *Annual Review of Public Health, 19,* 173–202.

Killion, C., & Wang, C. C. (2000). Linking African American mothers across life stage and station through photovoice. *Journal of Health Care for the Poor and Underserved, 11,* 310–325.

Kretzmann, J., & McKnight, J. (1993). *Building communities from the inside out: A path toward finding and mobilizing a community's assets.* Chicago: ACTA.

May, M. (2001, November 25). Sounding the alarm: East Bay's teenage "town criers" use cameras to bring new focus to AIDS. *San Francisco Chronicle.*

Minkler, M. (Ed.). (1997). *Community organizing and community building for health.* New Brunswick, NJ: Rutgers University Press.

Minkler, M. (1999). Personal responsibility for health? A review of the arguments at century's end. *Health Education and Behavior, 26,* 121–140.

Moss, T. (1999a). Photovoice. *Children First, 3*(26), 28–29.

Moss, T. (1999b). Photovoice: Youth put their world on view. *Children First, 3*(27), 32–35.

Ruby, J. S. (1991). Speaking for, speaking about, speaking with, speaking alongside: An anthropological and documentary dilemma. *Visual Anthropology Review, 7*(2), 50–67.

Shaffer, R. (1983). *Beyond the dispensary.* Nairobi, Kenya: Amref.

Sharpe, P. A., Greany, M. L., Lee, P. R., & Royce, S. W. (2000). Assets-oriented community assessment. *Public Health Reports, 113,* 205–211.

Smith, D. E. (1987). *The everyday world as problematic.* Boston: Northeastern University Press.

Spears, L. (1999, April 11). Picturing concerns: The idea is to take the messages to policy makers and to produce change. *Contra Costa Times,* pp. A27, A32.

Spence, J. (1995). *Cultural sniping: The art of transgression.* London: Routledge.

Thoits, P. A. (1986). Social support as coping assistance. *Journal of Consulting and Clinical Psychology, 45,* 416–423.

Toro, P. A., & McDonell, D. M. (1992). Beliefs, attitudes, and knowledge about homelessness: A survey of the general public. *American Journal of Community Psychology, 20,* 53–80.

Toro, P. A., Trickett, E. J., Wall, D. D., & Salem, D. A. (1991). Homelessness in the United States: An ecological perspective. *American Psychologist. 46,* 1208–1218.

Vanucci, G. J. (1999). Photography used to solve problems. *East Village, 37*(4), 4.

Vaughn, M. (1998, November 27). "Photovoice" project to capture everyday life. *Flint Journal,* p. C4.

Wallerstein, N. (1987). Empowerment education: Freire's ideas applied to youth. *Youth Policy, 9*(11), 11–15.

Wallerstein, N., & Bernstein, E. (1988). Empowerment education: Freire's ideas adapted to health education. *Health Education Quarterly, 15,* 379–394.

Wang, C. C. (1999). Photovoice: A participatory action research strategy applied to women's health. *Journal of Women's Health, 8,* 185–192.

Wang, C. C., & Burris, M. (1994). Empowerment through photo novella: Portraits of participation. *Health Education Quarterly, 21,* 171–186.

Wang, C. C., & Burris, M. (1997). Photovoice: Concept, methodology, and use for participatory needs assessment. *Health Education and Behavior, 24,* 369–387.

Wang, C. C., Burris, M., & Xiang, Y. P. (1996). Chinese village women as visual anthropologists: A participatory approach to reaching policymakers. *Social Science and Medicine, 42,* 1391–1400.

Wang, C. C., Cash, J. L., & Powers, L. S. (2000). Who knows the streets as well as the homeless? Promoting personal and community action through photovoice. *Health Promotion Practice, 1,* 81–89.

Wang, C. C., Morrel-Samuels, S., Bell, L., Hutchison, P., & Powers, L. S. (Eds.). (2000). *Strength to be: Community visions and voices.* Ann Arbor: University of Michigan.

Wang, C. C., & Redwood-Jones, Y. A. (2001). Photovoice ethics: Perspectives from Flint Photovoice. *Health Education and Behavior, 28,* 560–572.

Wang, C. C., Wu, K. Y., Zhan, W. T., & Carovano, K. (1998). Photovoice as a participatory health promotion strategy. *Health Promotion International, 13,* 75–86.

Wang, C. C., Yuan, Y. L., & Feng, M. L. (1996). Photovoice as a tool for participatory evaluation: The community's view of process and impact. *Journal of Contemporary Health, 4,* 47–49.

Wolf, K. A., Goldfader, R., & Lehan, C. (1997). Women speak: Healing the wounds of homelessness through writing. *Nursing and Health Care Perspectives on Community, 18*(2), 74–78.

Wolper, A. (1995). Making art, reclaiming lives: The artist and homeless collaborative. In N. Felshin (Ed.), *But is it art? The spirit of art as activism* (pp. 251–282). Seattle: Bay Press.

World Health Organization. (1986). *Ottawa charter for health promotion.* Copenhagen, Denmark: Author.

Wu, K. Y., Burris, M., Li, V., Wang, Y., Zhan, W. T., Xiang, Y. P., et al. (Eds.). (1995). *Visual voices: 100 photographs of village China by the women of Yunnan Province.* Yunnan: Yunnan People's Publishing House.

Zimmerman, M. A. (1989). The relationship between political efficacy and citizen participation: Construct validation studies. *Journal of Personality Assessment, 53,* 554–556.

METHODOLOGICAL AND ETHICAL CONSIDERATIONS IN PLANNING AND CONDUCTING COMMUNITY BASED PARTICIPATORY RESEARCH

A frequent criticism of participatory research is that it pays little attention to concepts such as validity and rigor and is indeed long on stories and short on discussion of the knotty methodological issues involved in its implementation. In Part Four, we address these issues head on, as well as some ethical and practical concerns, beginning with Hilary Bradbury and Peter Reason's detailed look at issues of quality and validity in the family of participatory and action-oriented approaches to inquiry that they term *action research* (Reason & Bradbury, 2001). Arguing that in such research, "*knowledge* is a verb rather than a noun," these authors help us move from the language of validity *criteria* popular in traditional social science research to the language of *choice points for improving quality* along multiple dimensions. From this broader perspective, they engage us in addressing such questions as whether our work is useful, helpful, and capable of making a difference; whether it is conceptually clear to all involved; the degree to which it is experientially grounded; and whether it can be sustained over the long haul once the original initiator has gone. In short, as Bradbury and Reason suggest, the choice points around which we need to consider issues of quality in action research have to do with "relationships, practical outcomes, extended ways of knowing, and purpose and enduring consequences." As their chapter powerfully suggests, and as Robin McTaggart (1998) and others have noted, rather than skirting issues of validity and quality, action research and other participatory approaches to inquiry by definition urge us to substantially "broaden the conversation" in this realm. In so doing, we carefully consider such issues throughout the research process and not merely in relation to a narrowly defined discussion of "research methods."

As Phil Brown (1992, p. 272) suggests with respect to his own field of popular epidemiology, "Lay involvement is not merely 'good politics.' It is also 'good science,' since it changes the nature of scientific inquiry." Yet as earlier chapters have demonstrated, the high level of community involvement sought in CBPR also raises difficult questions, related to the tensions that frequently exist between using data gathering and analysis methods in ways that help empower rather than intimidate community members and ensure that solid and credible research is in fact being conducted. In Chapter Eleven, Stephanie Farquhar and Steve Wing draw on two case studies to examine these and other issues in academic-community partnerships designed to document and expose health problems and related social and environmental racism in rural North Carolina. In the first of these, the usefulness of CBPR is demonstrated in the uncovering of patterns of environmental racism in the placement of industrialized hog production factories in low-income, predominantly African American communities and the links between these factories and health problems. The necessity of collaboration for undertaking such sensitive work, its potency for catalyzing change, and the real threats that occurred when the research was seen as challenging a powerful industry and its allies are among the issues explored in this case study.

As Virginia Olesen (1998, p. 317) has argued with respect to feminist qualitative research, "In a certain sense, participants are always 'doing' research, for they, along with the researchers, construct the meanings that become 'data'" for subsequent analysis. In qualitative CBPR, however, the distance between researcher and participants is closed still further, as illustrated in the second case in this chapter, documenting and analyzing the discriminatory practice and inadequate emergency environmental and housing policies in the aftermath of Hurricane Floyd and the actions that followed. The political fallout of CBPR in these two cases, the problems with charges of bias and "unscientific" research, and the accent on co-learning through the CBPR process are highlighted.

The final case study in Part Four comes from the disability community in the San Francisco Bay Area and involves the efforts of its members to study and broaden the dialogue around a particularly contentious issue in their community: "death with dignity," or physician-assisted suicide legislation. As Pamela Fadem and colleagues suggest, despite the high-level community involvement achieved in each stage of the research process, major ethical issues arose throughout. These included the politics of issue selection when the community is deeply divided over an issue, tensions between insiders and outsiders, and tough questions over the appropriate use of findings. In sharing their struggles with these often painful issues, the authors hope to stimulate others engaged in CBPR partnerships as they confront their own ethical and practical challenges.

As each of these case studies suggests, despite difficulties encountered along the way, authentic partnerships can often result in far richer understandings of a problem area than outsiders or community members can achieve working on their own. At the same time, such collaboration can pave the way for action, while leaving behind a community of people better able to mobilize around, systematically study, and act on their issues in the future.

One of the greatest challenges for those involved in community building and related work is how to evaluate the results of such efforts without disempowering communities and in other ways violating the most basic tenets of such work (Minkler, 1997). The development of the field and practice of participatory evaluation over the past two decades has consequently been especially important for those committed to individual and community capacity building. Also termed "empowerment evaluation," participatory evaluation retains a commitment to high-quality inquiry and outcomes while incorporating an equally strong emphasis on the principles of empowerment and capacity building (Fetterman, Kaftarian, & Wandersman, 1996; Wallerstein, 1999). Although a critical new avenue for participatory collaboration between community members and their outside partners, however, the conduct of participatory evaluation is fraught with many of the same ethical, practical, and methodological difficulties that confront other forms of CBPR. It further faces additional challenges that are unique to the "judging" of programs, projects, and policies whose future may be heavily influenced by the research outcomes. In Chapter Thirteen, Jane Springett traces the conceptual and practice roots of participatory evaluation, its relationship to participatory research, and its increasingly central role in the evaluation of health promotion initiatives. She then illustrates a number of tensions and issues that frequently emerge in the course of such collaborative approaches. The relationship between the evaluator and the evaluated, the selection of appropriate tools and methods, the emergent nature of the evaluative process itself, and the contradictions inherent when "different agendas are being overtly brought together" are among the thorny issues surfaced and explored. Springett concludes by arguing that although this approach can play a critical role as a change catalyst, considerably more work is needed if we are to move from consultative approaches to evaluation to those that are truly participatory in the fullest sense of that word.

References

Brown, P. (1992). Popular epidemiology and toxic waste contamination: Lay and professional ways of knowing. *Journal of Health and Social Behavior, 3,* 267–281.

Fetterman, D. M., Kaftarian, S. J., & Wandersman, A. (Eds.). (1996). *Empowerment evaluation: Knowledge and tools for self-assessment and accountability.* Thousand Oaks, CA: Sage.

McTaggart, R. (1998). Is validity really an issue for participatory action research? *Studies in Cultures, Organizations, and Societies, 4,* 211–236.

Minkler, M. (Ed.). (1997). *Community organizing and community building for health.* New Brunswick, NJ: Rutgers University Press.

Olesen, V. (1998). Feminisms and models of qualitative research. In N. K. Denzin & Y. S. Lincoln (Eds.), *The landscape of qualitative research* (pp. 300–332). Thousand Oaks, CA: Sage.

Reason, P., & Bradbury, H. (2001). *Handbook of action research: Participative inquiry and practice.* Thousand Oaks, CA: Sage.

Wallerstein, N. (1999). Power between evaluator and community: Research relationships within New Mexico's healthier communities. *Social Science and Medicine, 49,* 39–53.

CHAPTER TEN

Issues and Choice Points for Improving the Quality of Action Research

Hilary Bradbury
Peter Reason

We cannot regard truth as a goal of inquiry. The purpose of inquiry is to achieve agreement among human beings about what to do, to bring about consensus on the ends to be achieved and the means used to achieve those ends. Inquiry that does not achieve coordination of behavior is not inquiry but simply wordplay.
—Richard Rorty (2000, p. xxv)

We must keep on trying to understand better, change and reenchant our plural world.
—Orlando Fals-Borda (1997)

There is no "short answer" to the question "What is action research?" But let us say as a working definition for us that action research is a participatory, democratic process concerned with developing practical knowing in the pursuit of worthwhile human purposes, grounded in a participatory worldview. It seeks to reconnect action and reflection, theory and practice, in participation with others, in the pursuit of practical solutions to issues of pressing concern to people. More generally, it grows out of a concern for the flourishing of individuals and their communities.

We therefore see action research practitioners as necessarily concerned with three important purposes. The first purpose is to bring an action dimension back to the overly quietist tradition of knowledge generation that has developed in the modern era. The second is to loosen the grip over knowledge creation held traditionally by universities and other institutions of "higher

Note: The authors are listed alphabetically. This chapter was adapted from the Introduction and Conclusion they wrote for *The Handbook of Action Research: Participative Inquiry and Practice,* which they edited. Copyright © 2001 by P. Reason and H. Bradbury. Adapted by permission of the authors and of Sage Publications Ltd. For some of the more detailed arguments and illustrations, the reader is invited to refer to the originals.

learning." The third purpose is to contribute to the ongoing revision of the Western disposition—to add impetus to the movement away from a modernist worldview based on a positivist philosophy and a value system dominated by crude notions of economic progress in a universe devoid of transcendent meaning toward an emerging participatory perspective.

Thus for us action research is a practice for the systematic development of knowing and knowledge, but arising from a rather different form than that of traditional academic research. It has different purposes and is based in different relationships; it has different ways of conceiving of knowledge and its relation to practice. Though the field of action research is hugely varied and there are countless choices to be made in practice, there are five broadly shared features that characterize action research, as shown in Figure 10.1.

A significant purpose of action research is to produce practical knowledge that is useful to people in the everyday conduct of their lives. A wider purpose of action research is to contribute through this practical knowledge to the increased well-being—economic, political, psychological, and spiritual—of persons and communities and to a more equitable and sustainable relationship with the wider ecology of the planet of which we are an intrinsic part.

So action research is about working toward *practical outcomes* and also about creating new forms of understanding, since action without reflection and understanding is blind, just as theory without action is meaningless. And more broadly, theories that contribute to human emancipation, to the flourishing of community, which help us reflect on our place in the ecology of the planet and contemplate our spiritual purposes, can lead us to different ways of being together, as well as provide important guidance and inspiration for practice (a feminist perspective would invite us to consider whether an

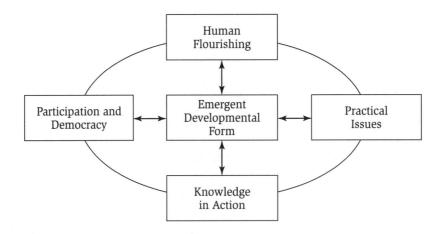

Figure 10.1 Characteristics of Action Research.

emphasis on *action* without a balancing consideration of ways of *being* is rather too heroic).

As we search for practical knowledge and liberating ways of knowing, working with people in their everyday lives, we can also see that action research is *participative research,* and all participative research must be action research. People are agents who act in the world on the basis of their own sense making; human community involves mutual sense making and collective action. Action research is only possible *with, for,* and *by* individuals and communities, ideally involving all stakeholders both in the questioning and sense making that informs the research and in the action that is its focus.

Since action research starts with everyday experience and is concerned with the development of living knowledge, in many ways the process of inquiry is as important as specific outcomes. Good action research emerges over time in an evolutionary and developmental process as individuals develop skills of inquiry and as communities of inquiry develop within communities of practice. Action research is emancipatory; it leads not just to new practical knowledge but also to new abilities to create knowledge. In action research, knowledge is a living, evolving process of coming-to-know rooted in everyday experience; *knowledge* is a verb rather than a noun. This means that action research cannot be programmatic and cannot be defined in terms of hard and fast methods but is, in Lyotard's (1984) sense, a work of art.

These five interdependent characteristics of action research emerge from our reflections on practice in this developing field. Together they imply an "action turn" in research practice that both harks back to the antique classical sense of holistic inquiry (Eikeland, 2001) while also building on and taking us beyond the "language turn" of recent years: the language turn drew our attention to the way knowledge is a social construction. In some ways, this awakening to our ability to create our world anew is simultaneously paralyzed by deep interdependence of self and language. Hilary Putnam (1992) points out that language and mind penetrate so deeply into reality that the very project of representing ourselves as language-independent is fatally compromised. Action research offers a fresh path from this quandary: the action turn draws our attention to how we can act in intelligent and informed ways in a world that we understand is not independent of our coconstruction.

We start from these assertions—which may seem contentious to some of the academic community while at the same time obvious to those of a more activist orientation—because the purpose of knowledge making is so rarely debated. The institutions of normal science and academia, which have created such a monopoly on the knowledge-making process, place a primary value on pure research, the creation of knowledge unencumbered by practical questions, driven simply by intellectual curiosity. In contrast, the primary purpose of action research is not to produce academic theories based on action; nor is it to produce theories about action; nor is it to produce theoretical or empirical knowledge that can be applied in action; it is to reweave knowing and doing so as to liberate the human body, mind, and spirit in the search for a better, freer world.

These characteristics of action research are not simply questions of methodology. To be sure, we can argue that they lead to "better" research because the practical and theoretical outcomes of the research process are grounded in the perspective and interests of those immediately concerned and not filtered through an outside researcher's preconceptions and interests. But far more than that, when we assert the practical purposes of action research and the importance of human interests; when we join knower with known in participative relationship; as we move away from operational measurement into a science of experiential qualities (Reason & Goodwin, 1999), we undercut the foundations of the empirical-positivist worldview that has been the foundation of Western inquiry since the Enlightenment (Toulmin, 1990) and start exploring the possibility that new worldviews are emerging. This in turn draws our attention to a broader bandwidth of choices that action research practitioners need to make in the course of their work, choices that have implications for the quality and validity of their inquiries.

BEYOND A TRADITIONAL VIEW: BROADENING THE BANDWIDTH OF VALIDITY

Our reflections on the practices of action research and a participatory worldview lead us to ask very different questions about the nature of high-quality practice in action research. How do action researchers, both individually and together with co-researchers, address the questions "Am *I* doing good work?" and "Are *we* doing good work?" We can use the five dimensions of the participatory worldview to interrogate our inquiry practice, and the questions and the subsequent choice points posed allow us to consider issues of validity and quality in action research work. We hope to build a bridge between academic concerns about validity and more reflexively practical questions about the work of action research.

For the academic community, we see our writing on the issue of quality as initiating and sustaining an engaging conversation among action researchers and between action researchers and other researchers. For although the issues and questions that provoke choice points in our work obviously inform the work of action research, we believe that they may also be extended to a conversation about validity in other types of research work. We hereby join the lively debate that has been referred to as the "fertile obsession" with validity (Lather, 1993). In joining this debate to add voices from action research, we hope to broaden the "bandwidth" of concerns associated with the question of what constitutes good knowledge research and practice.

We are aware that the possibility of even having standards or criteria of validity has been questioned in this era of postmodern loss of legitimacy (Lyotard, 1984). Kvale (1989) has questioned the validity of the very question of validity, that is to say, raised a question as to whether we are foolishly trying to fit the qualities of action research into a traditional discourse about validity whose concerns have little to do with those of action research. Wolcott (1990) has argued for dismissing validity altogether precisely because the discourse is inextricably bound to the ideals of positivism. Schwandt (1996) has also bid a "farewell to criteriology," where criteriology has meant a uniform set of measures. In light of those important concerns, we say that our purpose in this chapter is with continuing the discourse about validity predicated on our concern for continuing an ongoing and important dialogue. We hope that a shared and no doubt growing vocabulary providing clarity about common ground and disagreement can only improve both the quality of our work and collegial relationships in action research. To some measure, we hereby also stand on the shoulders of the scholars who have preceded us in their concern for continuing but shifting the dialogue about validity from a concern with idealist questions in search of "Truth" to concern for engagement, dialogue, pragmatic outcomes and an emergent, reflexive sense of what is important.

Lincoln (1995), in calling for a profusion of validities that emerge from the context of a given study, began a shift in the discourse about the *nature* of criteriology (what criteria for validity are) to their *function*. Lather (1997) has continued this trajectory as "a rehearsal for a new social imaginary out from under scientism." She writes, "Our framing is shifting validity from a discourse about quality as normative to a discourse of relational practices" (p. 2). Habermas (1979; see also Kemmis, 2001) posits that truth results from an emancipatory process that emerges as people strive toward conscious and reflexive emancipation, speaking, reasoning, and coordinating action together, unconstrained and uncoerced. And so we follow a number of scholars by taking up a point well made by Gustavsen (2001): our concern is not with getting the labels of the criteria "very right" but with drawing attention to important choices that an action researcher must make and thus with extending a useful conversation about getting valuable work done well.

A new set of validity criteria—we refer to them as choice points—is related to the participatory disposition that we believe is replacing the modernist worldview.

TOWARD A PARTICIPATORY WORLDVIEW

Many writers and commentators are suggesting that the modernist worldview or paradigm of Western civilization is reaching the end of its useful life. It is suggested that a fundamental shift is occurring in our understanding of the universe and our place in it, that new patterns of thought and belief are emerging that will transform our experience, our thinking, and our action. We have, since the Reformation, the beginning of the era of modern science, and the Industrial Revolution, made enormous strides in our material welfare and our control of our lives. Yet at the same time we can see the costs of this progress in ecological devastation, human and social fragmentation, and spiritual impoverishment. So if we fail to make a transition to new ways of thinking, our civilization will decline and decay. Gregory Bateson (1972/2000), one of the great original thinkers of our time, argued that the most important task we face is learning to think in new ways; he was deeply concerned with what he called the "epistemological errors" of our time, the errors built into our ways of thinking, and their consequences for justice and ecological sustainability. So the challenge of changing our worldview is central to our times.

The emergent worldview has been described as systemic, holistic, relational, feminine, and experiential, but its defining characteristic is that it is *participatory:* our world does not consist of separate things but of relationships that we coinvent. We participate in our world in such a way that the "reality" we experience is a mutual creation that involves the primal givenness of the cosmos and human feeling and construing. (For an extended reflection on the qualities of participation, see Reason & Torbert, 2001, and Torbert & Reason, 2001.) The participative metaphor is particularly apt for action research because as we participate in creating our world, we are already embodied and breathing beings *who are necessarily acting*—and this draws us to consider how to assess the *quality* of our acting.

A participatory worldview places persons and communities as part of their world—both human and more-than-human—embodied in their world, co-creating their world. A participatory perspective asks us to be both situated and reflexive, to be explicit about the perspective from which knowledge is created, to see inquiry as a process of coming to know, serving the democratic, practical ethos of action research.

A participatory view competes with both the positivism of modern times and the deconstructive postmodern alternative—and we would hold it to be a more adequate and creative paradigm for our times. However, we can also say that it also draws on and integrates both paradigms: it follows positivism in arguing that there is a "real" reality, a primeval givenness of being (of which we partake), and draws on the constructionist perspective in acknowledging that as soon as we attempt to articulate this, we enter a world of human language and cultural expression. Any account of the given cosmos in the spoken or written word is culturally framed, yet if we approach our inquiry with appropriate critical skills and discipline, our account may provide some perspective on what is universal and on the knowledge-creating process that frames this account.

The dimensions of a participatory worldview (shown in Figure 10.2) echo the characteristics of action research we identified earlier in Figure 10.1.

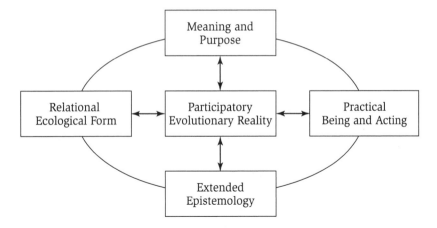

Figure 10.2 Dimensions of a Participatory Worldview.

On the Nature of the Given Cosmos

At the center of a participatory worldview lie our intimations of the *participatory nature* of the cosmos that we both inhabit and cocreate, whose form is *relational and ecological.* We live in a participatory world. There is a primordial givenness of being in which the human body and mind actively participate in a cocreative dance that gives rise to the reality we experience. Subject and object are interdependent. Thus participation is fundamental to the nature of our being, an *ontological given* (Heron, 1996a; Heron & Reason, 1997). Because we are a part of the whole, we are necessarily actors within it, which leads us to consider the fundamental importance of the practical.

On Practical Being and Acting

Given this fundamental participation in the whole, we humans are already engaged and thus are already acting (Skolimowski, 1994). Thus for the action researcher, practical knowing is the purpose, the consummation, the fulfillment of the knowledge quest (Heron, 1996b). All ways of knowing serve to support our skilful being-in-the-world from moment to moment to moment, our ability to act intelligently in the pursuit of worthwhile purposes. Human inquiry is necessarily practical, and a participatory form of inquiry is an *action science.*

On the Nature of Knowing

A participative worldview, with its notion of reality as both subjective and objective, involves an extended epistemology: we draw on diverse forms of knowing as we encounter and act in our world. Heron and Reason (2001; Heron, 1996a) argue that a knower participates in the known, articulating the world in at least four interdependent ways. *Experiential knowing* is through direct, face-to-face encounters with a person, place, or thing; it is knowing through empathy and resonance, that kind of in-depth knowing that is almost impossible to put into words. *Presentational knowing* grows out of experiential knowing and provides the first form of expression through story, drawing, sculpture, movement, and dance, drawing on aesthetic imagery. Propositional knowing draws on concepts and ideas, and *practical knowing* consummates the other forms of knowing in action in the world. Other theorists, writing from pragmatic, constructionist, critical, feminist, and developmental perspectives, have articulated different ways of framing an extended epistemology (Belenky, Clinchy, Goldberger, & Tarule, 1986; Greenwood & Levin, 1998; Park, 2001; Torbert, 1991).

On Relational Ecological Form

A participatory worldview is a political statement as well as a theory of knowledge. Just as the classical Cartesian worldview emerged in part from the political situation of the time (Toulmin, 1990) and found its expression not only in science and technology but also in our political structures and organizational forms, so a participatory worldview implies democratic peer relationships as the political form of inquiry.

This political dimension of participation affirms people's right and ability to have a say in decisions that affect them and that claim to generate knowledge about them. It asserts the importance of liberating the muted voices of those held down by class structures and neocolonialism, by poverty, sexism, racism, and homophobia. Action research practitioners from all perspectives have argued strongly in favor of the connections between power and knowledge.

Relationships do not exist only with other humans; we also have relationships with the more-than-human world. As we become increasingly aware that the damage being done to the planet's ecosystems and the resultant sustainability crisis (Brown, 1999) are in part the result of our failure to understand the systemic nature of the planet's ecosystems and humanity's role in the course of natural processes, we can also see that that participation is an *ecological imperative*.

On Purpose and Meaning: Spirit and Beauty

Action research practitioners may suggest slightly different emphases in describing the purpose of their work—they write of the "quest for life," "making the world better" or "more loving" or "freer"—but they broadly agree that the purpose of human inquiry is the flourishing of life, the life of persons, of human communities, and increasingly of the more-than-human world of which we are a part. A participative worldview invites us to inquire into what we mean by "flourishing" and into the meaning and purpose of our endeavors, and this, as we will argue, is a key dimension of quality in inquiry. As Berry (1999) asks us, what is the "great work" of humanity in our time, and how are our individual human projects aligned with it? Participative consciousness is part of a resacralization of the world, a kind of reenchantment (Berman, 1981; Berry, 1988; Skolimowski, 1993). Sacred experience is based in reverence, in awe and love for creation, valuing it for its own sake, in its own right as a living presence. To deny participation not only offends against human justice, not only leads to errors in epistemology, not only strains the limits of the natural world, but is also troublesome for human souls and for the *anima mundi.*

So a participatory worldview places the practical response to human problems in a necessarily wider spiritual context—human practical inquiry is a spiritual expression, a celebration of the flowering of humanity and of the cocreating cosmos, and as part of a sacred science, it is an expression of the beauty and joy of active existence.

CHOICE POINTS FOR ACTION RESEARCH

In offering a new set of criteria, which we prefer to call *choice points,* we make no pretence of being comprehensive—indeed, to do so would be to fall into the totalizing and essentialist trap of seeking to provide a new set of firm criteria for validity. Instead, we bring action researchers' attention to a smorgasbord of important issues and ask that they choose wisely and in conversation with other inquirers when deciding what is important in their research. Offering a perfect set of criteria is neither possible nor desirable because each piece of inquiry or practice is its own work of art articulating its own standards. What we hope we accomplish is to sketch out the basis for some of the choices and questions that need to be faced by an individual action researcher and by action research communities.

Each theory of the way the world is gives rise to particular ways of *seeing the world.* We have argued that action research emerges within a participative way of seeing or acting in the world in which we find ourselves always in relationship. As a starting point, we therefore need to be concerned with both the quality of our theory and our holistic, everyday, lived experience. Gustavsen (1996, p. 94) writes that "both our theoretical worlds and our life world [or lived experience] are necessary and cannot be substituted. More theory cannot fill the vacuum of a lack of experience, and more experience cannot bring more order into an uninterpreted world." Such concerns lead us into the following five broad issues, already discussed at the start of this chapter, within which we may begin to articulate choice points for good action research.

A participative worldview draws our attention to the qualities of the participative and relational practices in our work. Issues of interdependence, politics, power, and empowerment must be addressed at both micro and macro levels— that is, in inquiring relationships in face-to-face and small group interaction and in determining how the research is situated in its wider political context.

In particular, we must pay attention to the congruence between qualities of participation that we espouse and the actual work we accomplish, especially as our work involves us in networks of power dynamics that both limit and enable our work (Gaventa & Cornwall, 2001). A mark of quality in an action research project is that people will get energized and empowered by being involved, leading them to develop newly useful, reflexive insights as a result of a growing critical consciousness. They may ideally say, "That was our own research, and it helped us see ourselves and our context through new eyes and taught us to act in all sorts of new ways." We may therefore say that as action researchers, we must ask questions that inquire into and seek to ensure quality of participation and relationship in the work.

As we participate with people, oriented by our shared concerns and interests, the practical outcome of our work is important. Thus a series of pragmatic questions must be asked of action research work, such as "Is the work useful or helpful?" and "Do people whose reputations and livelihoods are affected act differently as a result of the inquiry?" We acknowledge that what is considered "helpful" or "useful" is itself not at all a straightforward issue—as Stephen Kemmis (2001) shows us by distinguishing between technical, practical, and emancipatory outcomes—and must be explored reflexively by those who are participating, and this reflection in turn informs the relational process. Ideally, people's response to action research work is "That worked" or "That was helpful." We may therefore say that as action researchers, we must ask pragmatic questions about outcome and practice in our work and consistently strive to be reflexive about this. So even though we may begin in a mode of "single-loop inquiry," seeking merely to get things accomplished, we must proceed appropriately to "double-loop inquiry" (Argyris & Schön, 1996), in which we ask questions about the value of the very things we are seeking to accomplish.

As we participate, our knowledge of the world includes—but is never limited to—conceptual or intellectualized forms of knowledge, most often associated with academic enterprise. Action research recognizes the importance of conceptual knowledge while also consciously engaging in extended epistemologies. We may ask how different ways of knowing, be they aesthetic or presentational, representational, experiential, or more theoretical or conceptual, have been drawn on or allowed to surface in our work. How have they informed the ways in which the work itself is represented?   Each particular way of knowing raises questions concerning quality in its own right. How well is an inquiry experientially grounded? How is it embodied in sensuous knowing? What is the appropriate form of presentation for this particular audience? Is it aesthetically elegant? Is it conceptually clear to all involved? Does it promote further knowing by raising new questions or by allowing us "see through" old conceptual frameworks so that these are newly experienced as more limiting than enabling? By drawing on and integrating diverse ways of knowing, people will ideally say of action research work, "That is true, that is right, that is interesting, engaging, thought-provoking." And as action researchers, we must ask about how the palette of extended ways of knowing is acknowledged in and by our work.

Inquiry methods may be seen as an outgrowth of epistemology in service to the research question. We must therefore ask why certain methods are chosen, how well they have been pursued, and whether they are indeed congruent with the participative orientation of the action research work. As Hall (2001) points out, participatory research is an attitude, a way of creating knowing in action, possibly even a way of life, not simply a method. So a question for action researchers is whether they have drawn on the different methodological traditions appropriately and creatively in the context of their own work.

Since our work together includes the commingled aspects of reflecting and acting, we must take time to ask questions about the value and worthiness of our work. It is not enough to do good work if the work itself is not of real importance—indeed, we believe it essential that researchers take the risk of asking big questions, even if that turns out to be as simple as stopping with one's colleagues to inquire "Why are we doing this work?" and Why are we doing it this way?" Sometimes it will be obvious what is important—preventing children from being poisoned or an ecology from being damaged; at other times it will be far more complex—for example, in the holistic medical cooperative inquiry (Reason, 1988), participants continually debated the relative significance of power sharing with patients, developing a complementary range of clinical treatments and bringing spiritual disciplines into medical practice, for there was not time to attend to everything.

We may ask as action researchers how our work calls forth a world worthy of human aspiration, so that ideally people will say, "That work is inspiring; it helps make me live a better life."

Our last broad issue concerns thinking through the developmental quality of our work through its history and into the future. Developing self-reflective practice, which, as described later in this chapter, we have called *first-person* research practice (Marshall, 1999, 2001; Torbert, 2001), is a lifetime's project. *Second-person* collaborative inquiry is something that has to be grown over time, moving from a tentative beginning to full cooperation. Participatory action research is emergent and evolutionary: you can't just go to a village or an organization or a professional group and "do it"; the work either evolves or doesn't as a result of mutual engagement and influence. Further, because we are participating in work of enduring consequences, we must attend to the question of viability in the longer term. We must therefore ask whether the ground on which the work proceeded was seeded in such a way that participation is sustained in the absence of the initiating researcher. We must create a living interest in the work.

Action research is a potent orientation to change and transformation. Before intentional change can be fostered, however, it helps to realize, at the individual, group, and community levels, that the reality we have cocreated, however unintentionally, can be repatterned in participative inquiry. In thinking of our institutions as emergent in our activities and therefore continuously changing, we suggest that the human world as we know it is produced and reproduced by the innumerable acts and conversations that we undertake daily. This is not to conflate large systems with aggregates of individual actors acting consciously; we must recognize that systems have their own logic. However, a structurationist view (Bourdieu, 1977; Giddens, 1984) offers a logic from which to commence the work of change by implicitly asserting that systems are not totalizing and that conscious, action-oriented people, especially those working and reasoning together, can indeed achieve systematic and systemic change over time. What seems important in action research, which leaves new institutional patterns in its wake, is its ability to integrate the three manifestations of work: for oneself ("first-person research practice"), work for partners ("second-person research practice"), and work for people within the wider context ("third-person research practice"). The integration of these three approaches to action research suggests a logic of continuous change, which supports the work of radical transformation of patterns of behavior that do not support a world worthy of human aspiration. Ideally, people involved in emerging and enduring work will say, "This work continues to develop and help us," and other people will say, "Can we use your work to help develop our own?" We may say that as action researchers, we must ask questions about how our work has emerged and developed over time, whether it is sustainable into the future, and how it will influence related work.

These five issues, about relationships, practical outcomes, extended ways of knowing, purpose, and enduring consequences, are quite demanding on action researchers. Before paralysis or emotional overload strikes, it is important to remember that action research is emergent and along the way is probably concerned with one broad issue more than another.

We can also say that in a pluralist community of inquiry—whether it be a face-to-face inquiry group, an organization, or a community—different individual members are likely to have different questions and different degrees of interest. Some will be most concerned with relationships, some with action, some with understanding, and some with raising awareness. The more that dialogue is encouraged regarding these different perspectives, the greater the quality of the inquiry will be. We would argue that it is important for the action research team or community of inquiry as a whole to take time regularly for reflection on the choice points encountered along the way and the possible need for reorientation from time to time.

Some action researchers (for example, Heron, 1996b) have argued for the primacy of one issue above all others—in Heron's case, it is to suggest the "primacy of the practical." We take the position that the issues are choice points and that the action researcher is therefore partial as a result of the material circumstances of each given situation.

In summary, the following five sets of questions "broaden the bandwidth" of issues to take into account in exploring the quality of action research.

Quality as Relational Praxis

A fundamental claim to quality in action research practice is that it is participative, fully involving others in the inquiry project. That means that in our research, we must endeavor to meet the others as subjects, equal to ourselves, in what Martin Buber famously called an "I-thou" relationship. In this relational stance, we move away from the "I-it" relationship of traditional science, which asks that a researcher not contaminate the relationship with the research objects by coming in "too close." This is not to say that distance is unimportant, as such distance can help with seeing what is hard to see when too close to a phenomenon. But that distancing is not exercised in the relationship with the co-inquirers. We must therefore generally ask ourselves whether the action research group is set up for (eventual) maximal participation; whether opportunities are used to allow all to feel free to be fully involved; whether when push comes to shove, serious decisions are made on the principle that the best decision is one that maximizes participation; and especially whether less powerful people are helped by their experience of participation in inquiry.

Quality as a Reflexive or Practical Outcome

Action research claims to make a difference in people's lives and practices. We are led to ask whether, in principle, our work has pragmatic consequences. Greenwood and Levin (1998) write of Dewey's "warranted assumptions": Are people with real material issues at stake (jobs, reputations, livelihoods) willing to act on what has been learned in the course of their research? An important question to ask, therefore, is whether the research is "validated" by participants' new ways of acting in light of the work. In the simplest sense, people should be able to say, "That was useful—I am using it!"

Quality as Plurality of Knowing

Here we discuss different forms of knowing in an effort to embrace more than the traditional focus on propositional, theoretical knowledge.

Quality Through Conceptual and Theoretical Integrity. Without theory, practice is impoverished. Action research practitioners are concerned with propositional and conceptual integrity and also that the efforts at theorizing be anchored in people's experience. Theory is used to bring more order to complex phenomena, with a goal of parsimonious description so that it is of use to the community of inquiry. And bringing theory may require iterative cycles of spectatorial distancing of researcher from co-inquirers to theorize and then discuss that theory with those whose experience is its basis. It was Kurt Lewin, in many respects the contemporary era's "father of action research," who said that theory is practical—not that it *should be* practical, merely that it *is* practical! In developing conceptual and theoretical integrity, we may wish to draw on current qualitative and ethnographic practices of making sense of data (Denzin & Lincoln, 2000). We might also ask if our new theory allows us to resee the world, or see past taken-for-granted conceptual categories that are oppressive or no longer helpful.

Quality Through Extending Our Ways of Knowing. Action research respects and works with many epistemologies. We have drawn on Heron's fourfold distinction but also note that the range of ways of knowing can be expressed in more vernacular form. "Ordinary women's talk" can hold an important place in inquiry (Barrett, 2001; Barrett & Taylor, 2002); song and dance are artful ways of expressing and continuing knowledge (Lewis, 2001); traditional forms can bring power to hitherto poorly educated people in that it allows them to successfully question the practices of the powerful. John Heron (1998, 2001) describes the primary outcomes of his spiritual inquiries not as descriptions or theories or pragmatic consequences but as transformations of personal being and associated skills brought about by the inquiry. In this view, practical knowing is the fulfillment and consummation of the knowledge quest.

In seeing that the outcome of inquiry can be a shift in ways of being in the world and in the development of new skills, we are liberated from the tyranny of having to "write up" everything. And in asking about how our work responds to the aesthetic representation issue, we are offered a chance to be creative and to liberate the creative impulses of those we work with. Conversation and paper writing are valuable tools, but the worlds of theater, dance, video, poetry, and photography invite us to be inspired in the service of better theory and practice.

Quality Through Methodological Appropriateness. In action research, the quality of inquiry practice lies far less in impersonal methodology and far more in the emergence of a self-aware, critical community of inquiry nested within a community of practice. However, this doesn't mean that judicious choice of method from the large range available is not important, although method is there to support the community of inquiry rather than to supplant it. If we are animated by a worldview of participation and seek to have congruence between our theory of reality and our practice, then our selected methods must also be relational and be able to describe a relational worldview (Bradbury & Lichtenstein, 2000). They will provide a systematic way of engaging people on issues of importance, drawing on many ways of knowing in an iterative fashion.

Quality as Engaging in Significant Work

We have argued that action research is a form of inquiry in pursuit of worthwhile human purposes, issues of significance.

It can of course be argued that any participative form of inquiry, well grounded in the everyday concerns of people, will necessarily be worthwhile. This is particularly so if it moves beyond addressing simple technically oriented questions toward emancipatory questions—in which case, people's capacity for asking questions of deeper significance is developed. It is arguable that as inquiry groups cycle between action and reflection over time, they move from surface concerns to more fundamental issues. And so we applaud critical attention to these questions. Since the action research community as a whole is committed to bringing an attitude of inquiry toward questions of fundamental importance, we would do well to find ways to address the question of what purposes are worthy of attention more directly.

In our reviews of action research projects, we are struck that while most practitioners are concerned to address questions they believe to have significant worth, few pay *explicit* attention to inquiring into what is worthy of attention, how we chose where to put our efforts. Significant exceptions are the action inquiry of Torbert (1999, 2001); the "appreciative" orientation of Cooperrider and his colleagues (Cooperrider, Sorensen, Whitney, & Yaeger, 2000; Ludema, Cooperrider, & Barrett, 2001); and the community systems approach of Senge (Senge & Scharmer, 2001).

Emergent Inquiry Toward Enduring Consequence

Action research is best seen as an emergent, evolutionary, and educational process of engaging with self, others, and communities that needs to be sustained for a significant period of time. For example, Marja-Liisa Swantz (Swantz, Ndedya, & Masaiganah, 2001) refers to the three decades of participatory research in Tanzania, involving people in their communities, academia, and government; she emphasizes the importance of a longer-term commitment from these different parties. More modestly, many projects continue over several months of developing engagement in which the quality and focus of engagement deepened over time. Action research in all its forms is a long-term, evolutionary, emergent form of inquiry.

As Peter Park (2001) argues, in addition to creating objective knowledge of social conditions, action research also strengthens community ties and heightens transformative potential through critical consciousness. The simultaneous pursuit of these three goals makes action research a holistic activity addressing key human social needs, making it unique among social change activities. Seeing social change as a research activity forces us to think of community ties and critical awareness as forms of knowledge.

We also note that action research practitioners repeatedly criticize institutional structures, especially universities, as being inappropriate vehicles for the kinds of inquiry practices we advocate and that good action research, in a way that truly differentiates it from traditional research, seems to leave repatterned institutional infrastructures in its wake, some of them embryonic but others surprisingly robust over the years.

BROADENING THE BANDWIDTH OF VALIDITY CONCERNS IN RESEARCH AND PRACTICE

No action research project can address all issues equally, and choices must be made about what is important in the emergent and messy work of each action research project. As we have suggested, making explicit the questions of what is important to attend to is itself often part of good action research. This might be done by reviewing the issues and the questions that they raise and deciding where to put the weight of attention. This may be the task of an individual action researcher acting alone; certainly we would expect a PhD thesis based on action research to contain a review of the strengths and weakness of the work in relation to these issues. In contrast, a facilitator of an action research project will wish to share this work with his or her inquiry colleagues; the role here is educative, to explore the issues with them so they can together decide which are most relevant. Of course, in a participative inquiry that has emerged in its fullest sense as research conducted not *on* people but *with* people, responsibility for exploring these issues will rest with the community as a whole.

We believe that it is helpful to address all questions, if only to elucidate why one is more important than another. Thus when next asked how big one's sample was or what to do about the fact that one's data must be considered contaminated by interests or that the co-inquirers were all self-selected, the action research may refer to the differing axiomatic assumptions in action research that arise from a worldview and lived experience of participation. We suggest that the action researcher seek to expand the conversation about validity to include the broader bandwidth of considerations that inhere in research and practice in search of a world worthy of human aspiration.

We have stated that there are five interrelated issues that together call forth seven choice points in action research. Questions of quality and validity in research involve encouraging debate and reflection about these issues among all participants. The following list is intended as a checklist for action researchers starting and continuing to develop a world worthy of human aspiration. These six questions will, we hope, provoke many others as appropriate to the needs and desired outcomes of the action research work undertaken.

Issues as Choice Points and Questions in Action Research

- Is the action research explicit in developing a praxis of relational participation?
- Is it guided by reflexive concern for pragmatic outcomes?
- Does it ensure conceptual and theoretical integrity?
- Does it include extended ways of knowing?
- Can it be considered significant?
- Does it lead toward a new and enduring infrastucture?

References

Argyris, C., & Schön, D. A. (1996). *Organizational learning II.* Reading, MA: Addison-Wesley.

Barrett, P. A. (2001). The Early Mothering project: What happened when the words "action research" came to life for a group of midwives. In P. Reason & H. Bradbury (Eds.), *Handbook of action research: Participative inquiry and practice* (pp. 294–300). Thousand Oaks, CA: Sage.

Barrett, P. A., & Taylor, B. J. (2002). Beyond reflection: Cake and cooperative inquiry. *Systemic Practice and Action Research, 15,* 237–248.

Bateson, G. (2000). Form, substance and difference. In G. Bateson, *Steps to an Ecology of Mind* (pp. 454–471). (Original work published 1972)

Belenky, M., Clinchy, B. M., Goldberger, N., & Tarule, J. (1986). *Women's ways of knowing: The development of self, voice, and mind.* New York: Basic Books.

Berman, M. (1981). *The reenchantment of the world.* Ithaca, NY: Cornell University Press.

Berry, T. (1988). *The dream of the earth.* San Francisco: Sierra Club.

Berry, T. (1999). *The great work: Our way into the future.* New York: Bell Tower.

Bourdieu, P. (1977). *Outline of a theory of practice.* Cambridge: Cambridge University Press.

Bradbury, H., & Lichtenstein, B. M. (2000). The space between: Operationalizing relationality in organizational research. *Organizational Science, 11,* 551–564.

Brown, L. (Ed.). (1999). *State of the world, 1999: A Worldwatch Institute report on progress towards a sustainable society.* London: Earthscan.

Cooperrider, D. L., Sorensen, P. F., Whitney, D., & Yaeger, T. F. (2000). *Appreciative inquiry: Rethinking human organization toward a positive theory of change.* Champaign, IL: Stipes.

Denzin, N. K., & Lincoln, Y. S. (Eds.). (2000). *Handbook of qualitative research* (2nd ed.). Thousand Oaks, CA: Sage.

Eikeland, O. (2001). Action research as the hidden curriculum of the Western tradition. In P. Reason & H. Bradbury (Eds.), *Handbook of action research: Participative inquiry and practice* (pp. 145–155). Thousand Oaks, CA: Sage.

Fals-Borda, O. (1997). Concluding remarks at the Eighth Participatory Action Research World Conference, Cartagena, Colombia.

Gaventa, J., & Cornwall, A. (2001). Power and knowledge. In P. Reason & H. Bradbury (Eds.), *Handbook of action research: Participative inquiry and practice* (pp. 70–80). Thousand Oaks, CA: Sage.

Giddens, A. (1984). *The constitution of society: Outline of the theory of structuration.* Berkeley: University of California Press.

Greenwood, D. J., & Levin, M. (1998). *Introduction to action research: Social research for social change.* Thousand Oaks, CA: Sage.

Gustavsen, B. (1996). Development and the social sciences: An uneasy relationship. In S. Toulmin & B. Gustavsen (Eds.), *Beyond theory: Changing organizations through participation.* Amsterdam: Benjamins.

Gustavsen, B. (2001). Theory and practice: The mediating discourse. In P. Reason & H. Bradbury (Eds.), *Handbook of action research: Participative inquiry and practice* (pp. 17–26). Thousand Oaks, CA: Sage.

Habermas, J. (1979). *Communication and the evolution of society* (T. McCarthy, Trans.). Boston: Beacon Press.

Hall, B. L. (2001). I wish this were a poem of practices of participatory research. In P. Reason & H. Bradbury (Eds.), *Handbook of action research: Participative inquiry and practice* (pp. 171–178). Thousand Oaks, CA: Sage.

Heron, J. (1996a). *Cooperative inquiry: Research into the human condition.* Thousand Oaks, CA: Sage.

Heron, J. (1996b). Quality as primacy of the practical. *Qualitative Inquiry, 2,* 41–56.

Heron, J. (1998). *Sacred science: Person-centred inquiry into the spiritual and the subtle.* Ross-on-Wye, England: PCCS Books.

Heron, J. (2001). Transpersonal cooperative inquiry. In P. Reason & H. Bradbury (Eds.), *Handbook of action research: Participative inquiry and practice* (pp. 333–339). Thousand Oaks, CA: Sage.

Heron, J., & Reason, P. (1997). A participatory inquiry paradigm. *Qualitative Inquiry, 3,* 274–294.

Heron, J., & Reason, P. (2001). The practice of cooperative inquiry: Research *with* rather than *on* people. In P. Reason & H. Bradbury (Eds.), *Handbook of action research: Participative inquiry and practice* (pp. 179–188). Thousand Oaks, CA: Sage.

Kemmis, S. (2001). Exploring the relevance of critical theory for action research: Emancipatory action research in the footsteps of Jürgen Habermas. In P. Reason & H. Bradbury (Eds.), *Handbook of action research: Participative inquiry and practice* (pp. 91–102). Thousand Oaks, CA: Sage.

Kvale, S. (1989). To validate is to question. In S. Kvale (Ed.), *Issues of validity in qualitative research* (pp. 73–92). Stockholm, Sweden: Studentliteratur.

Lather, P. A. (1993). Fertile obsession: Validity after poststructuralism. *Sociological Quarterly, 34,* 673–693.

Lather, P. A. (1997). Validity as an incitement to discourse: Qualitative research and the crisis of legitimation. In V. Richardson (Ed.), *Handbook of research on teaching* (4th ed.). Washington, DC: American Education Research Association.

Lewis, H. M. (2001). Participatory research and education for social change: Highlander Research and Education Center. In P. Reason & H. Bradbury (Eds.), *Handbook of action research: Participative inquiry and practice* (pp. 356–362). Thousand Oaks, CA: Sage.

Lincoln, Y. S. (1995). Emerging criteria for quality in qualitative and interpretive research. *Qualitative Inquiry, 1,* 275–289.

Ludema, J. D., Cooperrider, D. L., & Barrett, F. J. (2001). Appreciative inquiry: The power of the unconditional positive question. In P. Reason & H. Bradbury (Eds.), *Handbook of action research: Participative inquiry and practice* (pp. 189–199). Thousand Oaks, CA: Sage.

Lyotard, J.-F. (1984). *The postmodern condition: A report on knowledge* (J. Bennington & B. Massumi, Trans.). Minneapolis: University of Minnesota Press.

Marshall, J. (1999). Living life as inquiry. *Systematic Practice and Action Research, 12,* 155–171.

Marshall, J. (2001). Self-reflective inquiry practices. In P. Reason & H. Bradbury (Eds.), *Handbook of action research: Participative inquiry and practice* (pp. 433–439). Thousand Oaks, CA: Sage.

Park, P. (2001). Knowledge and participatory research. In P. Reason & H. Bradbury (Eds.), *Handbook of action research: Participative inquiry and practice* (pp. 81–90). Thousand Oaks, CA: Sage.

Putnam, H. (1992). *Renewing philosophy.* Cambridge, MA: Harvard University Press.

Reason, P. (1988). Whole person medical practice. In P. Reason (Ed.), *Human inquiry in action* (pp. 102–126). Thousand Oaks, CA: Sage.

Reason, P., & Goodwin, B. C. (1999). Toward a science of qualities in organizations: Lessons from complexity theory and postmodern biology. *Concepts and Transformations, 4,* 281–317.

Reason, P., & Torbert, W. R. (2001). Toward a Participatory Worldview (Pt. 2). *ReVision, 24*(2), 1–48.

Rorty, R. (2000). *Philosophy and social hope.* New York: Penguin.

Schwandt, T. A. (1996). Farewell to criteriology. *Qualitative Inquiry, 2,* 58–72.

Senge, S., & Scharmer, O. (2001). Community action research: Learning as a community of practitioners, consultants, and researchers. In In P. Reason & H. Bradbury (Eds.), *Handbook of action research: Participatory inquiry and practice* (pp. 238–249). Thousand Oaks, CA: Sage.

Skolimowski, H. (1993). *A sacred place to dwell.* Rockport, MA: Element.

Skolimowski, H. (1994). *The participatory mind.* London: Arkana.

Swantz, M.-L., Ndedya, E., & Masaiganah, M. S. (2001). Participatory action research in southern Tanzania, with special reference to women. In P. Reason & H. Bradbury (Eds.), *Handbook of action research: Participatory inquiry and practice* (pp. 386–395). Thousand Oaks, CA: Sage.

Torbert, W. R. (1991). *The power of balance: Transforming self, society, and scientific inquiry.* Newbury Park, CA: Sage.

Torbert, W. R. (1999). The distinctive questions developmental action inquiry asks. *Management Learning, 30,* 189–206.

Torbert, W. R. (2001). The practice of action inquiry. In P. Reason & H. Bradbury (Eds.), *Handbook of action research: Participative inquiry and practice* (pp. 250–260). Thousand Oaks, CA: Sage.

Torbert, W. R., & Reason, P. (2001). Toward a Participatory Worldview (Pt. 1). *ReVision, 24*(1), 1–48.

Toulmin, S. (1990). *Cosmopolis: The hidden agenda of modernity.* New York: Free Press.

Wolcott, H. (1990). On seeking—and rejecting—validity in qualitative research. In E. Eisner & A. Peshkin (Eds.), *Qualitative inquiry in education: The continuing debate* (pp. 121–152). New York: Teachers College Press.

CHAPTER ELEVEN

Methodological and Ethical Considerations in Community-Driven Environmental Justice Research

Two Case Studies from Rural North Carolina

Stephanie Ann Farquhar
Steve Wing

Inequalities in health between gender, race, and class groups are generated by social institutions that create disparities in exposure to adequate nutrition, hazardous agents, safe living and working conditions, educational opportunities, and personal medical services. Because governments and corporations cannot be expected to eliminate these disparities without pressure from those who are adversely affected, environmental justice is not only about harmful agents and access to basic services; it is also about the rights of all people to participate as equal partners in policy and decision making, regardless of class, race, ethnicity, or national origin (Kuehn, 1996; Environmental Protection Agency, 1998). However, participation in democracy requires access to knowledge, including research, and most environmental health research has been conducted to investigate problems identified by governments, industries, health professionals, and the scientific community. In contrast, communities that are most exposed to environmental hazards, especially low-income communities and communities of color, seldom have access to environmental researchers and have been underrepresented in the public health research professions (Lynn, 2000; St. George, Schoenbach, Reynolds, Nwangwu, & Adams-Campbell, 1997).

Note: Portions of this chapter have been adapted from "Social Responsibility and Research Ethics in Community-Driven Studies of Industrialized Hog Production," by Steve Wing, in *Environmental Health Perspectives, 110,* 437–444. Copyright © 2000.

Recently, some environmental health research has united communities and researchers to challenge some of the basic assumptions of traditional research. Environmental studies informed by community based principles of research can arise from mutually beneficial partnerships that define and address the environmental health problem (Lynn, 2000; Israel, Schulz, Parker, & Becker, 1998). The actual application of the methods and principles of community based participatory research (CBPR), as well as the definition of *community participation,* can vary among different researchers and public health disciplines (Israel et al., 1998). CBPR projects also differ in terms of the roles of researchers and community residents (see Chapters Five and Six), the goals and "products" of the research, the research methodology and data sources, and the targets of change (for example, pollution prevention and cleanup versus screening and self-protection).

Faber and McCarthy (2000) argue that researchers need to make visible the connections between environmental inequity, economic inequality, racism, and the lack of democracy. Research has the greatest potential to contribute to improved conditions for exposed populations when it is driven by community needs. Collaborative studies at the Love Canal, New York, and in Woburn, Massachusetts, are examples of community-academic partnerships that raised awareness and helped contribute to changes in environmental public policy (Brown & Mikkelsen, 1990; Levine, 1982; Shepard, 2000).

However, it can be difficult for community members to become involved in the research process, especially where there is a history of disempowerment and the necessity of expending most available time and energy on work and basic needs. Involvement in efforts that challenge the status quo can inflict an emotional burden and fear for jobs, especially when local employers and politicians are the focus of the research. Participating in the research process can leave community partners feeling vulnerable, exposed, and open to criticism from neighbors and family members who do not support their efforts. Despite these challenges, it is important to consider the central and valuable role of community members in defining the research questions, informing data collection protocols, influencing the application of study results, and creating change (Cornwall & Jewkes, 1995; Gaventa, 1993).

This chapter explores these and other issues of CBPR through an examination of two community based participatory public health projects initiated by residents of rural eastern North Carolina. Both projects provide examples of the collective efforts of community-academic partnerships that were organized to challenge environmental, social, and health disparities. The case studies involved different community members and researchers and used varying research methods, yet they faced similar obstacles and methodological dilemmas. Both depended on a history of effective community organizing and the existence of powerful community assets. The chapter concludes with a discussion of the similarities and differences of the projects, highlighting some of the universal challenges that many CBPR projects must address.

A SNAPSHOT OF EASTERN NORTH CAROLINA

The eastern region of North Carolina is located in the "Black Belt," where most of the nation's rural African Americans reside, with approximately one out of four residents living in poverty and 44 percent not served by a public sewer system (Eastern North Carolina Housing Summit, 1999). This area has been heavily affected by poverty, discrimination, and joblessness. With the rise of industrialized agriculture and the decline of independent family farmers, jobs in agriculture have declined dramatically and been replaced by low-paying factory jobs. These factories are notorious for unfair labor policies and antiunion sentiments (Le Duff, 1999). At the same time, land ownership, a significant building block for economically and socially stable African-American communities, is diminishing due in part to the growth of large agribusinesses (Edwards & Ladd, 2000) and discrimination in USDA loan programs. As a result of this lack of desirable jobs, there has been a sizable out-migration of working-age adults, leaving behind a large senior population.

In the face of these challenges, eastern rural North Carolina has for several decades successfully initiated local self-improvement efforts, including a farmers' cooperative, the region's first NAACP chapter, free health care clinics, and a nationally recognized pro-labor union association (Minkler, 2000). The two case studies presented in this chapter describe the process and results that occurred when these community building blocks partnered with researchers from a public university to define and address community issues.

CASE STUDY 1: COMMUNITY-DRIVEN STUDIES OF INDUSTRIALIZED HOG PRODUCTION

This case study was first recounted in Wing (2002).

Demographic Analysis of Disproportionate Exposure

Between the mid-1980s and the late 1990s, as the hog population of North Carolina expanded from under three million to approximately ten million, the number of operations decreased as smaller independent family farmers were replaced by industrial-style operations (Furuseth, 1997). Expansion of industrial operations occurred under regulatory controls that were influenced by hog producers and other agribusiness interests in the North Carolina general assembly. State legislation was enacted to prevent local and county governments from rezoning agricultural land, and state universities closely allied with agribusiness concerns provided research support (Cecelski & Kerr, 1992).

As rural residents learned about industrialized hog production, many became deeply concerned about the impact of the industry on their communities. They worried about air pollution and noxious odors associated with confinement of thousands of hogs and liquid waste management systems that included open fecal waste pits and spray fields. Noxious odors prevented some hog operation neighbors from enjoying their homes and the outdoors. Since odorant chemicals can penetrate clothing, curtains, and upholstery, they can affect people long after plumes of emissions pass and may subject them to ostracism at school or in public. Hog operation neighbors, most of whom depend on groundwater, feared that their wells could be contaminated in an area with sandy soils and high water tables and that surface water pollution from spray field runoff and lagoon failures would contaminate creeks and rivers. They were concerned about loss of independent family farmers and the land that they had farmed, as well as about the vitality of their churches, schools, and communities. Residents also felt that they had been targeted for this kind of "economic development" because their primarily African American, low-income communities lacked political power (Wing, 2002; Wing, Grant, Green, & Stewart, 1996).

The Concerned Citizens of Tillery (CCT), a grassroots organization in southeastern Halifax County in eastern North Carolina, worked with county officials to develop an intensive livestock ordinance that would impose stricter environmental controls than state regulations. In that effort, and in the course of providing assistance to other communities in the path of corporate pork production, CCT sought support from environmentalists, social activists, and researchers who could help document economic, social, environmental, and public health issues affecting communities living near industrialized hog operations. Although university scientists had conducted many studies related to agricultural technologies, veterinary health, and the health of agricultural workers, relatively little research had addressed environmental, social, and health concerns of communities affected by industrial hog production. One of the studies that had been conducted suggested that hog odors affect the mental health of nearby residents (Schiffman, Miller, Suggs, & Graham, 1995). Another suggested that neighbors experience respiratory effects similar to those seen among workers (Thu et al., 1997). Consistent with the latter findings, mothers in eastern North Carolina reported that their asthmatic children experienced episodes of wheezing in the presence of strong plumes from nearby hog operations.

In 1996, a partnership formed by CCT with the Halifax County Health Department and the University of North Carolina (UNC) School of Public Health received funding from the National Institute of Environmental Health Sciences (NIEHS) Environmental Justice: Partnerships for Communication program

(Thu et al., 1997). Along with environmental justice education and outreach to communities and medical providers, the partnership was funded to conduct research that could quantify systematically, using official records, the extent to which hog operations were located disproportionately in low-income areas and communities of color (primarily African American) in North Carolina. Aims of the project were to evaluate data for local communities, to consider possible alternative explanations for observed patterns, and to examine data on household water sources and potential groundwater contamination. The partnership, originally known as Southeast Halifax Environmental Reawakening, was later renamed Community Health and Environmental Reawakening (CHER) to reflect its statewide work (Wing, 2002).

In 1998, the CHER partnership obtained a list of all industrial livestock operations permitted by the North Carolina Division of Water Quality. Following intensive efforts to evaluate errors in these data and make corrections, the epidemiologist members linked information on the locations and sizes of industrial hog operations to data for U.S. Census Bureau block groups, areas that average about five hundred households. They compared the prevalence of operations in whiter and wealthier communities with the prevalence in poorer and more nonwhite areas. Because rural areas are often poor and nonwhite, and agricultural operations by definition take place in rural areas, the investigators recognized that findings of disparate impact might be dismissed by industry and government as merely reflecting the demographics of rural areas. They therefore developed a statistical model to adjust for population density in their comparisons of areas with different racial and income characteristics (Wing, Cole, & Grant, 2000).

Although the data analysis was undertaken at the university, the study questions originated in the exposed communities. Community members participated in evaluating data quality through their knowledge of local hog operations. Decisions about how to define the study population and data sources, choose and define variables for the analysis, and interpret results were made in consultation with community partners; researchers and community members become both teachers and learners (Israel, Checkoway, Schulz, & Zimmerman, 1994). The university based researchers augmented their statistical analyses with maps and charts. They found that hog operations were far more common in low-income communities and communities of color, that this concentration was more extreme for hog operations owned or operated by large corporations than for independent operations, and that the pattern was only partly explained by differences in population density. Furthermore, they found that hog operations were concentrated in areas where most people depend on household wells for drinking water (Wing et al., 2000).

University and community partners issued a press release about the research findings in conjunction with their presentation at a national meeting. The release was coordinated with the UNC News Service, which routinely prepares stories about topical research, and several major state newspapers ran stories on the findings, some including interviews with community members. The CHER partnership was invited to present the findings before the North Carolina general assembly's agriculture committee, and the study was considered in a policy paper on the future of the hog industry prepared by the governor's office.

Inclusion of Community in the Quantification of Health Effects

In addition to the environmental justice study, the CHER partnership conducted more traditional health effects research. In the fall of 1998, with support from the North Carolina State Health Department, the partnership initiated a survey of rural residents in eastern North Carolina. Reports of odor problems and respiratory effects had been coming in from hog operation neighbors across eastern North Carolina, and the health department was interested in obtaining more information. In consultation with community members and staff from the health department, the CHER partnership designed a survey to compare health and quality of life of residents of three communities, one in the neighborhood of a hog operation, one in the neighborhood of a cattle operation, and a third with no intensive livestock production.

There were a number of challenges in designing the study. The earlier environmental justice analyses had confirmed the observations made by community members that industrial hog operations are disproportionately located in low-income and African American communities. Members of the research partnership would need to ask for the participation of people whose previous experiences of discrimination led them to distrust health departments, medical providers, universities, and researchers. Strong relationships with community based organizations established through the CHER partnership would be essential for collecting reliable data and establishing a high response rate in defined populations in the three areas. At the same time, the research partnership knew the potential biases that could be introduced by community participation in areas divided between those with negative feelings about the hog industry and those whose livelihood depended on the industry. To collect valid data, they would need to insulate the data collection process from peer pressure or leading questioning. As in all environmental epidemiology, the power of the study to detect any real effects would be weakened by lack of good measurements of exposures and outcomes. Members of the partnership debated whether it would be ethical to conduct a study if they could not measure exposures and outcomes sufficiently well to detect a health effect if one existed, recognizing that the study design would be constrained by funding that could be provided by the state health department. The decision to proceed was influenced by evidence from previous studies and by community members and state officials who felt there was an urgent need for respiratory health data from North Carolina (Wing, 2002).

Health Survey Design and Administration

CHER partners developed a structured symptom questionnaire based on previous studies and input from eastern North Carolina residents who helped develop a culturally appropriate survey instrument. The study used the same questions in each of the three communities; there were no questions about odor, hogs, or livestock because one community had no livestock. Three communities were chosen with similar demographic characteristics according to census data. In each community, occupied dwellings were enumerated on a map and assigned a random identifying number (Wing & Wolf, 2000).

The partnership collaborated with a community based organization in each area. Community members helped researchers locate roads and houses, and they served as community consultants during the data collection. Trained interviewers from UNC visited households in each area accompanied by a community consultant who made the initial introduction of the interviewer. Interviews were conducted without the presence of the community consultant unless the participant requested that the consultant remain. The interviewer read aloud, and provided the study participant with a copy of, an "agreement to participate" that explained that the study was about environmental exposures and the health of rural residents. Participants were assured that their responses would be kept confidential and that their name would not be written on the questionnaire, although a link would be maintained between their address and their responses. UNC's Institutional Review Board gave permission to obtain oral consent since there were no interventions or sensitive questions.

Households nearest to the livestock operations were visited first. The interviewing teams then visited households in order, moving away from the livestock operations until the target sample size of fifty was reached. One adult in each household was interviewed in January and February 1999. Over 150 interviews were completed, with a refusal rate of just 14 percent. Respondents were 92 percent African American, 65 percent female, and 27 percent aged sixty-five or over (Wing & Wolf, 2000).

In keeping with a core principle of CBPR—returning research findings to the community (Cornwall & Jewkes, 1995; Gaventa, 1993; see also Chapter Three), the CHER team invited members of the three community based organizations to a meeting to discuss initial findings of the research prior to submitting the report to the state health department. Input from community members was obtained, and the university partners responded to community members' concerns about excesses of respiratory and digestive symptoms that had been reported by hog operation neighbors compared to residents of the other communities. Community members decided at this meeting that they did not want the names of their communities to be included in the report. Respecting and responding to this feedback, data on numbers of households, population size, race, and income characteristics of the census block groups in the study were removed from the report, along with information about the exact size of the hog and cattle operations.

State Reaction to Survey Results

A draft report was submitted to the state health department, presenting analyses that showed that the frequency of miscellaneous symptoms such as muscle aches and vision and hearing problems was similar in the three communities. In contrast, residents near the hog operations reported increased numbers of headaches, runny nose, sore throat, excessive coughing, diarrhea, and burning eyes. Residents also reported many more occasions when they could not open windows or go outside even in nice weather. The report was reviewed by health department staff, the chief statistician for the State Center for Health Statistics, the chair of the UNC Department of Epidemiology, and others, and the final report incorporated their comments.

The state health department issued a press statement releasing the study's report to the public on May 7, 1999. Later that day, attorneys for the North Carolina Pork Council wrote to the university members of the research partnership, demanding that they "make available for copying by this office any and all documentation in your possession (or that you are aware of in the possession of other State agencies or State personnel) that contain, represent, record, document, discuss, or otherwise reflect or memorialize the results of the Study."

The Pork Council request raised a number of ethical concerns, including the protection of the confidentiality of participants. In order to evaluate the quality, internal consistency, and analytical methods in the study, the industry would need to be able to conduct an independent reanalysis. However, although participants' names were not recorded, maps of the locations of their homes were linked to their responses. Even without the maps, information about participants, including age, race, sex, occupation, industry, number in household, water source, and responses to questions about health status, was sufficient to deductively disclose which individuals were in the study in these sparsely populated rural communities.

Breach of confidentiality was not only a concern from a legal and ethical standpoint. The community trust on which the CHER partnership depended would be seriously compromised, potentially destroying valued professional and personal relationships and threatening the continuation of research into exposures and health of neighbors of industrial swine operations. The need for protection of confidentiality would have to be considered in relation to a scientific culture in which reanalysis is essential and in relation to power inequalities between industry and the exposed communities.

The state's public records statute required release of the research documents, which were the property of the university, not the researchers who conducted the study. After much consultation and legal deliberation, the university and CHER researchers released records to the Pork Council, including computerized files of individual responses, interviewer training instructions, draft copies of the report, other statistical tabulations, and study-related correspondence, including electronic mail messages of project staff. To protect confidentiality of the participants and the communities, however, information that could lead to disclosure of where the study was done, including maps, driving instructions, phone records, travel records, and names of persons that would identify locations in the study, were withheld from the Pork Council. This was done under the assumption that individuals could not be identified from information in the survey unless the locations of the survey were known (Wing, 2002).

In the years since the Pork Council took legal action to acquire analytical data sets, CHER investigators have not learned of any published refutations or reanalyses of the health survey data. During the same time period, community members and researchers have used the study to help draw attention to public health concerns associated with industrial hog production. Results of the health survey have been considered by health departments, the Environmental Protection Agency's National Environmental Justice Advisory Council, and the U.S. Department of Agriculture and have supported applications for funding of additional research on environmental exposures from industrial hog operations as well as their biological effects.

The role of community members in defining the research questions and informing data collection and application is a vital component of CBPR. However, as illustrated in this case study, ethical, legal, and personal dilemmas may arise for both the researchers and the community members engaged in community-academic research partnerships.

CASE STUDY 2: "BLACKS STAYED ON THE FLOORS, WHITES STAYED IN HOPE HOUSE PLANTATION": DISCRIMINATION IN DISASTER RELIEF

This environmental and social justice study involves ethical and methodological challenges similar to those in Case Study 1.

The Effects of Hurricane Floyd: Intensified Community Challenges

On September 16, 1999, Hurricane Floyd hit rural eastern North Carolina. In its destructive path it left 7,000 homes destroyed, 17,000 uninhabitable, and more than 47,000 residents in public shelters (Segrest, 1999). This area of North Carolina, suffering from racial discrimination, poverty, unemployment, and inadequate housing (Segrest, 1999), is also highly segregated, with the communities most affected by Floyd and ensuing floodwaters being predominantly African American. The historic town of Princeville, for example, one of the most heavily damaged communities, is the oldest incorporated all-black town in the country and was founded by former slaves after the Civil War.

The flooding forced thousands of rural eastern North Carolina residents out of their homes and into temporary housing sites located in several counties. These sites, consisting largely of trailers and mobile homes, were established and continue to be maintained by the Federal Emergency Management Agency (FEMA) and state and local government agencies and organizations. Despite the initial response and assistance from citizens and charitable organizations, the long-term recovery efforts carried out by local, state, and federal governments were inadequate. Two years after the flooding, more than one thousand citizens were still without permanent housing. Nearly all of these displaced citizens were African American residents who had been turned down for financial assistance, had received misinformation about opportunities for recovery aid, and had been unable to secure affordable and decent housing due to a dearth of rental units (Lindenfeld, 2001). Survivors were largely excluded from influencing local and state decisions regarding community recovery efforts and the allocation of recovery funds, intensifying their feelings of vulnerability, discrimination, and disempowerment.

In an effort to help create conditions in which the survivors of Hurricane Floyd could be empowered and to help unify the survivors in the struggle for social and environmental equity, a coalition of local organizations was formed. The Workers and Community Relief and Aid Project (RAP) was comprised of flood survivors and partners from member organizations, including Black Workers for Justice (BWFJ), North Carolina Fair Share, North Carolina Low Income Housing, Concerned Citizens of Tillery, and the North Carolina Student Rural Health Coalition. From its inception, RAP conducted meetings at the temporary housing sites and encouraged survivors to contribute to the development and implementation of RAP's mandate and action plan. Although the process of mobilizing the survivors and partner organizations was not without its challenges, the usually slow and laborious process of developing a partnership of multiple individuals and organizations was accelerated. RAP was focused on the survivors' immediate and urgent recovery needs—such as threatened health and substandard housing—which demanded swift organizing and decision making. As noted earlier, the process of issue selection provides an opportunity for the participatory action research team to reflect and make decisions as a group. Throughout the process, the partnership attempted to balance the more immediate concerns (for example, pushing back FEMA deadlines) with the more fundamental issues of discrimination and inequity.

RAP benefited from the long history of successful community-academic partnerships formed through CHER. Because of CHER, a new public health researcher, Stephanie Ann Farquhar, from the University of North Carolina, was relatively quickly embraced by RAP. As discussed in earlier chapters, all CBPR projects must establish trust and address any past injustices between university and community to create successful partnerships. The extensive history of community organizing in eastern North Carolina helped RAP member organizations to bring together disparate groups, including university researchers, to address a common goal of disaster recovery in the context of larger struggles for social justice.

RAP collaborated with university researchers on two projects. One uncovered state records showing that hundreds of African American flood survivors had been relocated, without their knowledge, on an industrial coal ash landfill. The second documented experiences and needs of hundreds of survivors, highlighting cases of discrimination by local and state agency representatives. Both projects were initiated on the basis of input from the flood survivors. These projects followed the fundamental CBPR principle of "starting where the people are" (Nyswander, 1967), ensuring greater participation, project success, and sustainability of the partnership.

Unearthing State Landfill Data

In March 2000, Saladin Muhammad, a member of RAP and BWFJ, spoke on the topic "environmental injustice and the 1999 floods in North Carolina" in a new environmental justice class initiated by students at the UNC School of Public Health (Wing, 2000). He described a broad range of problems of disaster response in an area with a history of racial discrimination and economic underdevelopment, including deplorable environmental conditions and dehumanizing treatment at Fountain Industrial Park, a temporary housing site in Edgecombe County established by local, state, and federal officials. At the time, the Fountain site, nicknamed "Camp Depression," included 207 travel trailers and 64 mobile homes inhabited largely by residents of Princeville. Muhammad reported that residents and other community members were concerned that the temporary housing facility had been constructed on top of a landfill. Sooty material was evident around some of the trailers and mobile homes, and large mounds of material, some covered with grass and others looking like fresh ash, were near a playground and a pond where some residents fished.

A student in the class took on the task of finding documentation on the history of the site and its potential risks. Despite his access to telephones, libraries, the Internet, and other university resources that were not available to Camp Depression residents, this student had difficulty obtaining information from county and state officials. After initially being denied copies of public documents by the North Carolina Division of Emergency Management (in violation of the same State Public Records Act invoked by the North Carolina Pork Council in Case Study 1), he obtained site records and reports with the assistance of UNC faculty and state officials. These documents confirmed that the flood survivors had been relocated on an industrial coal ash landfill that had been in use up to the day of the hurricane and had not been tested or closed according to EPA standards required for coal ash to be used as fill material for housing. The student summarized published information on health hazards present in coal ash, including arsenic, chromium 6, lead, mercury, cadmium, barium, and thallium. Following presentation of his findings at Camp Depression, RAP held a press conference that was covered by local media, the North Carolina State Health Department arranged for soil testing and coverage of exposed coal ash with a layer of soil, and the pace of finding alternative housing for site residents was accelerated.

This was a mixed victory. Even though environmental sample results indicated that contaminants were not above actionable levels, officials had clearly failed to inform survivors about the landfill prior to relocation, denying survivors the "human right to make a conscious decision about placing their lives in another potentially dangerous situation" ("Environmental Racism," 2000). Yet despite the fact that residents were all African American, state officials denied that any issue of environmental racism was involved. Finally, the new site where many residents were offered housing presented other hazards: it was an area that had flooded badly in the rains following Hurricane Floyd, and the only entrance crossed railroad tracks with no crossing protections.

Although the victory was a partial one, however, it was very important, and achieving it clearly required the collaboration and shared resources of the community and the university. The university partners had contacts in state government and were knowledgeable about the public records statute and citizens' rights to view government documents. More important, and unlike recipients of agency assistance, university partners did not have to be concerned that their research would jeopardize their own financial or housing aid. Equally critical, however, the survivors and members of local organizations possessed important historical knowledge of the area, were familiar with local key players, and provided poignant accounts of the offensive and potentially harmful dust and odors. Working in partnership, the coalition successfully collected and applied the data necessary to raise awareness and demand action.

Combining Strengths to Document Discrimination and Need

One year after Hurricane Floyd, many flood survivors were still without permanent housing and unhappy with the flood recovery process. Through CHER, RAP organizations enlisted the help of Farquhar, who began attending bimonthly RAP meetings convened at a temporary housing site. During the meetings, survivors voiced their concerns and shared individual stories of discriminatory treatment by local and state-level government agencies, unmet needs, and great frustration with the recovery process to date. At the next several meetings, RAP members and their university partner discussed and reached consensus on the benefits of collecting and releasing survey data and survey objectives. Their shared goals were (1) to systematically document the survivors' experiences of relocation, living conditions, and potential threats to health and loss of community as a result of the flooding; (2) to begin to mobilize the survivors for action; and (3) to give the survivors a voice. The group also reached agreement on the content of and intended audience for a final report that would be released at a flood survivor summit.

A few participating community members, however, expressed some concern about their involvement with RAP. Some survivors worried that their financial or medical benefits might be reduced or discontinued by agencies whose recovery efforts were identified as substandard. Others were concerned about being labeled a "mole" by fellow survivors who were suspicious of their involvement with RAP's community organizations and its university partner. RAP was largely successful in assuring flood survivors that their affiliation with RAP would not threaten their benefits, as they would not be identified in the report or in RAP's organizational records. Further, since RAP was composed largely of local grassroots organizations and was established on the basis of survivors' expressed needs for organization and representation, few survivors perceived RAP as a threatening or exclusive organization. This accurate perception of RAP as "for the survivors and of the survivors" reduced concerns that affiliation would lead to ostracism by others.

RAP committed several meetings to specifically focus on the primary objectives of the flood survivor survey report. During these meetings, flood survivors struggled with research concepts such as statistics, scientific validity, confidentiality, and the methods of data analysis. The university partner shared knowledge and skills through discussion, interviewer training, and sharing examples of past research projects. Similarly, community members shared information about social norms, vernacular (such as use of the term "FEMAvilles" in reference to a temporary housing site set up in the aftermath of Hurricane Floyd), and past experiences with researchers and health agencies that was especially useful when thinking through the details of survey instruments and protocol. Valuing and using community expertise early in the project clearly contributed to a more successful partnership (Northridge et al., 2000; see also Chapter Six).

Yet attending to community issues and concerns can slow any process (Green & Mercer, 2001), and all members of the research team must have the patience to enable needed dialogue about areas of conflict. There were several instances, for example, in which the university partner and other members of RAP strongly disagreed with regard to survey design and administration. For example, some community members were reluctant to ask interviewers to read the informed consent paragraphs and to require interviewers to read questions exactly as written. Some RAP members considered these procedures too formal and "scientific" and felt that they distracted from the community orientation of the survey. During numerous discussions, the university partner talked about the need to be prepared to defend the data from those who would question its scientific validity. In each of these instances, the challenge for the researcher was to work with community members to frame questions and design procedures to produce answers that respect community concerns while at the same time investigating them with the best technical approaches possible. Results of these investigations would be useful to communities burdened by environmental problems because they can address topics that could not be investigated without the technical resources of institutions and because the findings can be used in situations where community observations are not highly valued. Rather than facing a conflict between standard procedures and alternatives that are acceptable to the community but viewed as "unscientific" by scientists, both researchers and community members benefit from negotiating the use of rigorous methods. A healthy partnership should encourage discussion of concerns and alternative points of view (Northridge et al., 2000). Furthermore, as discussed in Chapter Three, the processes and products of CBPR develop through the mutual engagement and influence of all members (academics, community, health department, service agencies) of a partnership. Such collaborative and engaged efforts are more likely to contribute to the sustained viability of an empowered and capable community than traditional research approaches (Israel et al., 1998).

Description of Survey Design and Administration

Flood survivors and members of RAP visited temporary housing sites to describe the purpose of the survey and ask survivors for their ideas concerning questions to include in the survey. Survey items generated during this process were categorized under the following general headings: flooding experience, housing situation, health status, children's well-being, finances and employment, environmental threats, interactions with agencies, and hopes for the future. For example, questions asked, "Has the flood affected your children's health?" and "Do you think community citizens should participate in decision making during an emergency situation such as this?" RAP's university partner formatted the survey based on general category themes and the survivors' language. Only a few survey items had to be reworded, as they were either leading or double-barreled. For example, one item was originally worded, "Are you unhappy living here and would you move to a house permanently?" Following dialogue about the importance of asking only one question per survey item, the question was reworded, "Would you like to move into permanent housing?" Members of

RAP reviewed the revised survey, and after minor modifications, the instrument was approved. A draft of the survey and a description of the survey protocol were submitted to and approved by the university's Institutional Review Board (IRB). The IRB process presented an ideal opportunity for helping community members and survivors better understand the research process and for again emphasizing the importance of confidentiality, informed consent, and voluntary participation.

Several RAP partners agreed to serve on a survey subcommittee that was responsible for designing and conducting the survey interviewer training. Two survivors from each site were invited to participate in all-day interviewer training. The training included a module that described survey methodology and issues of data reliability and validity. In an effort to increase the proportion of completed surveys, the trained interviewers surveyed survivors residing at their own sites, where they were familiar with the survivors and their daily schedules.

Despite such training, however, some obstacles to data collection remained. One of the challenging aspects of participatory research, for example, is the difficulty in tracking attempted versus completed interviews. The survey interviewers did not consistently record refusals, not-at-homes, passive refusals, and so on, making it difficult to calculate an overall response rate.

Survey data collection lasted approximately three weeks, during which 270 surveys were completed from ten temporary housing sites located in six different counties. The partnership determined that RAP's university partner would analyze the data, as she had the time and experience to conduct a quick turnaround and produce a summary report. Survey items had required that the respondent answer "yes" or "no," after which the interviewer invited the survivor to elaborate using his or her own words. This format required both qualitative and quantitative methods of analysis, allowing data to be presented as both words and numbers (Denzin & Lincoln, 1994). Early in the survey meetings, RAP partners recognized that different audiences respond to different forms of information delivery. For example, the media and emergency service representatives may be more affected by the survivors' words, while those who are writing policy may require numbers and percentages. Furthermore, the use of multiple methods can also increase the validity of the study's conclusions and the range of information collected (Cook & Reichardt, 1979; Steckler, McLeroy, Goodman, Bird, & McCormick, 1992).

Survey results were tested for validity through a series of member checks (Patton, 1990), during which survey data were summarized and shared with more than seventy survivors. As noted earlier, bringing the data back to the community is an important step in the CBPR process and one that encourages community ownership and control of the data. Although the overall feedback was positive, a few flood survivors expressed that they felt "lumped together" with all the other survivors and that this process of data summary ignored individual experiences. A final survey report and subsequent presentations were modified to acknowledge that the flood survivors are not a homogeneous group but rather many unique individuals. The next section presents some of the findings included in the survey report.

Preliminary Survey Results

Immediately after the flooding, many of the survivors were forced to seek shelter in motels, with relatives, and in local schools. Survivors who spent anywhere from one day to several weeks in a shelter were dissatisfied with the accommodations, describing them as "overcrowded," "hectic," and lacking privacy. Some survivors felt that the first cases of discriminatory relief and aid occurred at the shelters. As one survivor reported, "My family stayed [in the shelter] for three days. Blacks stayed at school on floors and blankets that they brought in the carts. Whites stayed in Hope House Plantation, a historical site."

Survey results indicated that almost 50 percent ($n = 119$) of the survivors were unable to find affordable housing in their communities or neighborhoods and that 110 survivors were turned down for housing loans or rentals because of poor credit histories or low income. Many survivors described the costs of housing and rentals as a major barrier to finding permanent housing, noting that "since the flood, all the realtors and landlords have been allowed to raise their rent" and "I don't make enough to afford these high-price apartments." Survivors also reported that there were multiple structural and administrative barriers to finding housing, such as complicated paperwork and restrictive eligibility criteria.

After the flooding, over one-third ($n = 96$) of the survivors reported that their health declined. Health problems associated with stress and living conditions included a decrease in appetite, depression, crying spells, loss of sleep, nightmares, worry, panic attacks, arthritis, chest pains, headaches, and stomachaches. Many survivors reported suffering from serious respiratory, sinus, and breathing problems related to exposure to mold, mildew, and wetness.

Eighty-six of the survivors reported that the flooding damaged their community's church or school. "Both the church and the school [were destroyed]. The church is being rebuilt. The school is operating. It's torn apart our neighbors." The collapse of pivotal community structures, such as school and church, is devastating beyond the physical and structural level. As Eng (1993) has noted, for example, the church is a unit of identity, affirmation, and solution in African American communities, so the loss of a church structure may consequently be experienced on several levels. The loss of meeting places and familiar sites can similarly result in a loss of personal identity, as well as a decreased sense of community cohesion (Chavis & Wandersman, 1990). Familiarity and community were also frequently cited as reasons why survivors chose not to relocate outside of their communities.

Dissemination of Survey Report

These and other findings were included in a ten-page report to communicate the experiences and perspectives of the flood survivors. RAP partners spent several meetings discussing how to apply these findings to create broader structural and systemic change at the local and state levels. It was agreed that the data should be presented in several different formats and to a variety of audiences. RAP members, including flood survivors, attended rallies and visited North Carolina legislators to advocate for the fair treatment of all flood survivors as they struggled to restore their lives. RAP members also met with the North Carolina budget director and the senior policy adviser of the North Carolina Department of Commerce, North Carolina Low Income Housing, North Carolina Fair Share, and other organizations to argue for the rebuilding of affordable low-income housing. Results from the survey were useful during these meetings to inform state-level decision makers of the flood survivors' needs and the inadequacies of the state's response. The experiences that survivors had gained participating in research helped them better communicate their own concerns and needs and tell the stories of other survivors.

Survey results were also presented to an audience of flood survivors, grassroots organizations, and agency representatives using slides and interview excerpts at the Hurricane Floyd Survivors' Summit. RAP organized and sponsored the summit at a local conference center with the goal of uniting the voices of the hundreds of flood survivors throughout North Carolina and planning a common agenda for unity and empowerment. To encourage coverage by the local news and print media, RAP partners worked together to create and widely circulate a press release. Several local newspapers and television and radio stations covered the summit. As a result of this coverage, the director of the state emergency management division was pushed to respond publicly and to grant survivors six additional months beyond the original deadline to locate permanent housing and remain at the temporary sites.

Some academics are reluctant to interact with the media. Researchers may feel that their findings are misrepresented and misunderstood, while interviews take considerable time and have little potential to influence scientific publications or grant funding, the criteria that matter most for career advancement. However, researchers working in partnership with communities have responsibilities regarding publication of scientific findings, making those findings public in appropriate ways, and participating in processes involving the media and policymakers (Sandman, 1991). Mass media campaigns and targeted media advocacy have the potential to reframe health and social issues, set policy agendas, and influence funding priorities (Wallack, 1990). Environmental health findings presented via mainstream media channels can help protect exposed community members, motivate participation in democratic processes, and influence public opinion and policymakers.

DISCUSSION

The two case studies presented in this chapter differ from each other in several important respects. Although both cases involved community-driven research partnerships, the industrial hog operation studies were more quantitative and used multivariable statistical analyses and principles of experimental design based on comparisons of exposed and unexposed groups. Trained university interviewers were employed in the rural health survey in order to standardize comparisons between communities. By contrast, the RAP study relied more heavily on narratives and qualitative methods to create a portrait of the flood survivors' situation. RAP determined that those individuals who were most affected by Hurricane Floyd—the flood survivors themselves—would be the most appropriate persons to collect and help analyze the data. Finally, whereas the rural health survey examined more specifically health and quality of life in relation to livestock operations, the RAP study examined more broadly the consequences of displacement and mistreatment of people and their associated basic needs.

Despite these differences, however, each case study illustrates the vulnerability of both researchers and communities to the agendas of politicians and decision makers. The research partnerships provide examples of the potential power such collaborative endeavors have in influencing political decision making and practice related to the public's health and well-being. Furthermore, both research partnerships faced ethical dilemmas and worked with the communities to identify potential solutions.

Of central importance to both studies was the question raised by Randy Stoecker in Chapter Five when he asks, "How can I become relevant as an academic and create real and meaningful social change?" Public health researchers have the opportunity, and the social responsibility, to be relevant by using their skills, wherever possible, to promote public health through democracy and social justice. Although many scientists remain unaware of or disinterested in the social construction of science, no research question, method, or results can be separated from its social context. Meaningful and influential community involvement in research studies can help public health researchers begin to address those structural and power issues that perpetuate inequity (Wing, 2001). More objective research—whether in support of democratic social change or commercial interests—can be achieved by relentlessly analyzing and revealing its policy and advocacy dimensions (Wing, 1998).

References

Brown, P., & Mikkelsen, E. J. (1990). *No safe place: Toxic waste, leukemia, and community action.* Berkeley: University of California Press.

Cecelski, D., & Kerr, M. L. (1992, February). "Hog wild." *Southern Exposure,* pp. 9–15.

Chavis, D. M., & Wandersman, A. (1990). Sense of community in the urban environment: A catalyst for participation and community development. *American Journal of Community Psychology, 18,* 55–81.

Cook, T. D., & Reichardt, C. S. (Eds.). (1979). *Qualitative and quantitative methods in evaluation research.* Beverly Hills, CA: Sage.

Cornwall, A., & Jewkes, R. (1995). What is participatory research? *Social Science and Medicine, 41,* 1667–1676.

Denzin, N. K., & Lincoln, Y. S. (Eds.). (1994). *Handbook of qualitative research.* Thousand Oaks, CA: Sage.

Eastern North Carolina Housing Summit. (1999, April). *The state of housing in eastern North Carolina: Final report.* New Bern: Eastern North Carolina Sustainable Community Economic Development Center.

Edwards, B., & Ladd, A. (2000). Environmental justice, swine production and farm loss in North Carolina. *Sociological Spectrum, 20,* 263–290.

Eng, E. (1993). The Save Our Sisters project. A social network strategy for reaching rural black women. *Cancer, 72*(3, Suppl.), 1071–1077.

Environmental Protection Agency. (1998). *Final guidance for incorporating environmental justice concerns in EPA's NEPA compliance analyses.* Washington, DC: Government Printing Office.

Environmental racism at FEMA camp. (2000, August–September). *Justice Speaks,* p. 6.

Faber, D. R., & McCarthy, D. (2000). *A different shade of green: A report on philanthropy and the environmental justice movement in the United States.* Washington, DC: Aspen Institute.

Furuseth, O. (1997). Restructuring of hog farming in North Carolina: Explosion and implosion. *Professional Geographer, 49,* 391–403.

Gaventa, J. (1993). The powerful, the powerless, and the experts: Knowledge struggles in an informational age. In P. Park, M. Brydon-Miller, B. L. Hall, & T. Jackson (Eds.), *Voices of change: Participatory research in the United States and Canada* (pp. 21–40). Westport, CT: Bergin & Garvey.

Green, L. W., & Mercer, S. (2001). Can public health researchers and agencies reconcile the push from funding bodies and the pull from communities? *American Journal of Public Health, 91,* 1926–1938.

Israel, B. A, Checkoway, B., Schulz, A. J., & Zimmerman, M. A. (1994). Health education and community empowerment: Conceptualizing and measuring perceptions of individual, organizational, and community control. *Health Education Quarterly, 21,* 149–170.

Israel, B. A., Schulz, A. J., Parker, E. A., & Becker, A. B. (1998). Review of community-based research: Assessing partnership approaches to improve public health. *Annual Review of Public Health, 19,* 173–202.

Kuehn, R. (1996). The environmental justice implications of quantitative risk assessment. *University of Illinois Law Review, 103,* 103–172.

Le Duff, C. (1999, July 16). At a slaughterhouse, some things never die: Who kills, who cuts, who bosses can depend on race. *New York Times.*

Levine, A. G. (1982). *Love Canal: Science, politics, and people.* Lexington, MA: Heath.

Lindenfeld, S. (2001, February 13). Floyd recovery in their own hands: Survivors "stand up." *Raleigh News and Observer,* p 1B.

Lynn, F. M. (2000). Community-scientist collaboration in environmental research. *American Behavioral Scientist, 44,* 649–663.

Minkler, M. (2000). Using participatory action to build healthy communities. *Public Health Reports, 115,* 191–198.

Northridge, M. E., Vallone, D., Merzel, C., Greene, D., Shepard, P., Cohall, A. T., & Healton, C. G. (2000). The adolescent years: An academic-community partnership in Harlem comes of age. *Journal of Public Health Management Practice, 6,* 53–60.

Nyswander, D. (1967). The open society: Its implications for health educators. *Health Education Monographs, 1,* 3–13.

Patton, M. Q. (1990). *Qualitative evaluation and research methods* (2nd ed.). Newbury Park, CA: Sage.

St. George, D. M., Schoenbach, V. J., Reynolds, G. H., Nwangwu, J., & Adams-Campbell, L. (1997). Recruitment of minority students to U.S. epidemiology degree programs. *Annals of Epidemiology, 7,* 304–310.

Sandman, P. M. (1991). Emerging communication responsibilities of epidemiologists. *Journal of Clinical Epidemiology, 44*(Suppl. 1), 41S–50S.

Schiffman, S. S., Miller, E. A., Suggs, M. S., & Graham, B. G. (1995). The effect of environmental odors emanating from commercial swine operations on the mood of nearby residents. *Brain Research Bulletin, 37,* 369–375.

Segrest, M. (1999). *Looking for higher ground: Disaster and response in North Carolina after Hurricane Floyd.* Durham, NC: Urban-Rural Mission USA.

Shepard, P. M. (2000). Achieving environmental objectives and reducing health disparities through community-based participatory research and interventions. In L. R. O'Fallon, F. L. Tyson, & A. Dearry (Eds.), *Successful models of community-based participatory research. Final report* (pp. 30–34). Washington, DC: National Institute for Environmental Health Science.

Steckler, A., McLeroy, K. R., Goodman, R. M., Bird, S. T., & McCormick, L. (1992). Toward integrating qualitative and quantitative methods: An introduction. *Health Education Quarterly, 19,* 1–8.

Thu, K., et al. (1997). A control study of the physical and mental health of residents living near a large-scale swine operation. *Journal of Agricultural Safety and Health, 3,* 13–26.

Wallack, L. (1990). Media advocacy: Promoting health through mass communication. In K. Glanz, F. M. Lewis, & B. K. Rimer (Eds.), *Health behavior and health education: Theory, research, and practice* (2nd ed.). San Francisco: Jossey-Bass.

Wing, S. (1998). Whose epidemiology, whose health? *International Journal of Health Services, 28,* 241–252.

Wing, S. (2000). Community-Driven Epidemiology and Environmental Justice: A course at the University of North Carolina. *Networker, 5*(5). [http://www.sehn.org/Volume_5-5_4.html].

Wing, S. (2001). Review: Challenging inequalities in health: From ethics to action. *New England Journal of Medicine, 345,*1857–1858.

Wing, S. (2002). Social responsibility and research ethics in community-driven studies of industrialized hog production. *Environmental Health Perspectives, 110,* 437–444.

Wing, S., Cole, D., & Grant, G. (2000). Environmental injustice in North Carolina's hog industry. *Environmental Health Perspectives, 108,* 225–231.

Wing, S., Grant, G., Green, M., & Stewart, C. (1996). Community-based collaboration for environmental justice: Southeast Halifax environmental reawakening. *Environment and Urbanization, 8,* 129–140.

Wing, S., & Wolf, S. (2000). Intensive livestock operations, health, and quality of life among eastern North Carolina residents. *Environmental Health Perspectives, 108,* 233–238.

CHAPTER TWELVE

Ethical Challenges in Community Based Participatory Research

A Case Study from the San Francisco Bay Area Disability Community

Pamela Fadem
Meredith Minkler
Martha Perry
Klaus Blum
Leroy Moore
Judith Rogers

With its emphasis on dialogue and participation and its commitment to education and social change as an integral part of the research process (Hall, 1981; Sohng, 1996), community based participatory research should be particularly well suited to studying and addressing controversial issues. Through dialogue and critical reflection, hard issues can receive the benefit of open and frank scrutiny and debate. The building of trust between inside and outside members of the research team, an emphasis on community rather than "outside expert"–driven study, and a commitment to community control of research findings to promote community well-being, should all ideally aid in

Note: Portions of this chapter were adapted from "Ethical Dilemmas in Participatory Action Research: A Case Study from the Disability Community," by M. Minkler, P. Fadem, M. Perry, K. Blum, L. Moore, & J. Rogers, *Health Education and Behavior, 29*(1), pp. 14–29. Copyright © 2002 by Sage Publications, Inc. Adapted by permission of Sage Publications, Inc.

The authors gratefully acknowledge other members of the Community Advisory Group, Mary Pugh-Dean, Lee Williams, and World Institute on Disability representative Devva Kavitz, for their major contributions to all aspects of this work. Thanks are also due to Tatra-Li Beuttler for help with data analysis, Eve Muller for her early contributions as a member of the project team, and Laura Spautz and Chris Roebuck for administrative assistance. We gratefully acknowledge the members of the Wallace Alexander Gerbode Foundation for their belief in and support of this project. Finally, our deepest thanks go to the participants in this study for sharing their life stories and deeply personal beliefs and contributing to a process that we hope will enrich and strengthen the community of people with disabilities.

the conduct of research in difficult terrain. Yet as the case study described in this chapter suggests, high-level community involvement and adherence to the principles of CBPR cannot prevent the tough ethical challenges that often emerge in the course of such work, and that must be openly acknowledged and addressed.

The CBPR project described here took place in the San Francisco Bay Area in 1999–2001 and was designed to uncover the attitudes of people with disabilities toward a particularly polarizing issue in their community—death with dignity legislation, or physician-assisted suicide. A central goal of the study was to broaden the discussion within the disability community on this difficult and contentious issue. By finding common ground for community members on both sides of the debate, it was hoped that the community would be in a better position to become an active participant in the ongoing legislative and policy debate on physician-assisted suicide.

The project was conducted by a university based research team, consisting of a faculty member and three students, and a six-member community advisory group (CAG), which was actively involved in every stage of the research process. All members of the CAG and two of the university team members were people with disabilities.

To provide a context for understanding the ethical issues that arose in this study, we begin with some background on death with dignity legislation and the debate within the disability community over this issue. We then briefly describe the genesis, goals, methods, and results of this CBPR project. Most of the chapter is then devoted to an examination of four of the key ethical dilemmas that emerged in the course of the project, all of which have relevance for people engaged in CBPR efforts: questions around issue selection when a community is deeply divided over a problem, inclusion and exclusion in both university research team makeup and sample selection, issues of power and misunderstanding related to the insider or outsider status of team members, and how best to use findings in ways that can unite and strengthen the community rather than weaken and further divide it.

Despite the ethical challenges faced, CBPR was found to be an empowering research approach, building individual and community capacity (Goodman et al., 1998) and increasing dialogue both within and beyond the community.

BACKGROUND

To date, only the state of Oregon has passed a Death with Dignity Act. The Oregon law (permitting doctors to prescribe a lethal dose of barbiturates to a terminally ill patient provided a series of conditions and guidelines have been met),[1] passed by voters in 1994, was followed by a series of legal challenges and did not go into effect until 1997 (Wolfe, 1997). The Oregon Department of Human Services (DHS) has issued an annual report monitoring compliance with the act (Oregon Health Division, 1999, 2000, 2001, 2002). California, Washington, and Maine have all considered and rejected ballot measures that would have legalized death with dignity (DWD) or physician-assisted suicide (PAS) legislation, and there has been fierce pubic debate about the issue in both Michigan and New York. Two 1997 U.S. Supreme Court cases firmly returned the debate over PAS from the federal courts to the individual states, (*Vacco* v. *Quill,* 1997; *Washington* v. *Glucksberg,* 1997). In November 2001, however, U. S. Attorney General John Ashcroft once again fueled the debate on a national level—and challenged the legality of the Oregon act—when he issued a new interpretation of the Controlled Substances Act prohibiting the use of federally controlled substances to hasten death (Verhovek, 2001).

Although DWD or PAS has been a deeply divisive issue in the United States in general, it has a particular history of polarization in the community of people with disabilities (Bickenbach, 1998). The organized disability rights community has historically taken a strong stand against such legislation, including mobilizing to defeat California's proposed Death with Dignity Act (Assembly Bill 1592) in 1999–2000 and vigorously opposing Oregon's Death with Dignity Act (Batavia, 1997; Bickenbach, 1998; Toy, 1999; Wolfe, 1997). Many of the leading disability institutions, including the World Institute on Disability, the National Council on Disability, and the American Association of People with Disabilities, as well as the issue-specific and widely publicized groups Not Dead Yet and ADAPT, have official positions opposing DWD or PAS legislation (Madorsky, 1997; National Council on Disability, 1997; Not Dead Yet/ADAPT, 1995). This opposition is based on recognition of the marginalized status of people with disabilities as a vulnerable population in our society due to well-documented historical and continuing stigmatization and discrimination. Although the Americans with Disabilities Act, signed into law in 1990, was designed to eliminate discrimination in employment and other arenas, there is still substantial work to be done in overcoming both attitudinal and structural barriers. Within this context, legislation permitting death with dignity or physician-assisted suicide is seen as inevitably leading down a slippery slope to denial of fair and equitable life choices and unwanted and unnecessary deaths among people who are disabled, poor, elderly, or otherwise vulnerable (Madorsky, 1997; National Council on Disability, 1997; Not Dead Yet/ADAPT, 1995).

Although a strong position opposing DWD/PAS legislation is frequently put forward as representing the views and interests of the disability community, this issue has engendered deeply polarized positions in the disability policy, advocacy, and community arenas (Batavia, 1997; Madorsky, 1997; National Council on Disability, 1997; Not Dead Yet/ADAPT, 1995; Toy, 1999; Wolfe, 1997). Some community members expressed concern that fear of criticism for failing to support the stated "official" community position on such legislation may have led to a stifling of open discussion within the community. A 1999 survey conducted by *New Mobility* magazine, for example, resulted in a huge volume of responses, with 37 percent of those who favored the legislation also reporting fear of censure from their own community if they voiced such opinions (Corbet, 1999a). This lack of open dialogue may potentially contribute to the exclusion of disability community representation in statewide and national policy development bodies.

The topic of this CBPR project came originally from one of us, who at the time was a graduate student and also deeply rooted in the local disability community. She and her professor discussed at length her concern about the difficulty her community was having in openly dialoguing about the very polarizing issue of death with dignity legislation. The professor then expressed her own interest in working with the student to develop a CBPR project that would address this community concern. As Peter Reason (1994) has pointed out, one of the great ironies in CBPR is that while the process is "radically egalitarian," "paradoxically, many PAR projects would not occur without the initiative of someone with time, skills and commitment, someone who will almost inevitably be a member of a privileged and educated group" (p. 334). As a person who occupied such a position of privilege and who was not a member of the community, the professor played the role of initiator, with the understanding that the project itself would be of and very largely by the student and her colleagues in the disability community.

STUDY METHODS AND ADHERENCE TO CBPR PRINCIPLES

This project attempted to follow the principles of CBPR (Hall, 1981; Israel, Schulz, Parker, & Becker, 1998; see also Chapter Three) in several ways. As will be described in more detail, the problem was identified by members of the disability community itself; the research was participatory, engaging community members and outside researchers in a collaborative, co-learning process that was community-driven; an emphasis was placed on community capacity building and empowerment; and a balance was sought between research and action (Israel et al., 1998).

Community Advisory Group and University Research Team Roles and Composition

A strong Community Advisory Group (CAG), composed of five natural helpers and informal leaders in the community (Israel, 1985) and a trained researcher who was also a member of the disability community, was formed at the project's inception and involved in all aspects of the research. As noted, two of the university research team members and all six members of the CAG have physical disabilities. The graduate student who was one of the project initiators subsequently worked as the project director.

Although we were unsuccessful in recruiting either Latinos or Asian Pacific Islanders to the CAG, it was in other respects a highly diverse group, divided evenly between African Americans and whites and women and men and including people of varied educational, religious or spiritual, disability, and other backgrounds. Finally, and although the university research team deliberately never asked potential CAG members about their own attitudes toward death with dignity legislation, a considerable range of opinions was held by those members who chose to share them.

The CAG met monthly with the university team for the length of the project and was actively engaged in determining the criteria for sample selection and identifying potential study participants; developing the research instrument; conducting interviews; doing data analysis; and preparing and presenting a final report to the study participants. Several CAG members and the project director have continued to work in the arena of education to broaden the dialogue and foster full inclusion of people with disabilities at the policy table.

Sampling

The project involved qualitative in-depth interviews with a diverse sample of forty-five people with physical disabilities.[2] In an effort to involve those who have often not been included in the discussion of this topic, focused outreach to communities of color was undertaken. A combination of methods was used to develop a sample that, while not random or representative, would include considerable diversity in terms of nature of disability, race/ethnicity, and socioeconomic status. Targeted sampling was used in which basic ethnographic mapping of the population helped determine representation (Watters & Biernacki, 1989). Through snowball sampling, respondents were asked for the names of other people with disabilities who might wish to participate, particularly those whom they believed might hold views toward DWD/PAS legislation different from their own. In addition, contacts were made with local disability community resources, such as independent living centers, outpatient rehabilitation services in local hospitals, disabled student services at college campuses, and county social services and senior centers. A special effort was made to contact agencies working disproportionately with people of color. Flyers describing the project were mailed or hand-delivered to all of the sites and posted.

Sixty percent of sample members were people of color, primarily African Americans and Asians, and sample members had considerable diversity as well along such dimensions as age (twenties through early nineties), educational level (no high school diploma through postgraduate degree), and length of disability. Sixty percent of sample members were women, and all but one had been disabled for at least four years (a detailed description of the sample appears in Fadem, 2001).

Questionnaire Construction and Interviewing

The university research team and the CAG worked together for three months to develop and pretest an instrument consisting of twenty-nine semistructured and open-ended questions. Background information on demographics, daily routine, social support, discrimination experienced, and relationships to health care providers was collected, as was information on end-of-life decision making and feelings, opinions, and experiences regarding death with dignity legislation. CAG members played a crucial role in this process. They suggested new question areas (regarding experience with chronic pain, for example), called for the simplification or definition of terms such as *accommodations,* and reminded interviewers to incorporate into their questions whatever terms the participants used in naming or referring to their disabilities.

The sixty- to ninety-minute interviews, for which participants each received a $50 honorarium, took place at sites most convenient for the participants. Although pairs of team members were present for each interview to facilitate subsequent interrater comparisons of coded responses, the interviews themselves were always conducted by a team member with a disability. Most of the transcribing of taped interviews was also undertaken by a team member with a disability.

Data Management and Analysis

A code book was developed by the university research team to numerically code those questionnaire responses that lent themselves to such analysis. Transcripts were each coded independently by two team members, and a high degree of interrater reliability was found, with any discrepancies discussed and reconciled. Although the nonrandom nature of the sample precluded any generalizing of findings, this process enabled the project team to uncover associations between attitudes toward DWD legislation and variables such as religion, race/ethnicity, educational level, gender, and whether or not respondents identified themselves as members of the disability community. CAG members were involved in helping identify possible associations for examination and subsequently in discussing their potential usefulness in providing contextual data for the qualitative analysis.

A qualitative data analysis software program, QSR NUD*IST 4.0, was used to generate reports based on coded words (such as "terminal"), phrases ("easy way out"), concepts ("autonomy"), and numbered question responses. Several members of the advisory group and the university research team worked together for three months to analyze the data and identify emerging themes and patterns.

Out of concern for confidentiality and respect for the time constraints of CAG members, the university research team members first examined all transcripts and computer printouts to remove any potential sample member identifiers and extraneous material. Some data potentially useful to CAG members in their analysis may have been excluded through this initial condensation process. However, the sheer volume of transcript data and our foremost concern with ensuring the confidentiality of study participants made this a necessary step in the process.

Returning Data to Study Participants

As Peter Reason (1998, p. 272) has suggested, "Community meetings and events of various kinds are an important part of PAR, serving to identify issues, to reclaim a sense of community and emphasize the potential for liberation" and "to make sense of the information collected." During the course of the interviews, a number of participants expressed their interest in meeting with others who had been involved in the project. To facilitate this, and to further the community building that is central to CBPR, the returning of findings to the community took place in the context of two luncheons, held for participants in Oakland and San Francisco. Roughly half of the participants took part in these luncheons, which included time for socializing as well as the discussion of study findings.

The major themes collaboratively identified by the CAG and the university research team were compiled in a booklet for study participants and distributed at these meetings. Following a summary presentation of findings by the project director and reflections on the process by other team members, participants were encouraged to comment on and question the findings, suggest alternate interpretations, and discuss ways to use the findings to further the needs and best interests of the disability community. As we will discuss later in this chapter, how—and indeed *whether*—findings from this project should be used arose as one of the central ethical debates in the course of this study and continues to be a source of struggle and reflection in the community.

Following a brief look at the findings that emerged through this collaborative study process, we return to the methods and implementation of our project to examine in more detail several critical ethical challenges that arose and how they were addressed.

FINDINGS

Seven key findings or themes emerged in this study and are described in detail elsewhere (Fadem, 2001; Minkler et al., 2002). We summarize them here.

1. *Great breadth and diversity of opinion with respect to attitudes toward DWD/PAS legislation.* In the words of one of the CAG members, "There seems to be one public position on behalf of people with disabilities about death with dignity legislation put forward by disability community spokespersons and groups, but when you go deeper into the community, there are many different

opinions. An individual's opinion seems to depend on [his or her] own character [and] personal experience [of self or a loved one] with near-death or death, among many other things."

2. *The importance attributed to self-determination and autonomy in the way people with disabilities live and die.* Regardless of where they stood on the topic of DWD legislation, all respondents reported wanting their independence and autonomy in life choices to be respected. All but one reported that if they were close to death, experiencing intractable pain or loss of cognition, they would want to have their own opinion about ending or continuing life respected.

3. *The pervasiveness of discrimination based on disability.* Close to 90 percent of respondents reported that they had experienced discrimination based on their disability, whether from employers or potential employers, teachers, health care practitioners, social service or government agencies, members of the community, or their own families. This experience of discrimination had a profound impact on participants' opinions about DWD legislation and on their trust in society to respect the life (and death) choices that people with disabilities may make.

4. *Contradictions between personal experiences and abstract or political beliefs shaping attitudes toward DWD/PAS legislation.* A sizable proportion of sample members reported having had personal experiences or anticipated changes in their own lives that would cause them to have opinions at odds with their abstract or political beliefs regarding DWD legislation. Abstract or political beliefs for many were largely based on perceptions of or direct experience with discrimination based on disability, race, or class.

5. *Misinformation about the Oregon law and its implementation.* Between 1998 and 2001, ninety-one people in Oregon used their prescriptions to end their own lives. Their average age was seventy, more than three-fourths had terminal cancer, and fully 80 percent were receiving both hospice care and pain control (Oregon Health Division, 2002). In stark contrast to these facts, many of the participants in this study harbored major misconceptions about the law, including beliefs that it was or potentially could be used to hasten death in people with disabilities. For many, misinformation about the Oregon experience appeared to color personal feelings about such legislation in general.

6. *Fear of criticism from other disabled people in relation to the expression of attitudes toward DWD legislation.* Over half of the participants either had experienced, knew someone who had experienced, or feared they would experience criticism if they spoke out in favor of DWD legislation, regardless of what their own opinion actually was.

7. *Lack of association between attitudes toward DWD legislation and other factors.* Many of the factors that the disability community and members of the project team felt would play a major role in shaping attitudes toward such

legislation did not bear a significant relationship to attitudes for the group as a whole. Contrary to a widely held assumption, for example, people who strongly identified with the disability community did *not* uniformly express the strong negative views about DWD legislation that have been put forward as the "official" disability community position on this issue. Of the almost two-thirds of the sample members who identified with the disability community, fully half reported having considerable ambivalence about the legislation. Other factors unrelated to attitude included religion, race/ethnicity, class, social support, and relationship with one's physician.

In sum, the findings of this study revealed a tremendous diversity of opinion within a community of people with physical disabilities on the highly controversial and divisive issue of death with dignity or physician-assisted suicide legislation. At the same time, they highlighted the pervasiveness of disability based discrimination and the very strong desire for autonomy among people with disabilities in matters of both living and dying.

ETHICAL ISSUES AND CHALLENGES

This project illustrated that CBPR using qualitative interviewing methods can be a powerful means of uncovering a breadth of opinions and attitudes on a controversial topic and the sources of those feelings and thoughts while also contributing to individual and community capacity building. Members of the CAG, for example, developed skills in research methods including sampling, questionnaire construction, and data analysis, as well as compiling and returning data to the community. One member with no prior research experience participated in the interview process. And perhaps even more important than the research experience gained, many project participants—including CAG and UCB team members—were given a chance to tell their own stories, be heard, and given the opportunity to reflect on their own experiences in relation to others in their community. This community capacity building, at the heart of CBPR, was, we believe, an important contribution to finding common ground that may potentially strengthen a community divided.

In accordance with a core principle of CBPR, members of the university research team also saw how much they gained as co-learners in the CBPR process and how the research component of the project was strengthened through this co-learning approach. As noted earlier, for example, the CAG members' emphasis on the importance of using participants' own vocabulary in relation to their disability provided a critical lesson for the able-bodied member of the team, and their participation in the identification of themes and patterns in the data greatly strengthened the study. Similarly, the project team paid special attention to giving voice to people beyond the white middle class, since low-income persons and people of color have often have been underrepresented in discussions of this topic. This is consistent with the emphasis that both participatory researchers of color and feminist participatory researchers place on the centrality of issues of race/ethnicity, gender, and social class (Bell, 2001; Maguire, 1987). The commitment to diversity in the CAG, as well as in the study sample, helped achieve the goal of diversity in the study and helped expand discussion of DWD legislation into often neglected sectors of the disability community.

Despite these successes, the use of CBPR, while always challenging, proved even more so in the project. We turn now to four of the major ethical dilemmas that emerged in the process of this project and our attempts to grapple with them.

Selecting an Issue When "The Community" Is Deeply Divided

A fundamental tenet of CBPR involves ensuring that the issue to be investigated and acted on comes from the community and not an outside professional or funding source (Gaventa, 1981; George, Daniel, & Green, 1998; Hagey, 1997). Three ethical principles that lie at the heart of CBPR—respect for self-determination, liberty, and action for social change—"reflect an inherent belief in people's ability to accurately assess their strengthens and needs and their right to act upon them" (Minkler & Pies, 1997, p. 121). Yet as Labonté (1997) has pointed out, communities are rarely homogeneous, and consequently there may be considerable disagreement over the merits of an issue selected for study and action.

The earlier mentioned history of controversy and debate over death with dignity legislation in the disability community made topic selection in this case a major ethical challenge. For while many major disability rights organizations had taken firm stands opposing such legislation, a growing number of individuals, including some of the authors, were concerned that those "official" views did not necessarily reflect the views of "ordinary folks" in their community. Like the nondisabled, they argued, people with disabilities have a wide array of attitudes and opinions on this topic, and they were concerned that fear of censure prevented open discourse (Corbet, 1999b).

To begin to address the dilemma of choosing an issue that was highly polarizing within the community, we arranged a meeting with colleagues at the World Institute on Disability (WID), a locally headquartered organization with a reputation for its research and advocacy with and on behalf of people with disabilities. Although we knew that WID was among the organizations to go on record opposing DWD legislation, we hoped to dialogue openly with its staff about our idea for a CBPR project and ideally to seek their collaboration as equal partners in such an undertaking.

A frank and sometimes difficult talk ensued, and the WID representatives ultimately concluded that although their organization could not officially cosponsor this project, they did not oppose its being undertaken. One representative suggested that it might indeed be good to open the conversation, and WID decided that it did want a representative on the Community Advisory Group. The WID staff member who volunteered brought not only an important organizational affiliation but also considerable knowledge and experience in participatory research within the disability community. Sadly, and for a variety of reasons, this individual did not participate actively on the CAG beyond attending a few meetings.

Hard questions around issue selection continued to arise throughout the course of this project. A prominent national disability leader, on being told of the study, responded, "Why would you look at that when there are so many more important issues?" In fact, this same opinion was voiced by a number of people interviewed in this project and may well reflect a contradiction between respect for the *idea* of open discussion of DWD/PAS and personal and professional concerns that open discussion may contribute to further stigmatization and discrimination.

In contrast to such views, a member of our study sample concluded the interview by saying, "This is so much more important than one more study of accessible transportation." The members of the CAG were recruited to work on the project based on their own interest and concern that this issue be aired in the community, regardless of what opinion, if any, they held about DWD legislation. CAG members were not asked what their own opinions were; some openly announced their views, and others never did. Our own conclusion, after much critical reflection and dialogue with members of the community, was that despite the contentious nature of the topic, there was sufficient sentiment in favor of more open dialogue to make venturing into this admittedly risky terrain worth any discomfort or difficulty.

This issue was a constant theme throughout the project, one to which we returned many times in discussing whether the findings would or would not be used in furthering the discussion both within and outside of the disability community.

Inclusion and Exclusion in Selecting Team Members and Study Participants

A second dilemma involved the ethics and the politics of inclusion and exclusion in the selecting of project team members and study participants. Because this was to be a study of and largely by people with disabilities, we expected to recruit student members of the project team who themselves had significant disabilities. Further, because the controversy over DWD legislation has been most pronounced in the community of people with physical disabilities, we wanted to limit students, advisory group members, and study participants to those with a primary physical disability, rather than a sensory or psychiatric disability or a disability secondary to AIDS or other conditions.

In recruiting members of the project team from the university, we ran into a disturbing example of one of the project findings regarding the pervasiveness of disability based discrimination. There simply weren't sufficient numbers of graduate students with physical disabilities at the university to enable us to identify several who could take part in this study. Students without physical disabilities but who worked in the field of disability expressed concerns about being categorically excluded. We ended up including on the team one nondisabled graduate student who had excellent qualitative research skills in addition to prior work experience in disability. However, this student was forced by a geographic move to leave the project early on so that the final university research team was made up of two students with disabilities (the project director and an undergraduate psychology student who is also a nurse) plus the able-bodied faculty member.

Just as some able-bodied students were unhappy at being excluded from participation on the research team, some prospective study participants with non-physical disabilities (such as blindness or HIV/AIDS) were disturbed on learning that their lack of a primary physical disability would exclude them from participation.[3] We carefully explained to each person the need for adhering to our sampling criteria, particularly with the small number of people to be involved, so that we could later determine which factors influenced a participant's opinions.

As noted earlier, a major concern in this study was with broadening the dialogue within the physically disabled community to include people who have historically been on the margins of the movement—people of color and low-income people with disabilities. This meant turning down some people with physical disabilities who wished to take part in the study but who were in the white, middle-class population that was already overrepresented in our sample. A number of people who were unhappy when they were excluded on the basis of race asserted that nonwhites would have a different position on the issue of DWD/PAS legislation. Our response was that this was one important reason to ensure diversity among project participants, so that we could ascertain whether race/ethnicity might be associated with opinions toward DWD legislation. We also assured all of those who had to be excluded from participating in the study that the results would be made available to the community in the broadest and most inclusive sense.

Concerns about diversity also played a part in selection of CAG members. Our primary focus was on recruitment of natural helpers and informal leaders with a wide range of backgrounds in class, education, employment, and race/ethnicity. This empowerment of people not usually recognized for their leadership helped ensure diversity in participant inclusion. However, we missed an important opportunity to add a CAG member from the Asian American community. One of the first people interviewed, this community member was so interested after the interview that she asked to participate on the CAG. Because her offer came four months into the process—after the CAG had already established sampling criteria, developed the interview instrument, and built considerable trust and rapport as a group—we turned down this request. In retrospect, bringing this person on board might well have helped increase participation among the Asian disabled community.

In most instances, the dialogue that is a central feature of CBPR proved an important vehicle for helping those excluded come to a better understanding of why this study was centered on creating a safe space for people with physical disabilities, especially those from underrepresented groups, to discuss their attitudes and feelings. We also took names and contact information from all who had hoped to be included and could not be and promised to make the project findings available for discussion. Despite these efforts, however, issues of inclusion and exclusion were difficult and reemerged at different points throughout the project.

Insider-Outsider Issues

The potential conflict between insiders and outsiders in community based research has been much discussed in the literature (Braithwaite, Biandi, & Taylor, 1994; Nyden & Wiewel, 1992; Sclove, 1997; Sullivan et al., 2001; Wallerstein, 1999). As Wallerstein (1999), has noted, even outsiders who pride themselves on being community allies and trusted friends frequently fail to realize the extent of the power imbued by their own, often multiple, sources of privilege and how it can adversely affect interactions and outcomes.

One simple manifestation of insider-outsider tensions involved the difficulty in conducting a participatory community project within the time frame of the academic and funding calendar. As Randy Stoecker notes in Chapter Five, "Real collaboration takes a lot of time—for meetings, for accountability processes, for working through the inevitable conflicts—that may be in especially short supply for community group members." The often conflicting time pressures and constraints between community members, community based organizations, and academic researchers frequently lead to frustrations on all sides (Nyden & Wiewel, 1992; Sullivan et al., 2001). As anthropologist Janice Perlman once remarked, community people are often "less interested in making history than in making life"—or in this case, putting a voluntary research project above the issues of day-to-day survival and fulfillment. As a case in point, two of our CAG members are noted creative artists, and their often demanding performance schedules not infrequently required a change in CAG meeting times.

Time demands were complicated still further by the realities of "DP" or "disabled people" time—the often inevitable delay in any life activity, including when interviews or CAG meetings could occur, due to bad weather, illness, or structural barriers (such as lack of accessible public transportation). The frequent need to change scheduled meetings or begin them more than an hour after the appointed time was understood as a fact of life in this project. But insider-outsider tensions sometimes emerged when the university and funding cycle deadlines proved difficult or impossible to meet. Although dialogue about DP time and other sources of conflicting time frames helped the able-bodied team member become more realistic in her expectations, conflicting time lines remained an issue. With the approval of the outside funding agency, the project was eventually extended for a year beyond the original termination date, thereby relieving some of the tensions around time pressure.

Differences in frame of reference between insiders and the academic outsider were also apparent in the sample selection phase of the project. The outside researcher's training in gerontology, for example, led her to push for the inclusion of a large number of older disabled people in the sample to be able to test her informal hypothesis that older individuals would be more favorably disposed toward DWD legislation than their younger counterparts. Inclusion of this population was not a high priority for most of the community members, however, whose insider knowledge suggested that the lived experience of people with long-term disability often forces them to confront issues of life and death numerous times over the life course—and sometimes when very young. Although a compromise was reached, including a minority of older persons in the study, different perceptions about the importance of specifically seeking out older sample members remained an issue of debate.

Finally, insider-outsider conflict also appeared in relation to analyzing the data. One example was in how to understand the disability experience of discrimination. Although many of the interviewees expressed a mistrust of doctors and the health care system, this mistrust existed within a broader social context of disability based discrimination and oppression. And the majority of respondents shared painful experiences in a wide range of social settings. The academic outsider perspective, which was shared by the insider team member who had training as a nurse, continued to emphasize health care related discrimination, even though close to two-thirds of sample members reported good patient-doctor relationships. For the project director and some members of the CAG, this was seen as reinforcing the traditional "medicalization" of people with disabilities. Through the continued dialogue and shared reflection that are hallmarks of participatory research (Sohng, 1996), the insider perspective prevailed, and discrimination at the hands of the medical care system was examined as simply one of many diverse and troubling forms in which prejudice against the disabled manifests itself in our society.

The potential conflict between insiders and outsiders in community based research is essentially about the difference between an academic or intellectual understanding and the lived experience of an issue. This conflict followed us into the final preparations for community presentations and in discussion about how broadly and in what way to disseminate the project findings. A particularly difficult but important role for the outside team member involved one of respectful disengagement when the project director and some members of the CAG decided that the final phase of the project (discussions and decision making about the use of findings in relation to policy and community education) should involve only the team members with disabilities. There is unfortunately much precedent for academics leaving a community soon after the data have been collected in what Michael Huberman (1991) describes as the "hello-goodbye approach." In the case of this study, however, the need to respect community based leadership was recognized as central to the action phase of the project. As Lorraine Gutierrez and Edith Lewis (1997) have pointed out, an important part of capacity building involves understanding and supporting the need communities of color—and in this case, the community of people with disabilities—may have for their own organizations and decision-making structures.

Dilemmas Around the Sharing and Use of the Findings

As noted, this project faced a difficult ethical and political challenge from the outset, since much of the formal leadership of the disability community was opposed to the presentation of anything but a united front against DWD/PAS legislation where the community was concerned (Coleman, 2000). Our findings revealed that many participants, including the majority of those who strongly identified with the disability community, did not share the blanket, negative view of such legislation and indeed held a varied and complex set of opinions. Such findings required that careful attention be directed to how best to use the study findings in ways that could unite and strengthen the community.

Among the many findings of this study, the most pronounced was the theme identified by the project director and her peers on the CAG as providing unique common ground for fostering a dialogue that could indeed offer a basis for strength and unity: the overwhelming agreement among study participants on the desire for autonomy and choice in how they live and how they die, regardless of where they stand on DWD legislation. By preparing a booklet of study findings for the participants that began with this critical point of unity, the project director and other team members played a key role in setting the stage for productive, strength based discussions.

Following the CBPR principle of community ownership of study findings (Israel et al., 1998; Roe, Minkler, & Saunders, 1995), the university research team and CAG began by giving back study findings to the participants, who were asked to share their reactions and comments, as well as their opinions about how the findings should be used. As noted earlier, roughly half of the study participants took part in the two community report-back luncheons, and many shared their belief that "getting the word out" was an important next step. As one young woman put it, "I think society at large has a very simplified view. [People] think just because we're all disabled, we have the same opinion. We're just as complex as any other body of people." Another participant remarked, "The study echoes over and over again the society we're part of." He added that "when you're in conversation with people you admire, you tend to agree with them. But when you're at home on your own pillow between the sheets, you think." In reference to the strong opposition to DWD legislation by the formal leadership in the disability community and the reluctance of many people with disabilities to voice an alternative opinion, still another participant said, "Nobody wants to rock the boat, to be on the fringes." Yet he also suggested the need to foster more open discussion.

Several participants spoke of the potential for using this study as a jumping-off point, both for a larger study and for increasing dialogue within the community through a variety of means. One young man suggested that the participants stay in contact and continue their own dialogue through the Internet. A contact list was circulated for this purpose, and a participant offered to coordinate this effort.

Alternative positions were also strongly expressed. One participant articulated his opinion that no discussion of DWD legislation was productive, since end-of-life decisions should be entirely "in God's hands." Another individual who had attended one of the meetings later confronted a member of the CAG to express her great displeasure with the study findings. And another participant told the project director that the disabled community would have no interest in the study findings, given that they contradicted the dominant view that is publicly presented.

The opinions of those who were unable to come or uninterested in attending the community report-backs were, of course, not known. Many of these individuals had requested copies of the report, and it was mailed to them with encouragement to share their copy with others and to give us any feedback they might have. In retrospect, a more proactive approach, including phone call follow-up to study participants who had not attended the report-backs, might have been a helpful means of eliciting their input on the study findings and their feelings about the potential use of the information uncovered.

Despite their own differing attitudes toward DWD legislation, Community Advisory Group members shared with the majority of community report-back participants a belief that the findings of this study provided a good mechanism for furthering dialogue on this topic. They supported making copies of the study findings widely available both within and beyond the disability community. Several also expressed a desire to meet with a local politician who had sponsored

California's unsuccessful Death with Dignity Act. Their hope was to discuss with her both the rich diversity of opinion concerning this issue and the fact that people with disabilities need and want to be included as full participants in any policy-level discussions of this contentious issue. Unfortunately, the state budget crisis and then the events of September 11, 2001, prevented this meeting from happening. Other presentations to disability, bioethics, and public health community groups and national professional societies have been made, with different results. Although two presentations before professional colleagues at the American Public Health Association generated considerable interest in and support for the study, for example, presentations to community groups received mixed reactions. Some groups have welcomed the opening up of dialogue, while others have been anxious to suppress the findings in the name of unity. At each of these meetings, project participants emphasized the complexity of the findings in our study, particularly the strong unifying principle of self-determination alongside a high degree of ambivalence toward DWD/PAS legislation. These findings contributed to the formation of a new disability organization, Autonomy (http://autonomy-now.org), in January 2002 that works to ensure the rights of all disabled to choice throughout the life course.

It is our hope that such activities will bolster the principle of full inclusion of people with disabilities at the policy table. However, it is also important to keep in mind that a CBPR project on so polarizing an issue for the disability community as death with dignity or physician-assisted suicide legislation cannot bridge the rifts around that issue.

IMPLICATIONS

In sharing our experiences in this very challenging project, we hope to have helped illuminate both some of the strengths and the challenges in community based participatory research. Most important, in our opinion, is for the community to be firmly in the driver's seat at every stage of the project. It is crucial to recognize the difference—and the impact in practice—between an academic, intellectual understanding of an issue and a community and the lived experience of that issue by that community. This has profound implications for the validity of CBPR and is a thread that linked several of the ethical dilemmas that we experienced and discussed in this chapter. Because of the disparity of skills and resources between professional, university based researchers and many community members, it is sometimes difficult to recognize and make best use of the strengths of both groups. Yet as Biggs (1989) suggests, truly collegiate research is characterized by interactions in which outside researchers and community members contribute different skills and work together in a mutual learning process over which community members have control. In retrospect, and building on Tierney (1994) and Wallerstein (1999), more open discussions of the hidden nature of power would have assisted us in our struggles to achieve this goal. In Wallerstein's words, "If we recognize that there are many realities in the phenomenon studied, including hidden voices that we may never know (Scott, 1990), then we must also recognize that there are many realities in the research relationship" (1999, p. 49).

A second thread linking ethical challenges in both issue selection and the sharing of findings involved the heterogeneity of "community" and the difficulties this can pose for a stigmatized community whose formal leaders may understandably wish to have its members "speak with one voice." In such cases, insider members of a CBPR team can play a critical role in dialoguing and reflecting with great care on the use (or nonuse) of study findings, with attention always focused on the goal of strengthening and building on sources of unity within the studied community.

Despite the challenges and frustrations faced, dealing with the ethical dilemmas that arise in the course of a project like this one can itself contribute to the building of stronger, more competent communities. By actively involving people with disabilities in all phases of this project and breaking down the barriers between the researchers and the researched (Gaventa, 1981), the study was able to contribute to both individual and community capacity building. As one CAG member remarked six months into the project. "When I come here to these meetings, it lets me be on another plane. Out there I am in survival mode, you know, looking around and behind me, watching out for everything. But when I come in here, I am on another plane and can function differently. And I thank you for that."

As Kathleen Roe and her colleagues (Roe, Berenstein, Goette, & Roe, 1997) have noted, "Strong communities know their history, understand how they are different [from] others, and find ways to honor their shared paths" (p. 313). By helping depolarize the issue of death with dignity legislation within the disability community and shining a spotlight on a critical point of unity and strength in that community, this study attempted to contribute to the process through which an already strong and varied community honors its shared path.

Notes

1. According to the Oregon law, a person must ask twice for the assistance, two weeks apart; must be eighteen or over; must be terminally ill; and must not be clinically depressed. Finally, the person must be able to self-administer the medication once it is prescribed.

2. Physical disability was defined as either congenital or acquired and requiring the use of accommodations or assistance with activities of daily living, such as bathing and dressing, or instrumental activities of daily living, such as cooking and housecleaning.

3. A number of people who met the criteria for physical disability but who currently were being treated for depression were also unhappy about being excluded, even though we explained that this was a requirement of our institutional review board agreement.

References

Batavia, A. (1997). Disability and physician-assisted suicide. *New England Journal of Medicine, 336,* 1671–1673.

Bell, E. E. (2001). Infusing race into the U.S. discourse on action research. In P. Reason & H. Bradbury (Eds.), *Handbook of action research: Participative inquiry and practice* (pp. 48–58). Thousand Oaks, CA: Sage.

Bickenbach, J. (1998). Disability and life-ending decisions. In M. P. Battin, R. Rhodes, & A. Silvers (Eds.), *Physician-assisted suicide: Expanding the debate* (pp. 123–132). New York: Routledge.

Biggs, S. (1989). *Resource-poor farmer participation in research: A synthesis of experiences from nine agricultural research systems.* The Hague, Netherlands: International Service for National Agricultural Research.

Braithwaite, R., Biandi, C., & Taylor, S. (1994). Ethnographic approach to community organizing and health empowerment. *Health Education Quarterly, 21,* 407–416.

Coleman, D. (2000). Assisted suicide and disability: Another perspective. *Human Rights, 27,* 6–8.

Corbet, B.(1999a, September). Editorial: Absolutely right. *New Mobility,* p. 4.

Corbet, B. (1999b, August). Editorial: Community assist. *New Mobility,* p. 4.

Fadem, P. (2001). *Attitudes of people with disabilities toward death with dignity/ physician-assisted suicide legislation: Broadening the dialogue.* Unpublished master's thesis, School of Public Health, University of California, Berkeley.

Gaventa, J. (1981). Participatory action research in North America. *Convergence, 14,* 30–42.

George, M., Daniel, M., & Green, L. (1998). Appraising and funding participatory research in health promotion. *International Quarterly of Community Health Education, 18,* 181–197.

Goodman, R. M., Speers, M. A., McLeroy, K., Fawcett, S., Kegler, M., Parker, E. A., et al. (1998). Identifying and defining the dimensions of community capacity to provide a basis for measurement. *Health Education and Behavior, 25,* 258–278.

Gutierrez, L., & Lewis, E. (1997). Education, participation, and capacity building in community organizing with women of color. In M. Minkler (Ed.), *Community organizing and community building for health* (pp. 216–229). New Brunswick, NJ: Rutgers University Press.

Hagey, R. S. (1997). Guest editorial: The use and abuse of participatory action research. *Chronic Diseases in Canada, 18*(1), 1–4.

Hall, B. L. (1981). Participatory research, popular knowledge, and power: A personal reflection. *Convergence, 14,* 6–19.

Huberman, M. (1991). Linkage between researchers and practitioners: A qualitative study. *American Educational Research Journal, 27,* 363–391.

Israel, B. A. (1985). Social networks and social support: Implications for natural helper and community level interventions. *Health Education Quarterly, 12,* 65–80.

Israel, B. A., Schulz, A. J., Parker, E. A., & Becker, A. B. (1998). Review of community-based research: Assessing partnership approaches to improve public health. *Annual Review of Public Health, 19,* 173–202.

Labonté, R. (1997). Community, community development, and the forming of authentic partnerships: Some critical reflections. In M. Minkler (Ed.), *Community organizing and community building for health* (pp. 88–102). New Brunswick, NJ: Rutgers University Press.

Madorsky, J. (1997). Is the slippery slope steeper for people with disabilities? *Western Journal of Medicine, 166,* 410–411.

Maguire, P. (1987). *Doing participatory research: A feminist approach.* Amherst: University of Massachusetts, Center for International Education.

Minkler, M., Fadem, P., Perry, M., Blum, K., Moore, L., & Rogers, J. (2002). Ethical dilemmas in participatory action research: A case study from the disability community. *Health Education and Behavior, 29,* 14–29.

Minkler, M., & Pies, C. (1997). Ethical issues in community organization and community participation. In M. Minkler (Ed.), *Community organizing and community building for health* (pp. 120–136). New Brunswick, NJ: Rutgers University Press.

National Council on Disability. (1997, March 24). *Assisted suicide: A disability perspective.* Position paper. Washington, DC: Author.

Not Dead Yet/ADAPT. (1995). *Amici curiae brief in support of petitioners in* Vacco v. Quill, 95 S. Ct. 1858.

Nyden, P. W., & Wiewel, W. (1992). Collaborative research: Harnessing the tensions between researcher and practitioner. *American Sociologist, 24,* 43–55.

Oregon Health Division. (1999). *Legalized physician-assisted suicide in Oregon: The first year's experience.* Eugene: Oregon State Department of Human Services.

Oregon Health Division. (2000). *Legalized physician-assisted suicide in Oregon: The second year.* Eugene: Oregon State Department of Human Services.

Oregon Health Division. (2001). *Legalized physician-assisted suicide in Oregon, 1998–2000.* Eugene: Oregon State Department of Human Services.

Oregon Health Division. (2002). *Fourth annual report on Oregon's Death with Dignity Act.* Eugene: Oregon State Department of Human Services.

Reason, P. (1994). *Participation in human inquiry.* Thousand Oaks, CA: Sage.

Reason, P. (1998). Three approaches to participative inquiry. In N. K. Denzin & Y. S. Lincoln (Eds.), *Strategies of qualitative inquiry* (pp. 261–291). Thousand Oaks CA: Sage.

Roe, K., Berenstein, C., Goette, C., & Roe, K. (1997). Community building through empowerment evaluation: A case study of HIV prevention community planning. In M. Minkler (Ed.), *Community organizing and community building for health* (pp. 308–322). New Brunswick, NJ: Rutgers University Press.

Roe, K., Minkler, M., & Saunders, F. (1995). Combining research, advocacy, and education: The methods of the Grandparent Caregiver Study. *Health Education Quarterly, 22,* 459–475.

Sclove, R. E. (1997). Research by the people, for the people. *Futures, 29,* 541–549.

Scott, J. (1990). *Domination and the arts of resistance: Hidden transcripts.* New Haven, CT: Yale University Press.

Sohng, S.S.L. (1996). Participatory research and community organizing. *Journal of Sociology and Social Welfare, 23,* 77–97.

Sullivan, M., Koné, A., Senturia, K. D., Chrisman, N. J., Ciske, S. J., & Krieger, J. W. (2001). Researcher and researched-community perspectives: Toward bridging the gap. *Health Education and Behavior, 28,* 130–149.

Tierney, W. (1994). On method and hope. In A. Gitlin (Ed.), *Power and method: Political activism and educational research* (pp. 97–115). New York: Routledge.

Toy, A. (1999, September). Assisted suicide: Issues of life and death. *New Mobility,* pp. 34–42.

Vacco v. Quill, 117 S. Ct. 2293 (1997).

Verhovek, S. W. (2001, November 7). Federal agents are directed to stop physicians who assist suicides. *New York Times,* p. 20.

Wallerstein, N. (1999). Power between evaluator and community: Research relationships within New Mexico's healthier communities. *Social Science and Medicine, 49,* 39–53.

Washington v. Glucksberg, 117 S. Ct. 2258 (1997).

Watters, J., & Biernacki, P. (1989). Targeted sampling: Options for study of hidden populations. *Social Problems, 36,* 416–430.

Wolfe, K. (1997, August). Choice or coercion? *New Mobility,* pp. 42–47.

CHAPTER THIRTEEN

Issues in Participatory Evaluation

Jane Springett

This chapter will examine participatory evaluation and the specific challenges it faces in the context of community based initiatives and community health promotion. The literature on participatory evaluation in the evaluation field is increasing, reflecting the growing disillusionment, at a number of levels, with approaches to evaluation derived from methodologies that originated in natural sciences. This literature represents a continuing philosophical debate that challenges thinking as to the way knowledge is created and by whom. On a practical level, it is a response to the great divide between research and practice and the tendency for the results of a majority of evaluation studies to be ignored by the parties who commissioned them (Weiss, 1988).

WHAT IS EVALUATION?

In recent years, there has been much discussion in community health promotion about the need for evidence based practice and more evaluation. This debate has in part been driven by the increasing demand for accountability in the public sector. (Henkel, 1991). It is also the sign of a maturing field as it seeks

Note: This chapter was adapted from "Participatory Approaches to Evaluation in Health Promotion," by Jane Springett, which appeared in *Evaluation in Health Promotion: Principles and Perspectives,* edited by I. Rootman et al., pp. 83–105. Copyright © 2001 by the World Health Organization. Adapted by permission of the World Health Organization.

to establish its underlying theoretical base and philosophy and begins to examine its effectiveness as a practice. Evaluation is something we do naturally all the time. It is essentially a process of reflection. It is also a process of learning from experience to inform future action. Kolb (1984), in his model of the adult experiential learning cycle, argues that for learning to take place, all elements of the cycle of thinking, deciding, doing, and reflecting must be accomplished. Thus evaluation must be seen as crucial for the development of the knowledge base of the field so that more is known about what works and, even more important, why and in what context.

Evaluation, however, is not the same as research. Although it uses the techniques and tools of research, it differs from research in a number of respects. A key difference lies in the word itself, the notion of value and its assessment. Although it is widely recognized—in social science, at least—that research is not value-free, the conventions of science attempt to limit, through a variety of checks and balances, the degree of deviation from so-called objectivity. By contrast, value lies at the center of evaluation. It always has a political dimension and is intimately tied up with societal priorities, resource allocation, and power (Greene, 1994). For at the heart of evaluation, the question has to be asked whose values are driving the evaluation and by whose standards the activities are being undertaken and assessed or being measured against. For health promotion and community based health interventions, this raises important issues, as quite often the values against which it is being assessed are not those of the field but those of medicine and disease prevention (Springett, 2001).

In summary, evaluation is a process of reflection whereby the value of certain actions in relation to projects, programs or policies is assessed. Evaluation can take many forms. Indeed, in the United States, over one hundred different types have been recognized (Patton, 1982). While some analysts distinguish one type of evaluation from another in terms of method, the trend in recent years has been toward a pluralistic approach that brings different models together. What is clear is that whatever the approach, methodology should not drive an evaluation. More important is the evaluation question, which is in turn dictated by the purpose of the evaluation. Is the purpose to find out if client needs are being met, to improve the intervention or program, to assess its outcomes, to find out how it is operating, to assess the efficiency, to assess its ability to facilitate empowerment, or to understand why a program of innovation works or does not work?

WHAT IS PARTICIPATORY EVALUATION?

Participatory approaches to evaluation attempt to involve in an evaluation all who have a stake in its outcomes, with a view to taking action and effecting change. If evaluation is going to change anything, it has to be useful and perceived as useful by everyone involved in a project or program, whether as a funder, a participant, or a project worker. The aim is an approach that encourages every voice to be heard and at the very least taken into consideration when deciding on the focus and design of the evaluation (Fuerstein, 1988).

Participatory evaluation, however, goes beyond just being aware of stakeholder interests, in that there is a joint responsibility for the evaluation by the participants, who play an active role in the nuts and bolts of evaluation. By being involved, participants can see the value of the information they are collecting. Involvement also ensures that the indicators actually measure the right things in the right way—in other words, that the indicators are meaningful to all concerned (Macgillavray, 1998). However, the benefits of such an approach go beyond ownership and clarity. Involving a range of people in each stage often generates innovative ways of measuring process, impact, and outcomes. These may include such innovations as the use of digital archiving, photovoice (see Chapter Nine), collage, storytelling, and oral history (Springett & Young, 2002). To generate and maintain enthusiasm and interest, a range of techniques, including celebration events, need to be employed (Springett & Dunkerton, 2001).

It could be argued that participatory evaluation is more a way of working based on a set of principles than an actual methodology. Indeed, the World Health Organization's recommendations to policymakers on the evaluation of health promotion (1998) specifically stipulate that evaluation should be participatory; this notion of participation at the center of health promotion evaluation was reinvoked in the Pan American Health Organization's principles for the evaluation of healthy municipalities, issued in 2001. In the evaluation field, variations have been called empowerment evaluation (Fetterman, Kaftarian, & Wandersman, 1996), democratic evaluation (Floch'hay & Plottu, 1998), and stakeholder evaluation. Involving stakeholders in some way in evaluation is now generally considered to be a good practice (Robson, 2000).

The philosophical and epistemological base of participatory evaluation itself lies in a hermeneutic tradition of knowledge creation (Dahlbom & Mathiassen, 1993). Its methodological and ideological roots lie in participatory action research, as described in other chapters. It is most commonly practiced at the community level in discrete localities and among disadvantaged groups where there is a grassroots tradition (De Koning & Martin, 1996; Eng & Parker, 1994; Sarri & Sarri, 1992; Standish, 1995).

Each of the three areas where participatory action research has been most commonly practiced—development research, management science, and education—has influenced the way participatory evaluation has developed. From its use in development work, there is the close association with Freirian approaches to popular education (Kroeger & Franken, 1981). This means an emphasis in participatory evaluation on learning and capacity building. Brown and Tandon (1983) argue, however, that one can distinguish within development work a difference between what they call a Southern focus and a Northern focus. The former emphasizes mobilization, "conscientizing," and empowering the oppressed to achieve community transformations and social justice. The latter is merely an attempt to involve local people in the evaluation of development projects initiated by development agencies, appearing, for example, in the guise of "beneficiary or user assessment" in the work of the World Bank (Salmen, 1992). The increased use of such approaches stems from a widespread awareness of the inherent weaknesses of conventional evaluation methods (Rovers, 1986), especially when clear objectives have not been set at the outset of a project. However, the persistence of notions of the project cycle in aid agency work, with its emphasis on relatively fixed procedures for the individual steps, is seen by some as a major constraint on full-scale adoption of participatory principles. Indeed, Mikkelson (1995) argues that participatory evaluation in such a context is more a matter of adjusting a project while it is in progress to meet conditions set by the indigenous participants. Evaluation is seen as a prerequisite to ensuring sustainability because of the focus on learning from experience. It serves, then, both as a management tool to enable people to improve their efficiency and effectiveness and as an educational process in which the participants increase their awareness and understanding of factors that affect their situation.

The influence of management science—a form of action learning that encourages the systematic collection of data and information for high-level organizational performance—underpins the notion of participatory evaluation to improve rather than evaluation to prove (Magerison, 1987). Thus participatory evaluation in organizational settings in communities is geared to solving major organization issues or problems on a group basis with a focus on decision makers as participants and moving from single-loop to double-loop learning (Argyris & Schön, 1978). Underpinning the rationale is the notion of learning and more particularly the notion of organizational learning. This reflects an increasing emphasis in management literature on the importance of participatory decision making in bringing about organizational change (Senge, 1990).

Participatory evaluation in the context of organization draws from this action research tradition, building on the notion of stakeholder involvement in evaluation. The approach is, however, distinguishable from the stakeholder tradition in evaluation practice (Fricke & Gill, 1989) in that it engages the primary users in all stages of the process. The other feature is that rather than being the principal investigator, the evaluator acts as a coordinator of the project, with responsibility for technical support training and quality control and joint responsibility for conducting the inquiry. The evaluator becomes a partner in an evaluation process where all involved have a commitment to change. The partnership is such that it may develop over a long period of time and not for the duration for one project. It also means that the external contract evaluator is less likely to be co-opted or manipulated by managers in favor of their own agenda (Cousins & Earl, 1995; Mathison, 1994).

It is in the area of education that participatory evaluation has been used most extensively. Here it has also traditionally had an organizational focus, but a greater feature has been the emphasis on practitioners' becoming evaluators in order to become more reflexive and improve practice (O'Hara & McNamara, 2001). The focus is on the systematic collection of evidence as well as collaborative and collective inquiry, motivated by the quest to improve and understand the world by changing it. It focuses as well on learning how to improve practice from the effect of the changes made, particularly in the classroom but also in the whole school. This strand of influence is encapsulated in the notion of reflective practice.

These traditions of thought have influenced evaluation theory and practice in general as more participatory approaches have come to be adopted in a whole range of fields with relevance to community health promotion, including policy analysis, social work, and urban planning. A common factor in this trend has been an increasing concern for the variability in evaluation utilization as well as the failure to develop useful indicators emphasizing conventional approaches. Another concern has been the high failure rate of policy implementation in the public services. For example, a study of the evaluation of urban regeneration policies undertaken in the 1980s in the United States found considerable disillusionment with large-scale external evaluation studies using sophisticated methods (for example, mathematical modeling), often answering questions that were not actually asked. Rarely were the evaluation studies system- or concept-driven, and often they developed inappropriate indicators that were difficult to collect and failed to influence policy. As a consequence, participatory approaches to evaluation involving learning networks have been developed. At the same time, the demand for universal indicators has receded, and the emphasis is now on involving users and managers in developing local sensitive indicators, often of a "soft" type (Barnekov, Hart, & Benfer, 1990). In the United States, in this area at least, narrowly defined empirical evaluation is on the retreat, with a movement toward an eclectic mix of methods involving those who manage programs.

In the research and evaluation literature, a subtle and perhaps semantic distinction is made between participatory research (PR) and participatory evaluation (PE). Some consider PE just one aspect of the PR cycle (Israel, Checkoway, Schulz, & Zimmerman, 1994); others see it as a distinctive approach to evaluation. PE shares with PR the key principles of the active involvement of various parties in the actual work and in decisions about the evaluation process, requiring the continuous exchange of knowledge, skills, and resources (Cousins & Earl, 1995). Some analysts, however, contend that there is no difference between the two if participation takes place throughout a project cycle (Mikkelsen, 1995).

Advocates of participatory evaluation often emphasize the distinction between evaluation and research (Springett & Dugdill, 1995), as well as the distinction from PAR, which is seen as "explicitly normative and ideological in form and function" (Mathison, 1994). Participatory evaluation is linked directly to participative decision making (Cousins & Earl, 1995). Its distinctiveness is that it changes the relationship between the evaluated and the evaluator (Gustavsen, 1992; Hazen, 1994; Vanderplaat, 1995). Thus it explicitly challenges evaluation based on the authority of the outside observer and independent assessor. This it shares with PAR, which challenges the traditional scientific notion of an independent and objective researcher (Peile, 1994).

Given these nuances, it is not surprising that there is confusion among practitioners as to what PR and PE actually are, leading to wide variation in practice (Green et al., 1995). Wadsworth tried to resolve the dilemma and combined the two, calling for an action evaluation research process. The basics of that process are laid out in a visual model that forms a useful wall chart accompanying her practical book *Everyday Evaluation on the Run* (1991). This model, however, can be seen as an ideal to reach for rather than a reality; except in very few circumstances, it has yet been achieved. There are widespread variations in levels of participation, and most agendas are still being determined by a small group of people. Current practice is consultative at best, rather than truly participatory (Baum, 1995). Opinion in this debate, however, is dependent on ideological perspective and context. Those concerned with the evaluation of community based projects will be attracted to the ideology underpinning the Southern tradition of PR, which developed to empower the oppressed (see Chapter Two). In contrast, those evaluating organizationally based programs and policies will lay emphasis on participatory decision-making aspects of participatory evaluation.

It is important to emphasize the fundamental differences between participatory evaluation and conventional evaluation undertaken in the field of community health promotion (see Table 13.1). Evaluation in this field continues to be dominated by epidemiologists, demographers, and biomedics with a positivist way of viewing the world that contrasts with the hermeneutic perspective that underpins action research. Moreover, there are some examples of so-called participatory research into health that bear little relationship to the underlying ideological, methodological, and epistemological bases of PAR, reflecting the reappropriation by positivist science of the terminology (Couto, 1987; Dockery, 1996; Lawell, Noriega, Martinez, & Villegars, 1992). Participation is more than just taking part; it is about engaging in a dialogue at all stages of the process of evaluation and shifting the power in favor of those who are being researched. It is, as Vanderplaat (1995), puts it "evaluation for empowerment."

Table 13.1. Differences Between Conventional Evaluation and Participatory Evaluation.

	Conventional Evaluation	Participatory Evaluation
Who	External experts	Community, project staff facilitator
What	Predetermined indicators of success, primarily cost and health outcomes or gains	People identify their own indicators of success, which may include health outcomes and gains
How	Focus on "scientific objectivity," distancing evaluators from other participants; uniform, complex procedures; delayed, limited access to results	Self-evaluation; simple methods adapted to local culture; open, immediate sharing of results through local involvement in evaluation processes
When	Usually completion; sometimes also midterm	Merging of monitoring and evaluation; hence frequent small-scale evaluations
Why	Accountability, usually summative, to determine if funding continues	To empower local people to initiate, control, and take corrective action

Source: Adapted from PROWWESS, 1990.

Participatory evaluation focuses on knowledge creation in the context of practice and the development of local theory (Greenwood, Whyte, & Harkavy, 1993) and capacity building. Such a perspective is based on a completely different conception of the relationship between science, knowledge, learning, and action than is found in positivist methods in social science (Peile, 1994). It assumes that people can generate knowledge as partners in a systematic inquiry process based on their own categories and frameworks. This, it can be argued, enhances scientific validity, producing richer and more accurate data; creates active support for the results of the process of inquiry; and therefore creates greater commitment to change as well as the greater likelihood that ideas will be diffused. In traditional research, the emphasis is on theory creation and testing, while in traditional practice, the emphasis is on action. In participatory evaluation, the production of knowledge results from collaboration between insider-practitioner and outsider-evaluator. The resultant reflection acknowledges both personal and collective engagement (Gatenby & Humphries, 2000). The aim is to encourage change and learning as a self-generating and self-maintaining process that continues after the evaluator-researcher has left. The process itself is seen as an important a product as any evaluation report.

Although this approach is particularly appropriate to community based projects, it also has value for the other end of the spectrum, policy development and implementation (Winje & Hewell, 1992). It would appear to be an excellent vehicle for breaking down the boundaries between research and policy. No longer would the production of knowledge be retained in the hands of experts and lodged on the shelves of offices and libraries as interesting but not relevant to day-to-day practical problems of the here and now. Rather, by being involved in the evaluation process, policymakers would own both the ideas of the evaluation and its results. They would thus be ready to implement the appropriate action because it is already an innate part of their consciousness and because the process of doing the evaluation has already begun to change the way they act and what they believe. The key to this process is dialogue (Hazen, 1994). Creating situations in which thoughts are communicated and exchanged begins to shape a new social reality (Habermas, 1984). The role of the evaluator is to create those situations through various techniques such as workshops and allow the joint product, a more integrated and higher form of consciousness, to emerge from the interplay between the actors (Reason, 1988). A new set of social relations is created, and the new knowledge is the result of that process. The essence of this type of evaluation is that it is an emergent process controlled by local conditions (Wallerstein, 1999). It encourages innovation and change (Cranton, 1996). Traditional evaluation approaches can easily undermine innovation. As people become aware of being judged, they perform to satisfy the measurement chosen instead of improving capability. The intrinsic motivation that drives learning and creates change is replaced by a desire to provide numbers for bureaucrats (Henkel, 1991; Seddon, 2000).

The strength of participatory evaluation is that it integrates evaluation into project work or an intervention, allowing a more natural emerging and evolving approach to the development (Springett & Leavey, 1995). It is not outcome-driven. It is people-centered and potentially empowering. Traditional approaches to evaluation reinforce marginalization and social exclusion. Problems are often seen to be located in a particular community or ethnic group, and the evaluation often focuses exclusively on that community, rather than on the context in which that group operates (Goodman, Wheeler, & Lee, 1993). Little is done to probe the experience and assumptions of the organizations that are the source of disempowerment or to bring the two groups together in a dialogue concerning the problem, the program, and how its success or failure will be evaluated and against whose criteria. Similarly, little is done to change the power relationships so that excluded groups can have a say and take control of the factors that promote good health. The most appropriate type of evaluation, therefore, is one that involves enhancing this control (Vanderplaat, 1995). In other words, participatory evaluation is a health-promoting intervention in itself.

THE USE OF PARTICIPATORY EVALUATION IN COMMUNITY HEALTH PROMOTION

Currently, there are relatively few published sources relating specifically to the participatory evaluation of community health promotion and community based initiatives. This is not surprising, given the general lack of evaluation in the health promotion and community health development field and the paucity of outlets, until recently, for reporting this type of research. Added to this is the time taken to undertake this type of study and the time lag between completing an evaluation and the publication of the results in the literature, given the precedence of the demands from funding agencies for a report. The dominance and power of medicine in health and the consequent sanctity of the randomized controlled trial, traditional epidemiology, and the conventional scientific method are, however, major factors. Issues such as lack of scientific rigor and generalizability, validity of the results, and replicability are put forward against the approach, all perceived as stemming from a failure to be objective (Susman & Evered, 1978).

Issues that do not stem from this perspective also have an impact on the amount of participatory evaluation that takes place. These include the time it takes to undertake PE, the resources it involves, and the messiness of the process. Even if the process of evaluation has clear steps, its inherent messiness seems counter to the search for clarity, the need to control and be logical and plan. Furthermore, funders have difficulty funding such an unpredictable process and its indefinable outcomes (Maclure, 1990). Moreover, researchers often lack the skills required, and the community generally falls short in terms of critical thinking capacity (Fuerstein, 1988). In a policy context and where multifaceted health promotion programs are involved, the potential complexity of the process to be handled can be problematic (Costongs & Springett, 1997). All these barriers are reinforced by the tradition in health promotion of project evaluation being imposed from outside and often in ways that are inappropriate (Kennedy, 1995).

Nonetheless, the value of PAR and participatory approaches to research in health promotion is increasingly recognized, and the number of projects taking place using this approach is growing. The approach is increasing substantially in popularity in the areas of primary care and public health and health promotion in developing countries and in nursing research, particularly at the community level (Abbott & Duncan, 1993). In Canada, the federal government has supported the approach, including funding a major report (Green et al., 1995) and providing a tool for project workers through its Web site (see Appendix C).

In the United Kingdom, a number of current initiatives are supporting the development of participatory approaches. In Wales, the National Assembly is funding a five-year series of community based health initiatives using the participatory evaluation model as part of its SHARP program, providing support for communities and researchers as they struggle with the process (National Assembly, 2001). In England, the Health Development Agency has funded the SARP program, which has followed a participatory action research approach. Interestingly enough, this latter initiative tried to fit the PAR model into a more conventional research framework that was abandoned as the development process progressed in each of the chosen sites (Health Development Agency, 2002). In Scotland, participatory evaluation has been the core approach to the Action on Smoking community based program (McKie, 2001). This mushrooming of participatory approaches has been given added momentum by the development of "Health Action Zones." This government-funded program was introduced in 1999 to tackle the huge health inequalities in the UK. In common with all government programs, a national evaluation was initiated. The model adopted by the team was a participatory model incorporating theories of change as used by the Aspen Institute in the United States (Fulbright-Anderson, Kubisch, & Connell, 1999). Individual Health Action Zones—especially those that had their origins in Healthy Cities and Health for All projects—adopted participatory evaluation approaches locally. A few, including Merseyside and Wakefield, made participatory evaluation an explicit part of the local strategy, with support for training in the approach (Baud & Judge, 2002; Cropper, 2001).

In the United States, an increasing number of programs and projects have used participatory evaluation. Some of the major foundations, such as the W. K. Kellogg Foundation, have been instrumental in encouraging such an approach. Among those with a specific community health focus is the Adolescent Social Action Program in New Mexico (Wallerstein & Bernstein, 1994), which has sought to empower youth from high-risk populations to make healthier choices using Freire's (1973) three-stage methodology of listening, dialogue, and action. Another is the Partners for Improved Nutrition and Health project implemented in 1988, as a five-year collaborative program by Freedom from Hunger, the Mississippi State Department of Health and the Mississippi Cooperative Extension Agency. In this program, decisions on what to evaluate were grounded in the experiences and visions of people living and working in the three areas of the project (Eng & Parker, 1996).

Participatory evaluation has also been used in evaluating health promotion programs in the workplace, especially those developed to deal with stress (Israel, Schurman, & House, 1989). The studies that have used this approach have tended to be organizational rather than program based approaches to health promotion. The main argument used for such an approach is that so many changes can take place in such organizations (for example, layoffs and changes in product line and personnel, which can undermine the use of control and experimental groups) that an action research approach is fundamental.

In such studies, statistical control techniques have been used, as well as a time-series designs, demonstrating that participatory evaluation does not just mean qualitative techniques but rather the eclectic use of appropriate methods. Participation under such approaches, which include both action and intervention in the workplace setting, is limited by the culture of the organization. Evaluation projects can easily become associated with co-optation and manipulation rather than true participation (Baker, Israel, & Schurman, 1993).

Despite the inherent democratic nature of participatory evaluation, growth in the use of participatory methods has been less in the area of policy development. There have been some successful attempts, however. Bang and Bang (1991) contrasted the lack of impact on public health of a traditional epidemiological study of sickle-cell disease in the Gadchioli district of India with a PAR alcoholism prevention program in the same district. The latter approach led to collective action at both the local and state levels. A participatory evaluation approach to healthy public policy presents quite a challenge because of the inherent complexity. This is well illustrated by the development of an evaluation and monitoring framework and indicators for the City Health Plan in Liverpool (Springett, 1998). An attempt was made to satisfy a range of stakeholders while incorporating evaluation into the implementation process. The result is a pragmatic approach, which is the product of interplay between an ideal model and reality in a particular context.

ISSUES IN PARTICIPATORY EVALUATION IN COMMUNITY HEALTH PROMOTION

It is the assumption of this chapter that participatory evaluation is a cyclical process based on the action research cycle that consists of a series of steps that in turn involve a series of decisions in which all stakeholders participate (see Exhibit 13.1). These steps can be used as a checklist when engaging in the process, and there are now a wide range of toolboxes and manuals to help people through the process (see Chapter Eight). Although it can be argued that participatory evaluation is a process, not a technique, there are methodological issues involved that are concerned with how you engage in the process, ensure that it is systematic, and adhere to basic principles. A key focus, too, is the way you create opportunities for dialogue (Mathison, 1994). Many issues stem from the need to balance the requirements of participation; the use of appropriate, rigorous, verifiable, and valid tools and techniques; and the practical demands of the real world while retaining the values of social action (Hoggart, Jeffries, & Harrison, 1994). There is currently confusion among practitioners and others as to what true participatory evaluation is, with the result that there

Exhibit 13.1. Steps in Participatory Evaluation.

1. All those involved in the program decide jointly to use a participatory approach.

2. They decide exactly what the objectives of the evaluation are. This can turn out to be far harder than originally thought.

3. When agreement on objectives is reached, a small group of evaluation coordinators is elected to plan and organize the details of the evaluation.

4. The methods that are best for attaining the evaluation objectives are now chosen. The choice of method will also be influenced by the capabilities of the people involved and how much time and resources are available.

5. As these decisions are made, the written evaluation plan is formed, showing why, how, when, and where the evaluation will take place and who will be involved.

6. Next, the methods are prepared and tested. Selected participants will need training in such matters as interviewing, and all participants need explanations as to objectives and methods. The more they understand, the more they will participate when asked.

7. The methods, having been tested, are now used to collect facts and information.

8. The information is analyzed by participants, the major part being done by the coordinators.

9. The results are prepared in written, oral, or visual form.

10. Finally, program participants decide how the results will be used and how they can improve the effectiveness and performance of the program.

Source: Adapted from Fuerstein, 1988.

is considerable variation in practice. Since participatory evaluation is context-driven anyway, variation is to be expected to some degree. Nonetheless, a number of issues need to be overtly addressed when engaging in participatory evaluation.

The first issue concerns the level and nature of participation and the cyclical characteristics of that participation. It is a spiraling process rather than a series of static episodes. In practice, who participates is the product of the negotiated situation. While the ideal is total participation by all, who participates will be a product of the existing distribution of power and resources between the potential stakeholders, the time available to undertake the evaluation, and the resources available. Inevitably, difficult decisions will have to be made, since who participates will have an impact on both the process and the results of the evaluation (Greenwood, Whyte, & Harkavy, 1993).

Couto (1987) notes that the balancing act can have different outcomes in different contexts, and often in the health context, because of medical hegemony, it is likely that the balance will move in favor of traditional approaches. Participation may also change during the process. The larger the reach of a project, the more difficult it is to ensure a democratic process. A great deal of creativity is required to do this. Small-scale community based programs are thus easier to manage. In all cases, it is quite important to involve managers and funders in the process. Often managers will try to limit the extent of participation, preferring to exercise control. But sometimes they fail to see the need to be involved in the process and send representatives to workshops and meetings or fail to attend at all. This means that they may not accept or even understand the results at the end of the process.

The development of an indicator tool for evaluating multisectoral collaboration in the UK provides a good example of how the characteristics of those involved in the process have an impact on the outcome. The research involved two hundred people and was conducted in three stages. Stage 1 consisted of a telephone survey, conducted through the snowball technique to gain an overview of "Healthy Alliance work." This was followed by six workshops, involving representatives from Healthy Communities networks to generate definitions of the characteristics of Healthy Alliances and how success could be measured. The results were used to develop a process and outcome indicator pack. Stage 2 involved a refinement of the indicator pack through pilot testing at three test sites. Results were discussed in a workshop of twenty participants that included representatives on the purchaser side of the purchaser-provider divide in health care provision, after which the pack was modified (Furnell, Oldfield, & Speller, 1995). The resulting final pack reflected the views of the dominant group in the process, and since these were all practitioners, it was firmly based in experience.

There were several limitations, however. Opportunities for dialogue between the practitioner group and management decision makers and resource holders did not occur until the end of the process and then only to a limited extent, which meant that the pack did not include task and managerial indicators. Moreover, when tested in the three case study areas, the pack was found to be inappropriate for small-scale community based projects, particularly those in the early stages of development, and was criticized by community participants. Its main advantage was that the pack helped provide a framework for discussion of more locally based and relevant indicators. Despite these drawbacks, it was an unusually well funded attempt at being truly participatory in indicator development.

Another difficulty in this context is the rapid turnover of project managers and other staff. This can particularly be the case when you are dealing with a civil-service-type bureaucracy such as a government department. A recent evaluation of the potential for introducing more community participation in decision making in federal government policy on health and human service delivery in Australia noted the high turnover of career staff as a major barrier to change (F. Baum, personal communication). The facilitator of the evaluation needs to ensure that arenas for dialogue are created and there is feedback at every stage of the process. The facilitator also needs to be aware of the inequalities in power between the participants and take action to reduce it. Arenas for dialogue should be varied and include workshops and other interactive as well as formal meetings. The latter can sometimes act as a barrier to effective communication but are nonetheless necessary.

A second issue is the relationship between the evaluator and the evaluated and the balance between expert and lay involvement and particularly between insider and outsider evaluation. There are advantages and disadvantages on both sides (see Table 13.2). The use of an outside evaluator still carries the greatest credibility. At a minimum, an external evaluator can serve as facilitator at workshops, writer of the report, and quality controller. Both layperson and expert have something to offer. Indeed., the value of a participatory research approach is that it combines the technical expertise of the evaluator with the local knowledge of the lay participants so that the sum is greater than the parts. Tied up with this issue is the need to gain the commitment of busy professionals and the need to negotiate who owns the findings in the end. This is a particular problem for academics. The question arises in writing research papers

Table 13.2. Advantages and Disadvantages of External and Internal Evaluators.

External	Internal
Can take a fresh look at the program	Knows the program well
Not personally involved	Finds it hardest to be objective
Is not part of the normal power structure	Is part of the power and authority structure
Gains nothing from the programs but may gain prestige from the evaluation	May be motivated by hopes of personal gain
Trained in evaluation methods; may have experiences in other evaluations; regarded as an expert by the program	May not be trained in evaluation methods; has no more (or very little more) training than others in the program
An outsider who may not understand the program or the people involved	Is familiar with and understands the program and can interpret personal behavior and attitudes
An outsider who may not understand the program or the people involved	Known to the program, so poses no threat of anxiety or disruption; final recommendations may appear less threatening

Source: Adapted from Fuerstein, 1986.

as to who should be listed as authors on an academic publication when everyone has been involved. If any participant is excluded, this flies in the face of the ideology underpinning the concept and reinforces academic hegemony (Gaventa, 1993). All these issues need to be negotiated at the beginning and recorded in written agreements so that all participants are clear with respect to their roles and responsibilities.

The role of the external evaluator can change (Cohen, 2001), and as in any development project, there is a skill in knowing when to take a leadership, facilitative, or backseat role without disempowering participants. In one community-led participatory evaluation project in Salford, England, a researcher as part of the reflection process realized that in trying not to dominate the agenda and to allow the participants to drive the process, she had failed to realize that her expertise had an equal part to play in the process. Volunteers expressed frustration that she had not come forward in the early stages and filled a gap in their knowledge. Interestingly enough, in the same project, one participant withdrew from the process on the grounds that the decision makers would ignore the findings no matter how participatory the process (Young, 2001)!

Without a key facilitator, participants can sometimes get so carried away with the notion of having fun that evaluation can lack true critical reflection. Without some structure provided by an external facilitator, direction can be lost. Too often there is a tendency to lose sight of the bigger picture. In the Netherton Health Action Zone in England, for example, participants easily fell back into evaluating their own projects rather than looking for common themes across them (Springett & Dunkerton, 2001). Also, unless a special effort is made, there is no feedback loop into policy structures and decision making leading to broader changes in the policy context (Winje & Hewell, 1992).

Critical reflection also requires a safe environment as well as a certain degree of skill and honesty (Mezirow, 1990). Looking at what is wrong is often challenging in organizations that are experiencing difficulties, leading to defensive reactions that can undermine the participatory ethos (Levin, 1999). Ironically, the organizations that need to change most and could benefit from the approach are most often the most resistant. In these situations, people may refuse to participate at any stage of the process and managers may refuse to engage directly with staff. To ignore the emotional response to evaluation and to see it only as a technical event is to ignore a fundamental element of the human experience. The importance of the emotional response to decision making is beginning to be an acknowledged dimension in social science (Anderson & Smith, 2001; Dimasio, 1994).

Thus a third issue that needs to be faced is the inherent contradiction that is a feature of participatory evaluation's dialectical nature. Different agendas are being overtly brought together. This inevitably results in conflict and power struggles, since it is the creation of knowledge on its own battleground

(Rebien, 1996). Skills in conflict resolution therefore become as important for a good evaluator as knowledge of data collection and analysis techniques. Managing conflict becomes a necessary skill for a participatory evaluator, as does the ability to become pragmatic while trying to keep to the participatory evaluation ethos and principles. Evaluators have competing and often contradictory tasks to fulfill. For example, when evaluating health promotion policy and its implementation, on the one hand, the evaluation must be useful to the policy initiative itself. On the other hand, however, it has to be relevant to external interest groups and policymakers. The evaluator should be involved with the policy initiative in order to collaborate effectively with local workers, but at the same time he or she must keep enough distance to be critical and ask the right questions (Quellet, Durand, & Forget, 1994). Also, the evaluator must find the balance between the public's right to know and the individual's right to privacy and discretion (Greene, 1994). Therefore, a range of communication, negotiation, creativity, motivation, political, and facilitative skills is needed among evaluators. Long and Wilkinson (1984) have pointed out that evaluators must cope with complex social programs and personality conflicts in often difficult environments. Means and Smith (1988) found this when they involved stakeholders in their research into a regional alcohol education program in southwestern England.

In addition, evaluators should play a more active role in the policy-process (Greene, 1994); they must go beyond their evaluation to sell their ideas to policymakers (Ham, 1991). Simply publishing in journals is not enough. This is especially true with qualitative evaluations, which are often underread in comparison with the compact tables and summaries of quantitative work (Richardson, 1994). The evaluator has to present his or her ideas and recommendations clearly and attractively to make an impact. Ham (1991) remarks that communication and salesmanship must go hand in hand with good academic techniques if the evaluator wants to influence policy.

A fourth issue is the emergent nature of the process, which can have a number of effects. First, there is a feeling among funders and evaluators of a lack of control (Van Eyk, Baum, & Blandford, 2001). Participatory evaluation does not always fit into a neat project cycle, and funds can be cut off at crucial moments and reports not available on time. A committed project manager in the funding agency helps. Second, and particularly relevant to health promotion, is the fact that most projects are single-issue-based, reflecting the disease and lifestyle model that still dominates the sector. Thus projects have to be applied for on the basis of these diseases—for example, the prevention of coronary heart disease, the reduction of alcoholism, or smoking cessation. Yet the lay perspective is very different and reflects a more holistic approach to life. The outcomes of such projects may include issues such as raised self-worth and better quality of life while still retaining high levels of smoking. The aims and objectives that the participants in a project might see as important and the consequent outcomes may therefore be very different from the original aims and objectives. Moreover, with action and change being central, the whole project might move in a different direction. This again illustrates that it is vital that funders and the initiators of the evaluation be part of the process. Keeping the process going and ensuring communication and feedback at all stages of the process in an appropriate form are key. Attempting to achieve all these goals while engaged in participatory evaluation in a complex environment of different interest groups and multiple causes is understandably difficult (Costongs & Springett, 1997).

A fifth issue concerns funding. This form of evaluation is funded relatively poorly, compared to projects that adopt a more traditional paradigm. There is a general lack of expertise among funders, and their chief demand is for short-term task-oriented approaches to evaluation (Green et al., 1995). This is despite the value added through the potential for change that participation produces because the evaluation results are actually implemented. The evaluator is dependent for effective follow-through on a sympathetic funding project officer who understands the unpredictability of the process and is willing to go along with it. So forming a good relationship at the beginning is crucial.

The evaluator's task is frequently made more difficult by the fact that health promotion project workers only start to think about evaluation when the end of a project is in sight. That is too late for adopting a truly participatory evaluation approach and needs careful thought. An added problem is that health promotion is often poorly resourced to begin with. Some organizations and funders of projects, however, are now approving such projects only if a sum is allocated to evaluation. This is now done on health projects in Australia funded by a tax on tobacco.

A sixth issue is a more traditional methodological one that has a particular action research slant. It concerns choosing the appropriate tools and techniques both for data collection and for dissemination of results at each stage in the feedback cycle. Tools should be simple but effective, understandable but relevant. Often a community group may be forced to defend its findings before those trained in traditional epidemiology, as the Yellow Creek Concerned Citizens, working with the Highlander Center in Kentucky, did in the evaluation of the impact of waste dumping on health. This resulted in the use of quantitative methods using a "scientific" framework (Couto, 1987). The emphasis is on eclecticism and appropriateness (Baum, 1992; Everitt, 1996). Training almost certainly will be required and should be included in the budget. The aim is to create a process that is sustainable and leaves added knowledge at the end of the process. As is discussed in Chapter Nine, a health project undertaken in China used photographs as a form of data collection that provided a valuable and effective alternative to the graphs and data presentation methods demanded by decision makers who wanted concrete measures (Wang & Burris, 1994).

Often, however, the information gained from the evaluation process will have to be presented in more than one form, and this needs to be taken into account in the work plan. In both Nooralunga, Australia, and Drumchapel, Scotland, for example, a variety of methods including artwork were used for dissemination (Baum & Cook, 1990; Kennedy, 1995).

The final issue is that of empowerment. The use of participatory evaluation for evaluating community based programs stems directly from empowerment's playing a central role in community health promotion and community health development. The evaluation process itself is seen to play a role in empowerment and can contribute to the elimination of social inequality, the intended outcome of many projects. It openly addresses issues of power, bringing social action and community development methods to evaluation. It also makes explicit the values and interests that are inherent in evaluation, thus confronting the issue as to whose values the evaluation serves. It allows those values and interests to engage in democratic dialogue and in so doing creates new social knowledge (Barnes, 1993). Advantages arise in other ways as well. If people are involved in decision making, the results of any evaluation are more likely to be used. This, according to Patton (1982), is the strongest argument for participation, alongside avoidance of orthodoxy and the need to encourage the use of a range of methods and tools in data collection and analysis. Participation also creates in people a critical awareness of their problems, and this is seen as playing an important health promotion role in capacity building. In effect, the process is the creation of knowledge on its own battleground (Rahman, 1993).

There are benefits to be gained in the sharing of lay and expert knowledge, the pooling of resources, and the sharing of strengths. For example, if people are involved in decision making, they may even undertake the questionnaire survey themselves, thus reducing evaluation costs. Relevance is also important in bringing about sustainable behavioral and social change at the individual and community levels. As Pyle (1982) has suggested, "When long-term behavioral change, self-sustaining capacity and universal coverage is desired, community participation is essential" (p. 64).

The failure to ground evaluation indicators in the needs of local workers and their community led the people of Drumchapel to develop their own evaluation of their project. Disillusioned with the externally commissioned evaluation driven by the agenda of a university, they adopted a truly participatory approach, which enabled a whole range of innovative methods to be used. These included alternative ways of reporting the results through art and a video (Kennedy, 1995). The video made by the people explores the stories of the different community members and how the evaluation process enhanced their sense of self-worth and self-efficacy as well as their health.

There is great potential here. Just as participatory evaluation encourages empowerment within the community, which is one of the aims of health promotion, a collaborative problem-solving approach to evaluation in itself also encourages intersectoral collaboration. It forces those involved as project workers to make conscious choices on how to collaborate and reflect on practice (Clark, Baker, Chawla, & Maru, 1993). In Netherton, a deprived neighborhood in Merseyside, twelve separate projects, all aimed at some aspect of developing the community with funding from a variety of sources, were brought together to explore and develop their evaluation frameworks. Supported by a trainer and an academic, the process was so successful that the approach was incorporated in the development funding of a "regeneration" program for a much wider area. (Springett & Dunkerton, 2001). This was possible because local decision makers were actively encouraging a participatory evaluation approach. However, such an approach is not being encouraged by the regional government agencies who are responsible for overseeing the funding through top-down monitoring. How to incorporate empowerment through evaluation at the local level within the broader governmental and political system remains a key challenge. Even where it is supported by the political system, encouraging empowerment through participatory evaluation requires all parties involved to be constantly vigilant about how they relate to others. This means ensuring that the practice remains consistent with the rhetoric and underlying philosophy are truly antioppressive.

The use of participatory action research methods in evaluation in community health development is increasing, but there is a long way to go before it is as widely accepted as it is in areas such as education, management, and development work. The dominance of medical science, with its methods rooted in the natural sciences, is a major factor in the slow adoption of this potentially fruitful approach to change. The irony is that participatory evaluation is the central feature, although it is not named as such, of clinical audit. The review by Cornwall and Jewkes (1995) demonstrating the strong influence of development work on individuals working in primary health care and public health in developing countries, the Royal Society of Canada study (Green et al., 1995), the work of the Pan American Health Organization, and the work of the evaluators involved in Health Action Zones and other recent community based health initiatives in the UK should give a much needed impetus to the acceptance of this form of evaluation in the developed world, where the structural barriers to adoption appear greater than elsewhere.

For this to happen, there needs to be greater support for this type of approach through funding and more direct participation by policymakers themselves in evaluation. However, there is still a widespread need for skills training for researchers, practitioners, and policymakers. There needs to be recognition of the long-term and capability-building value of this type of approach and its contribution to knowledge development and effective change rather than the completion of specific and often inappropriate short-term tasks. It is important, too, to accept that a participatory approach is inherently and overtly political. In it lies the potential to affect the broader social structures that are the source of disempowerment (Papineau & Kiely, 1996). Ensuring that evaluation is participatory is fundamental to addressing the real accountability issue, which is accountability to the community groups whose health any health-promoting intervention should serve.

There is still a long way to go before so-called participatory evaluations are truly such; the majority still are controlled by the funders and evaluators and are more consultative than participatory. At its best, participatory evaluation provides a solution to the practical problem of crossing the boundaries between theory and practice and the competing cultures of research and policymaking. As an approach, it can be a real catalyst for change (Charles, Schalm, & Seredek, 1994; Ledwith, 1998). At the same time, it is profoundly challenging in its execution.

References

Abbott, K., & Duncan, S. (1993, January). Participatory research. *Canadian Nurse*, pp. 25–27.

Anderson, K., & Smith, S. J. (2001). Emotional geographies. *Transactions of the Institute of British Geographers, New Series, 26*(1), 7–10.

Argyris, C., & Schön, D. (1978). *Organizational learning: A theory of action perspective.* Reading, MA: Addison-Wesley.

Baker, E. A., Israel, B. A., & Schurman, S. J. (1993). A participatory approach to worksite health promotion. *Journal of Ambulatory Care Management, 17*(2): 68–81.

Bang, A. T., & Bang, R. A. (1991). Community participation in research and action against alcoholism. *World Health, 12,* 104–109.

Barnekov, T., Hart, D., & Benfer, W. (1990). *U.S. experience in evaluating urban regeneration.* Lanham, MD: Unipub.

Barnes, M. (1993). Introducing new stakeholders: User and researcher interests in evaluative research. *Policy and Politics, 21,* 47–58.

Baud, L., & Judge, K. (Eds.). (2002). *Learning from Health Action Zones.* London: Aeneas Press.

Baum, F. (1992). Research for Healthy Cities: Some experiences from Down Under. In E. de Leeuw, M. O'Neill, M. Goumans, & F. de Bruijn, F. (Eds.), *Healthy Cities research agenda: Proceedings of an expert panel* (pp. 45–54). RHC Monograph Series No. 2. Maastricht, Netherlands: University of Maastricht.

Baum, F. (1995). Research and policy to promote health: What's the relationship? In N. Bruce, J. Springett, J. Hodgkiss, & A. Scott Samuel (Eds.), *Research and change in urban community health* (pp. 11–31). Aldershot, England: Avebury.

Baum, F., & Cook, D. (1990). *Healthy Cities Nooralunga Project evaluation.* Adelaide: South Australian Community Health Research Unit.

Brown, L. D., & Tandon, R. (1983). Ideology and political economy in inquiry: Action research and participatory action research. *Journal of Applied Behavioral Science, 3,* 277–294.

Charles, C., Schalm, C., & Seredek, J. (1994). Involving stakeholders in health services research: Developing Alberta's resident classification system for long-term care facilities. *International Journal of Health Services, 24,* 749–761.

Clark, N. M., Baker, E. A., Chawla, A., & Maru, M. (1993). Sustaining collaborative problem solving: Strategies from a study of six Asian countries. *Health Education Research, Theory and Practice, 8,* 385–402.

Cohen, R. (2001, December 6). *Call in a doctor or a plumber? Participatory empowerment evaluation in a South London food project.* Paper presented at the annual meeting of the UK Evaluation Society, London.

Cornwall, A., & Jewkes, R. (1995). What is participatory research? *Social Science and Medicine, 41,* 1667–1676.

Costongs, C., & Springett, J. (1997). Toward a framework for the evaluation of health related policies in cities. *Evaluation, 3,* 345–362.

Cousins, J. B., & Earl, L. M. (Eds.). (1995). *Participatory evaluation in education: Studies in evaluation use and organisational learning.* Washington, DC: Falmer.

Couto, R. A. (1987). Participatory research: Methodology and critique. *Clinical Sociology Review, 5,* 83–90.

Cranton, P. (1996). *Professional development as transformative learning: New perspectives for teachers of adults.* San Francisco: Jossey-Bass.

Cropper, A. (2001). *Learning from change: An evaluation strategy for Merseyside Health Action Zone.* Liverpool, England: Merseyside Health Action Zone.

Dahlbom, B., & Mathiassen, L. (1993). *Computers in context: The philosophy and practice of systems design.* New York: Blackwell.

De Koning, K., & Martin, M. (Eds.). (1996). *Participatory research in health: Issues and experience.* London: Zed Books.

Dimasio, A. R. (1994). *Descartes' error: Emotion, reason, and the human brain.* New York: Putnam.

Dockery, G. (1996). Rhetoric or reality? Participatory research in the National Health Service, UK. In K. De Koning & M. Martin (Eds.), *Participatory research in health: Issues and experience* (2nd ed., pp. 164–175). London: Zed Books.

Eng, E., & Parker, E. A. (1994). Measuring community competence in the Mississippi Delta: The interface between program evaluation and empowerment. *Health Education Quarterly, 21,* 199–220.

Everitt, A. (1996). Values and evidence in evaluating community health. *Critical Public Health, 6*(3): 56–65.

Fetterman, D. M., Kaftarian, S. J., & Wandersman, A. (Eds.). (1996). *Empowerment evaluation: Knowledge and tools for self-assessment and accountability.* Thousand Oaks, CA: Sage.

Floch'hay, B., & Plottu, E. (1998). Democratic evaluation: From empowerment evaluation to public decision making. *Evaluation, 4,* 261–277.

Freire, P. (1973). *Education for critical consciousness.* New York: Seabury Press.

Fricke, J. G ., & Gill, R. (1989). Participative evaluation. *Canadian Journal of Program Evaluation, 4,* 11–25.

Fuerstein, M. T. (1986). *Partners in evaluation.* London: Macmillan.

Fuerstein, M. T. (1988). Finding methods to fit the people: Training for participatory evaluation. *Community Development Journal, 23,*16–25.

Fulbright-Anderson, K., Kubisch, A. C., & Connell, J. P. (1999). *New approaches to evaluating community initiatives: Vol. 2. Theory measurement and analysis.* Washington, DC: Aspen Institute.

Furnell, R., Oldfield, K., & Speller, V. (1995). *Toward healthier alliances: A tool for planning, evaluating, and developing healthier alliances.* London: Health Education Authority/Wessex Institute of Public Health Medicine.

Gatenby, B., & Humphries, M. (2000). Feminist participatory action research: Methodological and ethical issues. *Women's International Forum, 23,* 89–105.

Gaventa, J. (1993). The powerful, the powerless, and the experts: Knowledge struggles in an information age. In P. Park, M. Brydon-Miller, B. L. Hall, & T. Jackson (Eds.), *Voices of change: Participatory research in the United States and Canada* (pp. 21–40). Westport, CT: Bergin & Garvey.

Goodman, R. M., Wheeler, F. C., & Lee, P. R. (1993). Evaluation of the Heart to Heart project: Lessons from a community based chronic disease prevention program. *American Journal of Health Promotion, 9,* 443–455.

Green, L. W., George, M. A., Daniel, M., Frankish, C. J., Herbert, C. P., Bowie, W. R., & O'Neill, M. (1995). *Study of participatory research in health promotion: Review and recommendations for the development of participatory research in health promotion in Canada.* Vancouver, British Columbia: Royal Society of Canada.

Greene, J. C. (1994). Qualitative program evaluation, practice, and promise. In N. K. Denzin & Y. S. Lincoln (Eds.), *Handbook of qualitative research* (pp. 530–544). Thousand Oaks, CA: Sage.

Greenwood, D., Whyte, W. F., & Harkavy, I. (1993). Participatory action research as a process and as a goal. *Human Relations, 46,* 171–191.

Gustavsen, B. (1992). *Dialogue and development: Theory of communication, action research and the restructuring of working life.* Assen, Netherlands: Van Gorcum.

Habermas, J. (1984). *The theory of communicative action* (Vols. 1 and 2) (T. McCarthy, Trans.). Boston: Beacon Press.

Ham, C. (1991). Analysis of health policy: Principles and practice. *Scandinavian Journal of Social Medicine, 46*(Suppl.), 62–66.

Hazen, M. A. (1994). A radical humanist perspective of interorganizational relationships. *Human Relations, 47,* 393–415.

Health Development Agency. (2002). *Involving lay publics in developing Policies and services: Lessons from Salford SARP.* London: Author.

Henkel, M. (1991). The new evaluative state. *Public Administration, 69,* 121–136.

Hoggart, R., Jeffries, S., & Harrison, L. (1994). Reflexivity and uncertainty in the research process. *Policy and Politics, 22,* 59–70.

Israel, B. A, Checkoway, B., Schulz, A. J., & Zimmerman, M. A. (1994). Health education and community empowerment: Conceptualizing and measuring perceptions of individual, organizational, and community control. *Health Education Quarterly, 21,* 149–170.

Israel, B. A., Schurman, S. J., & House, J. S. (1989). Action research in occupational stress: Involving workers and researchers. *International Journal of Health Services, 19,* 135–155.

Kennedy, A. (1995). Measuring health for all: A feasibility study of a Glasgow community. In N. Bruce, J. Springett, J. Hodgkiss, & A. Scott Samuel (Eds.), *Research and change in urban community health* (pp. 199–217). Aldershot, England: Avebury.

Kolb, D. A. (1984). *Experiential learning: Experience as a source of learning and development.* Englewood Cliff, NJ: Prentice Hall.

Kroeger, A., & Franken, H. P. (1981). The educational value of participatory evaluation of primary health care programmes: An experience with four indigenous populations in Ecuador. *Social Science and Medicine, 15B,* 535–539.

Lawell, A. C., Noriega, M., Martinez, S., & Villegars, J. (1992). Participatory research on worker health. *Social Science and Medicine, 34,* 603–613.

Ledwith, M. (1998). *Participating in transformation: Towards a working model of community empowerment.* London: Venture Press.

Levin, R. (1999). Participatory evaluation researchers and service providers as collaborators versus adversaries. *Violence Against Women, 5,* 1213–1227.

Long, R. J., & Wilkinson, W. E. (1984, May). A theoretical framework for occupational health program evaluation. *Occupational Health Nursing,* pp. 257–259.

Macgillavray, A. (1998). Turning the sustainable corner: How to indicate right. In D. Warburton (Ed.), *Community and sustainable development: Participation in the future* (pp. 81–95). London: Earthscan.

Maclure, R. (1990). The challenge of participatory research and its implications for funding agencies. *International Journal of Sociology and Social Policy, 10,* 1–21.

Magerison, C. J. (1987). Integrating action research and action learning in organisational development. *Organisational Development,* pp. 88–91.

Mathison, S. (1994). Rethinking the evaluator role: Partnerships between organizations and evaluators. *Evaluation and Planning, 17,* 299–304.

McKie, L. (2001, December). *Developing a community resource on evaluation.* Paper presented at the annual meeting of the UK Evaluation Society, London.

Means, R., & Smith, R. (1988). Implementing a pluralistic approach to evaluation in health education. *Policy and Politics, 16,*17–28.

Mezirow, J. (Ed.). (1990). *Fostering critical reflection in adulthood: A guide to transformative and emancipatory learning.* San Francisco: Jossey-Bass.

Mikkelsen, B. (1995). *Methods for development work and research: A guide for practitioners.* Thousand Oaks, CA: Sage.

National Assembly for Wales. (2001). *Sustainable Health Action Research Programme* [http://www.hpw.wales.gov.uk/research/research_e.htm].

O'Hara, J., & McNamara, G. (2001). Process and product issues in the evaluation of school development planning. *Evaluation, 7,* 99–109.

Pan American Health Organization. (2001). *Report of the Healthy Municipality Meeting, Antigua, Guatemala.* Washington, DC: Author.

Papineau, D., & Kiely, M. (1996). Participatory evaluation in a community organization: Fostering stakeholder empowerment and utilization. *Evaluation and Program Planning, 19,* 79–93.

Patton, M. Q. (1982). *Practical evaluation.* Beverly Hills, CA: Sage.

Peile, C. (1994). Theory, practice, research: Casual acquaintances or a seamless whole? *Australian Social Work, 47*(2), 17–23.

PROWWESS. (1990). *Taking the pulse for community management in water and sanitation.* New York: United Nations Development Program.

Pyle, D. F. (1982). *Framework for the evaluation of health sector activities by private voluntary organizations receiving matching grants.* Washington, DC: Agency for International Development.

Quellet, F., Durand, D., & Forget, G. (1994). Preliminary results of an evaluation of three Healthy Cities initiatives in the Montreal area. *Health Promotion International, 9,* 153–159.

Rahman, M. A. (1993). *People's self-development: Perspectives on participatory action research.* London: Zed Books.

Reason, P. (Ed.). (1988). *Human inquiry in action: Developments in new paradigm research.* Newbury Park, CA: Sage.

Rebien, C. (1996). Participatory evaluation of development assistance. *Evaluation, 2,* 151–171.

Richardson, L. (1994). Writing: A method of inquiry . In N. K. Denzin & Y. S. Lincoln (Eds.), *Handbook of qualitative research* (pp. 516–529). Thousand Oaks, CA: Sage.

Robson, C. (2000). *Small-scale evaluation: Principles and practice.* Thousand Oaks, CA: Sage.

Rovers, R. (1986). The merging of participatory and analytical approaches to evaluation: Implications for nurses in primary health care programs. *Nursing Studies, 23,* 211–219.

Salmen, L. F. (1992). *Beneficiary assessment: An approach described.* Washington, DC: World Bank.

Sarri, R. C., & Sarri, C. M. (1992). Organizational and community change through participatory action research. *Administration in Social Work, 16,* 99–122.

Seddon, J. (2000, August 27). On target to nothing. *Observer,* p. 36.

Senge, P. M. (1990). *The fifth discipline: The art and practice of organizational learning.* New York: Doubleday.

Springett, J. (1998). Quality and effectiveness in evaluation of healthy cities. In J. K. Davies & G. MacDonald (Eds.), *Quality, evidence, and effectiveness in health promotion: Striving for certainties.* New York: Routledge.

Springett, J. (2001). Appropriate approaches for the evaluation of health promotion. *Critical Public Health, 11,* 139–151.

Springett, J., & Dugdill, L. (1995). Workplace health promotion programme: Towards a framework for evaluation. *Health Education Journal, 55,* 91–103.

Springett, J., & Dunkerton, L. (2001). *Evaluating together: Netherton Health Action Zone report.* Liverpool: Institute for Health, John Moores University.

Springett, J., & Leavey, C. (1995). Participatory action research: The development of a paradigm: Dilemmas and prospects. In N. Bruce, J. Springett, J. Hodgkiss, & A. Scott Samuel (Eds.), *Research and change in urban community health* (pp. 57–66). Aldershot, England: Avebury.

Springett, J., & Young, A. (2002). Comparing theories of change and participatory approaches to the evaluation of projects within Health Action Zones: Two views from the North West on engaging community level projects in evaluation. In L. Baud & K. Judge (Eds.), *Learning from Health Action Zones.* London: Aeneas Press.

Standish, M. (1995). A view from the tightrope: A working attempt to integrate research & evaluation with community development. In N. Bruce, J. Springett, J. Hodgkiss, & A. Scott Samuel (Eds.), *Research and change in urban community health* (pp. 259–262). Aldershot, England: Avebury.

Susman, G. I., & Evered, R. D. (1978). An assessment of the scientific merits of action research. *Administrative Science Quarterly, 23,* 582–602.

Vanderplaat, M. (1995). Beyond technique: Issues in evaluating for empowerment. *Evaluation, 1,* 81–96.

Van Eyk, H., Baum, F., & Blandford, J. (2001). Evaluating healthcare reform: The challenge of evaluating changing policy. *Evaluation, 7,* 487–503.

Wadsworth, Y. (1991). *Everyday evaluation on the run.* Melbourne, Australia: Action Research Issues.

Wallerstein, N. (1999). Power between evaluator and the community: Research relationships within New Mexico healthier communities. *Social Science and Medicine, 49,* 39–54.

Wallerstein, N., & Bernstein, E. (1994). Empowerment education: Friere's ideas adapted to health education. *Health Education Quarterly, 15,* 379–394.

Wang, C., & Burris, M. A. (1994). Empowerment through photo novella: Portraits of participation. *Health Promotion Quarterly, 21,* 171–196.

Weiss, C. H. (1988). Evaluation for decisions: Is there anybody there? Does anybody care? *Education Practice, 9,* 15–20.

Winje, G., & Hewell, H. (1992). Influencing public health policy through action research. *Journal of Drug Issues, 22,* 169–178.

World Health Organization. (1998). *Health promotion evaluation: Recommendations to policymakers.* Copenhagen, Denmark: Author.

Young, A. (2001). *The PEG report.* Salford, England: Institute for Public Health Research and Policy/Salford University Press.

PART FIVE

COMMUNITY BASED PARTICIPATORY RESEARCH WITH AND BY DIVERSE POPULATIONS

A s Lawrence Green and Shawna Mercer (2001) have pointed out, most community based participatory research has tended to take place in and with communities of color. Both the origins of participatory research in Third World nations (see Chapters One and Two) and its commitment to "involving oppressed people in the analysis of and solution to social problems" (Yeich & Levine, 1992, p. 1895) make such a focus a logical and important one. Yet as discussed in earlier chapters, because the initiators of CBPR efforts are often members of more privileged groups (Couto, 1987; Reason, 1994), issues of power and conflict can arise in cross-cultural CBPR.

In Part Five, we present three case studies that explore in more detail collaborative research across class, racial or ethnic, and gender identity divides. In Chapter Fourteen, Amy Schulz and her community and university partners describe and analyze the East Side Village Health Worker Partnership in Detroit, Michigan, and its efforts to actively engage neighborhood women as lay health workers and CBPR participants in their community. Grounding their analysis in both feminist and CBPR principles, the authors describe the strong accent placed on cultural sensitivity and respect and on addressing such "real world" barriers as health problems and lack of transportation and child care that can significantly constrain local women's ability to participate. The authors also stress throughout, however, the strong emphasis the project placed on identifying and building on the women's individual and collective strengths and the contributions of this strength-based perspective throughout the research process.

In Chapter Fifteen, we explore the special challenges involved in conducting a CBPR effort with and by young people. Preparing to examine the work with Cambodian girls undertaken by Asian Pacific Islanders for Reproductive Health (APIRH), Ann Cheatam and Eveline Shen describe the extensive social support work and community building that was necessary to give the effort a chance to succeed. The role of Freirian theory, feminist principles, and concepts from community building and community organizing in APIRH's approach to CBPR are clearly articulated, as are the ethical and practical problems faced in working collaboratively with youth of color. The chapter graphically illustrates how problem-posing dialogue and tools such as Arnold and colleagues' "power flower" (1991) can be used to help youth explore dimensions of power and powerlessness in their own lives, identify a collective issue, collect data, and use the findings to bring about institution-level changes to address their concerns.

A growing body of collaborative and participatory research has been conducted in and with the gay, lesbian, and bisexual communities, much of it focused on the problem of HIV/AIDS (Sanstad, Stall, & Doll, 1999). In Chapter Sixteen, however, we are introduced to the first CBPR project specifically designed to uncover the nature and prevalence of problems such as HIV in one of the nation's most highly stigmatized groups—the transgender population. Using as a conceptual framework the CBPR principles outlined by Barbara Israel and colleagues (Israel, Schulz, Parker, & Becker, 1998), Kristen Clements and Ari Bachrach explore how a high-quality epidemiologic study not only involved members of this hidden population throughout the research process but also depended on its members' extensive involvement for success. The San Francisco Transgender Community Health Project documented very high levels of HIV/AIDS, depression, suicide attempts and other health and social problems in this extremely marginalized population. But it also clearly demonstrated community strengths, epitomized in the central role community members of the research team played in achieving changes in policy and practice. As noted in Chapter Sixteen, this study led to changes in the way data are reported so that transgender people are no longer an invisible part of the population. It also helped pressure the health department to cover sexual reassignment surgery, setting the stage for other health care providers to follow suit. And in a particularly important development since the writing of this chapter, the study led the powerful American Medical Association to seek the help of the San Francisco Health Department in its forthcoming resolution on how to more sensitively handle the health care needs of transgender people (K. Clements, personal communication, 2002).

References

Arnold, R., Burke, B., James, C., Martin, D., & Thomas, B. (1991). *Educating for a change.* Toronto: Between the Lines Press.

Couto, R. (1987). Participatory research: Methodology and critique. *Clinical Sociology Review, 5,* 83–90.

Green, L. W., & Mercer, S. (2001). Can public health researchers and agencies reconcile the push from funding bodies and the pull from communities? *American Journal of Public Health, 91,* 1926–1929.

Israel, B. A., Schulz, A. J., Parker, E. A., & Becker, A. B. (1998). Review of community-based research: Assessing partnership approaches to improve public health. *Annual Review of Public Health, 19,* 173–202.

Reason, P. (Ed.). (1994). *Participation in human inquiry.* Thousand Oaks, CA: Sage.

Sanstad, K. H., Stall, R., & Doll, L. S. (Eds.). (1999). Collaborative community research partnerships between research and practice [Special issue]. *Health Education and Behavior, 26*(2).

Yeich, S., & Levine, R. (1992). Participatory research's contribution to a conceptualization of empowerment. *Journal of Applied Psychology, 24,* 1894–1908.

CHAPTER FOURTEEN

Engaging Women in Community Based Participatory Research for Health

The East Side Village Health Worker Partnership

Amy J. Schulz
Barbara A. Israel
Edith A. Parker
Murlisa Lockett
Yolanda R. Hill
Rochelle Wills

*It's not enough to come into a community and do research. The community is
not about research—that's a university or academic perspective. The community
is about solving problems or challenges that it's facing. . . . The research can
aid in that process, so as much as possible, we have to push beyond
the research.*
—Zachary Rowe, member, East Side Village Health Worker Steering Committee

Note: Portions of this chapter were adapted from "Community Based Participatory Research: Integrating Research with Action to Reduce Health Disparities," by A. J. Schulz, B. A. Israel, E. A. Parker, M. Lockett, Y. R. Hill, and R. Wills, *Public Health Reports*, vol. 117. Copyright © 2002 by Oxford University Press. Adapted with permission of the publisher.

The authors wish to acknowledge the contributions of the East Side Village Health Worker Partnership. The Partnership is made up of community members who are Village Health Workers, as well as representatives from the Butzel Family Center, Detroit Health Department, East Side Parish Nurses, Friends of Parkside, Henry Ford Health System, Islandview Development Coalition, Kettering/Butzel Health Initiative, University of Michigan School of Public Health, and Warren Conner Development Coalition. It is a project of the Detroit Community-Academic Urban Research Center and is funded by the Centers for Disease Control and Prevention. The research reported here was supported in part through a cooperative agreement with the Centers for Disease Control and Prevention, Grant No. U48/CCU515775. The authors thank Sue Andersen for her contributions to the preparation of this manuscript and Adam Becker, Juliana van Olphen, and Stephanie Ann Farquhar for assistance with data collection and analysis.

293

A mong the most persistent challenges to the public's health are those linked to racial and socioeconomic inequalities. These challenges are readily apparent in urban census tracts with the highest concentrations of poverty, where residents are disproportionately members of labeled racial or ethnic groups (Jargowsky, 1999; Massey & Denton, 1993), with mortality rates substantially higher than those of the country as a whole (Collins & Williams, 1999; Freudenberg, 1998; Geronimus, Bound, & Waidmann, 1999; House et al., 2000). Community based partnerships have emerged as one mechanism through which community members and public health professionals can work together to identify and implement actions to improve health. Ideally, this is done by combining the knowledge base and skills of public health researchers and practitioners with community residents' in-depth understanding of their communities and the resources within them, as well as their skills in community building. Advocates of community based participatory approaches within public health have argued that such approaches have the potential to enhance the quality, relevance, and application of research and interventions to more effectively address community-identified needs (Baker, Homan, Schonhoff, & Kreuter, 1999; Green et al., 1995; Hatch, Moss, Saran, Presley-Cantrell, & Mallory, 1993; Israel et al., 1998).

Challenges and potential benefits of community based participatory research approaches in public health have been explored elsewhere in the literature (Green et al., 1995; Israel et al., 1998; Lantz, Viruell-Fuentes, Israel, Softley, & Guzman, 2001; Northridge et al., 2000). Similarly, a considerable literature has examined women's participation and influence within their communities, as well as the ongoing challenges, tensions, and dilemmas that arise in those efforts, particularly when those efforts involve collaboration across power differentials commonly associated with race, gender, or class (Collins, 1990, 1991; Gilkes, 1988; Gutierrez & Lewis, 1999; Lugones & Spelman, 1983). However, relatively little attention in the literature has been focused specifically on the experience of African American women as they engage in community based participatory research efforts in their communities.

In this chapter, we draw on the experience of Village Health Workers to examine a series of questions related to the experience of women who become involved with community based participatory research in their communities. Specifically, we ask, What brings women to participate in a CBPR effort such as the East Side Village Health Worker Partnership? What challenges do they encounter in the course of their participation? And how has the partnership attempted to recognize and grapple with those challenges, for example, to address inequalities of power and resources? Our aim in the following discussion is to enhance our understanding of challenges women encounter as well as to offer some suggestions for addressing those challenges in community based participatory research partnerships.

BACKGROUND

Following a brief review of the literature on challenges and motivations of women community residents who are engaged in their communities, we provide background on the East Side Village Health Worker Partnership and its work to address social determinants of health on Detroit's East Side.

Literature Review

As noted in earlier chapters, community based participatory research involves the integration of research and action for community change and has roots in participatory research and critical and liberatory schools of social science (Maguire, 1990, 2001; Park, 1993; Stoecker & Bonacich, 1992). Participatory forms of research are grounded in critical social science theories that challenge the assumptions of objectivity and value neutrality in Cartesian social science, arguing instead that knowledge is shaped by *who* participates and *how* in the process of creating knowledge (Hall, 1975). Proponents of participatory forms of research suggest that the active engagement of those who will be affected by the research is necessary in order to challenge power differentials that currently exclude some from the process of creating knowledge (Stoecker & Bonacich, 1992). Participatory forms of research are also grounded in the assumption that knowledge that is connected to people's lived experience is more readily translated into action than knowledge that is disconnected from practice (International Council for Adult Education, 1980). The integration of research and action in participatory research is generally described as occurring through a cyclical and overlapping process involving data collection, analysis, critical interpretation, definition and implementation of action steps, and evaluation and refinement of those actions (Israel et al., 1998).

A number of challenges faced by members of community based participatory research efforts have been discussed in the literature (see, for example, Green et al., 1995; Hatch et al., 1993; Israel et al., 1998). These challenges include differing emphases on task and process, differing perspectives and priorities, the time-consuming nature of participatory processes, conflicts over funding, lack of trust and respect, and inequalities in power and access to resources. These challenges are often related to the differing social locations and experiences that members bring to their partnership efforts—for example, as representatives from academic institutions, community based organizations, health service providers, or community residents.

Yet relatively little has been written about the challenges or the motivations and potential rewards for community residents who engage in community based participatory research efforts, particularly women, who are often major players in such partnerships. A considerable body of literature examines challenges confronted by women as they engage in community-building and social change efforts, yet that literature is seldom invoked in writing about community based participatory research (see Maguire, 2001). The literature on, for example, African American women's engagement in community and social change efforts identifies challenges such as women's multiple obligations and competing demands of family, work, and community (Collins, 1990); working in both formal and informal systems of relationships (Collins, 1990, 1991; Gilkes, 1988; Morgen & Bookman, 1988); finding or creating spaces within which to share experiences and develop a shared vision of change (Collins, 1990); the implications of multiple oppressions for access to resources and power (Dill & Baca Zinn, 1997; Gutierrez & Lewis, 1999); and challenges associated with both transforming and re-creating relationships of power through community engagement (Ramirez-Valles, 1999; Schulz, Parker, Israel, & Fisher, 2001). Furthermore, feminist literature has been at the forefront in efforts to understand the implications of interlocking identities, examining, for example, the implications of the intersections of race, class, and gender in shaping women's experience (Collins, 1991; Crenshaw, 1995; Maguire, 1990, 2001).

Thus while recognizing that categories such as "women" or even "African American women" may capture some commonalities in perspectives, lived experience, and access to power and privilege, feminist writers have repeatedly pointed to the ways that the categories themselves oversimplify the complexity of experience and identities, obscuring differences among women (Crenshaw, 1995; Lugones & Spelman, 1983). For example, the title of this chapter, "Engaging Women in Community Based Participatory Research," suggests that there is a relatively homogeneous group—"women"—about whose engagement we can write. However, women as well as men from a variety of social backgrounds have been involved with the partnership from its inception, from East Side neighborhoods, academic institutions, community based organizations, and health service providers. Three of the coauthors of this chapter are residents of Detroit (two reside on the East Side); two are representatives from a health practice organization in Detroit; one is a Village Health Worker; three are representatives from an academic institution; three identify as African American, three as white; three are mothers; all are daughters. The overlap among these categories (for example, daughter and researcher, community member and health service employee) begins to illustrate the overlapping nature of identities and to disrupt overly simplistic attempts at categorization; they challenge the notion that there is a unified, homogeneous "woman's experience."

We have narrowed the focus in this chapter to Village Health Workers— women who are residents of Detroit's East Side, the majority (93 percent) of whom identify as African American and who share a history of active engagement in and commitment to their communities. Village Health Workers differ in religious background (Catholic, Protestant, Muslim), political affiliation, age (from their twenties to eighty years of age), educational histories (less than high school to college graduates), and economic circumstances. These differing backgrounds shape their social position within their communities and in relation to the partnership. Despite these differences, some common themes arise as Village Health Workers describe their involvement in the partnership and offer insights into the experiences of VHWs as members of the partnership. Before turning to a discussion of those themes, we offer a brief chronology of the partnership and the community based participatory research process in which we have been involved.

East Side Village Health Worker Partnership Research and Action Process

The East Side Village Health Worker Partnership (ESVHWP) is a community based participatory research partnership that uses a lay health adviser model to address social determinants of health on Detroit's East Side (Parker, Schulz, Israel, & Hollis, 1998). It is a project of the Centers for Disease Control and Prevention–funded Detroit Community-Academic Urban Research Center (Israel et al., 2001; Lantz et al., 2001). The CBPR principles that guide the work of the partnership emphasize the integration of research and intervention as well as the active participation and influence of community partners in all major phases of both the research and the intervention aspects of the partnership (see Chapter Three). This model of research and action brings together participants who represent a variety of perspectives and experiences to identify shared concerns and to plan, implement, and evaluate actions taken to address those concerns (Hatch et al., 1993; Israel et al., 1998; Stoecker & Bonacich, 1992).

The structure and the process of the ESVHWP build on the many resources that exist within the city of Detroit. For example, the work of the partnership is guided by a steering committee made up of Village Health Workers (community residents), representatives from community based organizations (including a local family center, a faith based nurses' organization, and a neighborhood coalition), health service providers, and academic institutions. Each of these brings unique resources and perspectives to the work of the partnership. In addition, fifty-six community residents have joined the partnership as Village Health Workers, of whom fifty-one (91 percent) are women.

The purpose of the partnership is to mobilize resources to address social factors that affect the health of East Side residents. The active engagement of residents of Detroit's East Side and the integration of their own knowledge of their communities with information contributed through more academic forms of research are central to this process. When the partnership began in 1996, the steering committee worked for six months to refine the research questions, evaluation design, and data collection methods (see Schulz et al., 1998, 2002c). As the steering committee developed the research and evaluation questions, it sought to identify strengths and resources as well as risk factors affecting the health of community residents.

During this time, the steering committee also focused on identifying and recruiting Village Health Workers. The first cohort of Village Health Workers joined the ESVHWP after the steering committee had been working for nine months, shortly before data from the community survey became available. The survey results were analyzed by academic partners and discussed by the VHWs and the steering committee as a whole. Themes identified in the analysis of in-depth interviews with Village Health Workers and steering committee members conducted as part of the evaluation of the partnership were later presented to and discussed by partnership staff, steering committee members, and Village Health Workers at monthly partnership meetings.[1] In addition, these results were examined as part of discussions and long-range planning activities at annual ESVHWP retreats, long-range planning workshops, and other ESVHWP events. Further analysis, interpretation, and integration of findings into partnership activities continues to occur through discussions that ensue in the process of working together to develop presentations and publications. For example, the process of writing this chapter was an opportunity for the coauthors to critically examine aspects of our process and their implications, contributing to an ongoing process of co-learning.

The processes just described illustrate the engagement of community partners in the research process, with steering committee members involved in the initial definition of the research and evaluation questions and the design of the research instruments. As Village Health Workers joined the partnership, they shaped later revisions of the research and evaluation (for example, the revised survey instrument used in a follow-up survey conducted in 2001). Similarly, while members of the steering committee were actively engaged in planning the survey data collection process and in identifying community members who became interviewers for the community survey, the steering committee members did not conduct the interviews themselves. Academic partners were responsible for preliminary analysis of the survey data and for bringing those results back to the steering committee and the Village Health Workers (who by that point had joined the partnership) for interpretation and discussion. Similarly, academic partners conducted the in-depth interviews with VHWs and steering committee members and then presented preliminary coded results to those members of the ESVHWP for discussion, interpretation, and application to the partnership's efforts. These presentations offered opportunities for co-learning among members of the partnership, as well as integration of the knowledge generated through the research and evaluation into the action components of the partnership. Thus while community partners were engaged in the research, they were engaged in different ways at different points. Not all community partners were involved in every stage of that process. The emphasis was on the engagement of community partners in shaping the research questions, determining how those questions would be asked, and interpreting the results and integrating them into the action components of the partnership. In the next section, we examine these processes in light of what Village Health Workers say about their reasons for being involved in the partnership.

"I'M NOT THE ONLY ONE OUT HERE TRYING TO STRUGGLE": BECOMING A VILLAGE HEALTH WORKER

What is it that motivates women with multiple commitments, with limited time and resources, to become and remain involved with a community based participatory research effort such as the ESVHWP? Central to community based participatory research is an understanding that all partners come with particular motivations, interests, and reasons for being around the table. Developing an understanding of what brings community women to the partnership and their reasons for remaining engaged is an important aspect of building partnerships enriched by members' intimate knowledge of their communities. As Village Health Workers describe their participation in the ESVHWP, they offer insights into their decision to become and remain involved in the partnership. As suggested by the quote with which this chapter begins, those motivations do not have to do with research per se but are centered around the desire to be actively engaged in creating solutions to challenges within their communities. Village Health Workers' descriptions of what brought them to the partnership and what kept them engaged emphasize their desire to address concrete challenges within their communities.

Village Health Workers frequently described opportunities offered within the Partnership to develop new skills and expand their base of knowledge. For example, Janelle[2] described the staff involved with the project as "just a walking resource book! They've always got answers to the personal part of your being." And Teresa said, "[The training] has helped to find the leaders who want to show leadership, show a change in their block, to formulate a block club, and how to go talk to your police commanders in your precinct. . . . These are some of the things that the training has helped me with—they gave me a lot of tangible skills." The type of knowledge described in these examples is knowledge that supports their community efforts, facilitates leadership development, and enhances skills in working with community systems and organizations. Such knowledge contributes to VHWs' individual and collective problem-solving capacity, one important dimension of community empowerment (Eng & Parker, 1994; Wallerstein, 1992).

Village Health Workers also valued the partnership for bringing together community members committed to their neighborhoods. Anita described other Village Health Workers, saying, "They're so resourceful and friendly. . . . When

I come [to the meetings], I get so much knowledge from these people. I sit back and listen to everything they have to say because they are such a resource base." Black feminist writers have described the critical importance of spaces within which African American women can come together, as well as the importance of the relationships that women develop among themselves within those spaces, as aspects of empowerment (Collins, 1990; Giddings, 1988; Gilkes, 1988). Both the spaces and the relationships that develop within them provide opportunities to exchange information, to share challenges as well as strengths and resources, and thus not only to see the skills and talents of others but also to recognize them in themselves. For example, Carmen noted, "[The training] let us know that we were all capable. We all had talents, you know. Like [the trainer] said . . ., 'You *do* have something to offer the community.'" For residents who often hear about the "deficits" of their community, opportunities to focus on the talents, skills, and resources within it, including themselves, can contribute to both personal and community empowerment.

Village Health Workers identified support from other Village Health Workers, as well as from friends and family, as another important aspect of their active engagement within the partnership. For example, Melina noted that the children in her neighborhood "come to see if I'm doing anything within the community. [They ask,] 'Do you have any flyers to pass out?' They get on their bikes, and they will run around and put the flyers in the mailbox or on the car." Others focused on the importance of the support that they received from each other. For example, Tenecia said, "You become just more than Village Health Workers. There's sort of a sisterhood that you develop among the women." This support took concrete and tangible forms, as when Ariel noted, "The Village Health Workers have been there for me—about maybe ten or fifteen showed up for the community party, and about four or five for the prayer breakfast" (two community events this VHW had organized). Other Village Health Workers felt supported simply through the knowledge that others were also working on issues of shared concern. For example, "You know, you sit there and you go, 'Hey, I'm not the only one out here trying to struggle.' You know they [other VHWs] are too, and you feel really great that everyone in that meeting is doing something to help." This knowledge often translated into increased confidence in community efforts, as noted by Nora: "I really do more than probably what I used to, and because I have you all to back me up. Because I say, 'I know if I don't know [the answer to a question], I can call somebody and I can actually get the information. . . .' That helps my self-esteem and my ability to talk to anybody out there in the street."

The sense that by working together with the partnership they could do more than they could as individuals, the opportunity to come together to talk and think about their communities and strategies for change, and the support that women provided and received in that process are key aspects of community or collective empowerment (Gutierrez & Lewis, 1999; Israel, Checkoway, Schulz, & Zimmerman, 1994; Kieffer, 1984; Wallerstein, 1992). For many Village Health Workers, the belief that collectively they could make a difference supported their continued engagement (see Schultz, Israel, Parker, & Becker, 2002a) even in the face of challenges. Notably absent from their descriptions of why they became or remained involved with the ESVHWP was anything related to formal research. Rather, Village Health Workers emphasized that they were engaged because of the intervention aspect of the partnership, which they felt supported their efforts to address real, everyday issues and concerns within their communities. As indicated by the quote at the beginning of this chapter, the research was useful to the extent that it contributed toward that end.

ADDRESSING DILEMMAS AND CHALLENGES OF PARTICIPATION IN COMMUNITY BASED PARTICIPATORY RESEARCH

The opportunity to bring one's own strengths and resources to a collective and to work together to address community concerns was, as we have seen, central to the women's engagement as Village Health Workers. But building collaborative relationships, those in which members share a common vision, work together, and support each other in the process of moving toward that vision, also bring a set of challenges and dilemmas. Village Health Workers described challenges associated with time and multiple commitments; women's own health concerns, as well as those of their families; limited resources and influence to tackle the underlying social inequalities that contribute to health concerns within their communities; building mutual support; mistrust of research; and differing agendas and priorities among members of the partnership. As we describe each of these challenges, we also discuss actions taken by the partnership to address them—some of which have been more successful than others.

Time and Multiple Commitments

Village Health Workers repeatedly voiced challenges related to time and multiple commitments. Women who become involved as Village Health Workers, often recruited specifically because they are known as trusted individuals to whom others in their community turn for support (Eng & Parker, 2002; Service, Salber, & Jackson, 1979), frequently have multiple community as well as family commitments. One VHW noted that "it's not easy for me to go to a lot of things that they have because I have children. And to drag [the] kids is too hard." It is not unusual for VHWs to arrive at the monthly ESVHWP meetings with children they have just picked up from after-school activities and to leave early in order to make it to another community meeting later that evening.

Women's multiple commitments—to work, family, and community—present challenges but also position women within multiple interlocking systems, disrupting the dichotomies often used to characterize women's activism (for example, the public realm of work and politics and the private realm of the family) (Collins, 1990; Gilkes, 1988).

In recognition of these multiple commitments, children are welcomed at VHW monthly meetings, and food is always offered for both children and their parents who attend meetings. The partnership has attempted to provide supervised activities for children whose parents are attending VHW meetings or events. In reality, however, that support has been sporadic. Most recently, with the support of the a local coalition, one of the members of the steering committee, a young adult from the East Side, has been available during VHW monthly meetings to supervise young people who attend with their parents. At the request of the VHWs, meetings are scheduled in the early evening to facilitate attendance by those who work days and who have family and other responsibilities in the evening. Many VHWS are involved with other community activities, so decisions about which nights to hold meetings are made collectively, with an eye toward avoiding nights when there are other regularly scheduled community meetings. Finally, VHW meetings are always scheduled on the same night (fourth Tuesday of each month) to facilitate regular participation by VHWs.

Efforts are also made to make the best use of the time that the VHWs spend together during their monthly meetings. As noted earlier, VHWs value the monthly meetings as opportunities to meet and talk with each other, learn about each other's activities, exchange information and mutual support (with each other and with the project coordinator), plan collective activities, and improve their knowledge and skills. The project coordinator has worked to structure and restructure meeting agendas to address these diverse priorities. The current meeting structure begins with food, informal conversation, and announcements by VHWs of upcoming community events or activities, allowing time for mutual support and informational exchange among the VHWs. A formal business meeting follows, with agenda items related to overall partnership business and events. Most meetings include informational presentations or speakers on topics of interest and relevance to the work of the VHWs or else time for VHWs to meet in "action groups" (to be described in more detail shortly) to plan intervention efforts. Maintaining a balance between structured time and flexibility to meet newly emergent agendas and recognizing the multiple commitments and other life events that constrain the amount of time VHWs are available are ongoing challenges.

Health Concerns

Among the other life events that influence VHWs participation are health problems. For residents of Detroit's East Side, health disparities are far from an abstract or academic concept. They are visible in the high rates of diabetes, hypertension, arthritis, and other chronic conditions among East Side residents and appear with stunning clarity in the lives of the Village Health Workers. One VHW described her own sporadic attendance at partnership meetings over an extended period of time due to health problems, saying, "To be flat on my back and not able to do things—even though it's been two years—it's still something that I can't admit . . . because I'm used to being very active."

In addition to their own health problems, Village Health Workers are often called on to care for mothers, fathers, aunts, uncles, cousins, sisters, brothers, children, grandchildren, and other members of their social networks. One Village Health Worker was the primary caretaker for her husband through his protracted terminal illness and was unable to participate regularly in VHW activities for some time. Making a rare appearance at a VHW event, she said, "[Another Village Health Worker] stopped by to give me a ride" to the meeting and noted that the same VHW also checked in on her frequently to see if she needed anything. Health problems frequently shaped women's day-to-day lives and their ability to participate in the partnership. But they also shaped VHWs' commitment to address the underlying social factors that affect health in their communities. Despite—or perhaps because of—the health challenges they confronted on a regular basis, they found or made the time to participate in the partnership. The support that Village Health Workers offered each other often enabled them to remain involved in community activities when faced with their own health challenges and those of family members.

Limited Resources and Influence

Challenges related to limited resources and influence arise in the context of discussions about the partnership and in discussions about the VHWs' efforts to address the underlying social conditions that affect health in their communities. Challenges voiced by VHWs related to their own ability to influence the direction of the partnership were regularly fed back to the project coordinator and to the steering committee and raised for discussion at monthly VHW meetings. Furthermore, the partnership worked to create structures through which VHWs could influence decisions made by the partnership—for example, two VHWs are selected by their peers as representatives to the steering committee, VHWs are members of subcommittees created to move forward specific agendas within the partnership, and major decisions affecting the partnership are discussed at VHW meetings to gain input before those decisions are made.

The nature and number of health concerns in this community are sometimes overwhelming, and the social and economic processes that underlie those health problems are a challenge for the VHWs, as well as for the partnership as a whole. For example, Thelma, describing the limited financial and human resources available to the partnership, noted, "One of the weaknesses is that we just can't cover all the pains. With our limited resources and funding, you can only do so much." Compounding such challenges are those associated with working with local organizations and institutions, as well as with local government officials. Darlene described her efforts to work with local schools, saying, "They don't want the community involved in the schools. They turn you off—they don't want you there."

As Village Health Workers described their struggles to be heard, to build credibility, and to establish relationships that would enable them to influence local decision makers, they demonstrated considerable perseverance and creativity in those efforts. For example, Nora said, "[In] August of last year, I wrote a letter to the mayor. No one did anything in December, and I started putting the pressure on in January because they kept procrastinating and giving me the runaround. So I met one of his assistants, . . . and she said if I had any problems to call her. Well, I asked her to help me, and she was able to [help]."

Finding ways to influence the systems that can maintain—or undermine—health in their communities is an ongoing challenge for the VHWs themselves and for the partnership as a whole. These challenges of credibility and the ability to influence systems that affect community life have been detailed by feminist scholars and by writers on community based participatory research and reflect multiple, interlocking processes that serve to constrain influence along dimensions of race, class, and gender (Collins, 1990; Dill & Baca Zinn, 1997; Hall, 1992; Israel et al., 1998; Maguire, 2001).

Building Mutual Support

In partnership approaches, one potential mechanism for addressing the problem of limited influence is to build mutual support and combine resources. Village Health Workers described challenges related to the development of mutually supportive relationships, in which there is a sense of trust and of working together toward commonly defined goals, that are at the core of such partnerships. The ESVHWP sought to build mutually supportive relationships among Village Health Workers and between Village Health Workers and members of the steering committee (Schulz et al., 2002b).

During the first few years of the partnership, a number of challenges arose with regard to relationships among the VHWs. For example, many VHWs did not know each other and had no basis for trusting and supporting each other. After a year of participation in the partnership, Arlene noted that there were VHWs whose names she did not know, much less anything about their perspectives or visions for their communities. Furthermore, VHWs entered the partnership with distinct expectations, diverse agendas, differing priorities, and different perceptions of viable solutions. Disagreements among the VHWs emerged as the women sought to determine their priorities and their expectations for themselves as a group, for each other, and for their meetings together.

The partnership took several actions designed to build mutual support and shared expectations among the VHWs. The project coordinator asked the VHWs to define group norms for themselves, walking them through an exercise in which they identified characteristics of groups that they enjoyed being a part of and using that exercise to come to agreement on norms for working together as a group. Norms that the VHWs identified included respecting each other's opinions, supporting each other, and agreeing to disagree. Once defined, these norms were revisited and refined as new members joined the group or as otherwise necessary: they helped clarify the aspects of group process that the VHWs value and make them explicit (Schulz et al., 2002b).

Second, the project coordinator restructured meeting agendas in an effort to provide opportunities for VHWs to work together in smaller action groups toward shared goals. VHWs first identified a set of priorities (using a process described in more detail later in the chapter), and each VHW then selected one priority area in which she wanted to focus her efforts. As VHWs worked together to address these priority areas, they began to build the relationships and shared visions that are central to mutual support. Though differences of opinion and priorities inevitably continue to emerge within the group, Anita said her participation in the partnership had been "more than what I've expected, because Village Health Workers are like a sister and a brother. We sort of embrace each other. Like I was saying about [names several VHWs]—they all are there for you, supporting you in whatever it is you're going to do."

The partnership also sought to build relationships between the VHWs and the members of the steering committee, to expand networks and the pool of resources (social as well as material) available to members of those networks. During the first two years of the partnership, the steering committee and the VHWs met separately to discuss partnership business, with staff acting as a liaison between the two groups. Perhaps not surprisingly, given this structure, results from in-depth interviews conducted with VHWs and steering committee members in the second year of the partnership indicated that although some VHWs appreciated the steering committee, there was significant confusion about what the committee was, the organizations that were members, and the committee's role within the partnership. As the steering committee and VHWs discussed these results (part of the formative evaluation of the project), they decided to take a number of actions to build closer relationships between the VHWs and the steering committee members. These included initiation of an annual picnic for VHWs and steering committee members, initiation of an annual overnight ESVHWP retreat for VHWs and steering committee members to discuss plans for the upcoming year, and a change in the steering committee structure to include two VHWs, elected as representatives to the committee by the VHWs as a whole.

The second wave of in-depth interviews conducted with VHWs two years later suggested that these efforts had modest success in terms of building stronger connections between VHWs and steering committee members. For example, Anita said, "The organizations and institutions [that make up the steering committee] are a nice foundation for the project—a good collaboration. Good things have and will continue to come out of it." And Thelma remarked, "The ESVHWP brings the resources [to us, and] we can take them back out into the community." However, these positive statements were tempered by others indicating that VHWs wanted the steering committee to be even more visibly engaged in the partnerships' efforts. For example, Tonya said, "We could do more if we saw the steering committee members more often." Building and sustaining relationships between members of the steering committee and the Village Health Workers remains a challenge for the ESVHWP.

Mistrust of Research

The mistrust of academic researchers felt by many community members was illustrated early in this project as VHWs requested a meeting with the project coordinator—a resident of the city—without academic partners present, to discuss the role and intentions of the academic partners. The history of this mistrust has been described elsewhere (Jones, 1981; Hatch et al., 1993), and the importance of building trust between academic researchers and community members is an explicit aspect of community based participatory approaches to research and intervention. Over the course of the partnership, as described in the following examples, members have worked toward the goal of establishing positive relationships, recognizing the power differentials that contribute to this challenge (Schulz et al., 2002b).

Opportunities to build trust occurred as researchers and Village Health Workers worked together to develop interventions and find ways to apply the research and the evaluation results to support and strengthen the work of the partnership. For example, researchers demonstrated their commitment to the principle of using the research to benefit the community by working with the partnership to integrate research and evaluation results into partnership activities. Furthermore, by sharing research and evaluation results with VHWs and steering committee members—often leading to spirited discussions and alternative interpretations among the VHWs—researchers can demonstrate their commitment to sharing the knowledge gained through the research and evaluation with community members. Trust is built through such interactions as members of the partnership demonstrate mutual respect, acknowledging differing interpretations and perspectives.

Discussions of research results by all members of the partnership contribute to the analysis and interpretation of the data, trigger discussions about the implications for practice, and sometimes lead to direct action as well. For example, following a presentation of results from ESVHWP data that suggested that social support provided by members of one's place of worship had positive implications for health outcomes, one Village Health Worker organized an overnight retreat for women at her church, designed to build and strengthen social networks and to provide social support to participants. Furthermore, trust is built as members of the partnership demonstrate trustworthiness—for example, as researchers acknowledge and validate the essential contributions of community members to the generation of knowledge through the partnership and demonstrate their commitment to using that knowledge to benefit the community. Results generated through the formal research and evaluation components of the partnership can also serve to validate and support community partners' experience. For example, as Arlene noted, "Now it's in black-and-white, and one can't tell us [residents] that it's not like that in the community."

Data from the second wave of in-depth interviews suggested that some progress had been made toward the goal of building trust between VHWs and academic researchers but that challenges remained. One VHW indicated to a partner from an academic institution that she remained involved in the partnership in part because "I know that you guys are up at school trying to work with us to make a change—that you are meeting people that are trying, with their education, to make a difference. And when we see that you're involved, it makes us more comfortable to say, 'Hey, well, we can do it.'" Such indicators, visible after several years of building relationships, speak to the potential for demonstrating trustworthiness and hence building trust among academic and community partners.

Differing Agendas and Priorities

We have already noted that the VHWs are a diverse group who bring many different agendas, priorities, and perspectives to their work with the partnership. Add to this the various perspectives and agendas of the members of the steering committee, and the challenges for working together are compounded. For example, reflecting on the first year of the partnership, Ina said, "I thought [there] should be more of a common group effort, [but instead] everybody was involved in their own personal agendas" (Schulz et al., 2002b). Challenges associated with creating a common vision of change appear throughout the literature on community change and suggest the importance of dialogue, mutual respect, and recognition of differences as well as commonalities in the process of forging a shared agenda from those individual visions (Johnson-Reagon, 1983; Lugones & Spelman, 1983).

Efforts to build a shared vision for the work of the partnership have explicitly drawn on the personal agendas and perspectives of VHWs and steering committee members, using multiple strategies—including visual imagery, drawings, small group work, and presentations and dialogue within the larger group.

We will now provide an example of processes the partnership used to develop a shared framework for understanding social factors that influence health and actions taken by community members to maintain or improve health within that context. This example illustrates the integration of a conceptual framework commonly used to guide formal research, with Village Health Workers' in-depth knowledge of their communities as one mechanism for creating a common vision among partnership members who bring different agendas and priorities.

Community members with an interest in becoming a Village Health Worker participate in an eight-week training sequence designed to introduce them to lay health adviser models, and to the ESVHWP more specifically; build relationships; extend their knowledge of health issues and resources within their communities; and extend their community organizing skills. One training session is built around a stress process model (see Schulz et al., 1998, 2002b), engaging VHW trainees in discussions about the particular stressors they and others in their communities confront. Discussions in this session focus on relationships between underlying social conditions and health outcomes, placing individual health behaviors within the context of broader social conditions that influence them (for example, placing individual food choices within the context of economic conditions that shape access to fresh produce). Opportunities for women to talk about the things that they do on a day-to-day basis to promote their own health and that of other community members often turn to discussions of potential actions that might be taken by the ESVHWP to address neighborhood stressors such as safety (for example, participate in police precinct meetings; develop relationships with community police officers; mobilize neighbors to work with city officials in obtaining prompt replacement of burned-out street lights). Similarly, as participants talk, they identify actions that they and other members of their communities take or might take in the future to modify the relationships between stressors and health outcomes (for example, the provision of tangible and emotional social support). Through these discussions, women have identified potential interventions that build on existing community relationships and patterns of action, such as strengthening social networks among community residents or extending those networks to incorporate new members.

The different agendas and priorities that other VHWs and steering committee members brought to the partnership were also a challenge as the partnership sought to come to agreement on its priorities and as members built support for each other in working toward those priorities. In 1999, VHWs and representatives from the steering committee gathered to determine priorities for the partnership for the next four years. Based on results from the community survey, descriptive data indicating the extent to which women living on Detroit's East Side reported a range of stressors, and partial correlations indicating the strength of the relationships between stressors and mental and physical health outcomes were incorporated into this dialogue (Schulz et al. 2001, 2002c). Results were also presented from in-depth interviews with community members illustrating stressors and community resources or conditioning factors described in those interviews. These results contributed to the ensuing discussion of partnership priorities, eventually leading to identification of priorities that would guide the work of the partnership for the next four years. Ongoing opportunities for dialogue and participation in decision making help integrate research with other sources of knowledge as well as with the values and priorities of members of the partnership in the process of developing a shared vision. By working together to define the priorities of the partnership and by drawing on multiple sources of information in this process (including the survey and lived experiences), members of the partnership were able to reach consensus. Furthermore, as all worked together in this process, an opportunity was provided for members of the partnership to act on their commitment to shared power and influence within the partnership itself. As one VHW noted, "We have input and influence, especially when we have retreats or planning meetings. That's a good place for VHWs' voices to be heard and to come to some sort of consensus in planning."

DISCUSSION

We have described both the reasons that Village Health Workers give for their involvement and the challenges they face in this CBPR partnership. Contributions of community members, who are often women, are integral to community based participatory research. These contributions rest on women's interest in and willingness to share their experiences and in-depth knowledge of community processes, norms, and resources and the integration of those experiences with resources and knowledge brought by other members of the partnership. Furthermore, partnerships seeking to effectively engage community members must both understand why community residents participate in such efforts and attempt to address the challenges they encounter (see also Chapter Six). As illustrated here, a major reason Village Health Workers gave for becoming and remaining engaged in the ESVHWP was their interest in promoting community change—contributing to or being involved with research was not a primary goal, and indeed, mistrust of the research agenda was an important challenge, particularly in the early years of the partnership. As the partnership continued and relationships were built among members, VHWs and others came to view research and evaluation as resources available within the partnership.

Some of the challenges described in this chapter (for example, those related to time, trust, and differing agendas) are consistent with those described in earlier chapters and in the literature on challenges to participation in CBPR partnerships (Green et al., 1995; Israel et al., 1998). Others—such as challenges associated with health—are not as apparent in the literature. Understanding and making explicit efforts to address these challenges means attending to structures and processes that encourage shared power and influence. For example, efforts to develop a common vision that reflects the multiple agendas that partners bring to the table, that recognizes and validates different sources of knowledge (for example, lived experience as well as survey and in-depth interview data), and that provides opportunities for partnership members to demonstrate trustworthiness and to build trust are essential. Feminist scholars and other writers on participatory action research have pointed to the importance of eliciting multiple perspectives and forms of knowledge in this process (Hall, 1981; Lugones & Spelman, 1983; Maguire, 2001; Park, 1993). Efforts to build a common language and a shared vision within a partnership rest on the ability to recognize and value the different priorities and perspectives that each member brings to the partnership. These challenges are never "taken care of" once and for all but continue to surface, evolve, and resurface as the partnership continues to develop.

Engaging community residents in the design, implementation, and evaluation of interventions in their communities can make substantial contributions to efforts to improve health. The strategies that CBPR partnerships use to support and encourage the engagement of community members must not only recognize the particular challenges and motivations of the partners involved but also realize that those challenges and motivations are not static but will change over time. Our focus here on the women who are Village Health Workers in this partnership must be considered a partial perspective on the challenges women face in community based participatory partnerships, as well as a partial perspective on challenges faced by Village Health Workers. Women from academic institutions or community based organizations bring a different set of contexts, expectations, challenges, and resources from those faced by many women who are residents of this community. Similarly, men who are Village Health Workers may have experiences that are similar to or different from those presented here.

Feminist theorists and participatory action researchers have long argued that critical attention to conceptualizations of power and influence is essential to the analysis of collective change efforts. The analysis provided in this chapter illustrates the substantial commitment of the women who participate as VHWs creating, shaping and sustaining a community that supports its residents—in this case, as members of a CBPR effort. It also makes explicit that Village Health Workers come to the partnership because they view it as having the potential to influence community events in ways that promote health. Realizing that potential requires careful analysis of race, class, and gender inequities and attention to the ways those inequities appear as differentials in power and influence within the partnership itself as well as in the broader community.

Toward that end, CBPR efforts must examine the assumptions about knowledge and the place of research in community change efforts that all partners bring to their work. On the one hand, research that reflects accepted standards of peer review can be a powerful tool for community change. On the other hand, an overemphasis on academic research may unintentionally obscure the perspectives, values, and lived experiences of community residents, with important implications for the partnerships' efforts to address the inequalities that underlie health disparities. Finding ways to balance or integrate research and action agendas can help partnerships set up structures that are both *empowering* for community members and enable community members to work in an *empowered* manner to foster change in the community. Realization of these dual goals requires attention to processes and relationships within the partnership. Furthermore, it requires that partnership resist dogmatic interpretations of, for example, principles for community based participatory research, recognizing that these principles are guidelines intended to assist partners in reaching the underlying objectives of participation, shared power, mutual influence, and the integration of research with action. As emphasized in Chapter Three, each partnership must examine these principles critically, with an eye toward its own context, goals, and power relationships.

Partnerships that seek to support and enhance the power of community residents must have as a first priority building and sustaining the relationships that provide an infrastructure or framework for a sense of common identity and reciprocal influence—a sense of community—within the partnership. These relationships—and the challenges, conflicts, and differences, as well as commonalities embedded in them—provide the foundation for each partnership to determine how to most effectively integrate research with action to attain the fundamental goals of addressing social inequalities that underlie health disparities.

Notes

1. All interviews were transcribed and analyzed by academic partners in the steering committee, using a focused coding process (Patton, 1990; Zimmerman, Israel, Freudenberg, Becker, & Janz, 1995) that identified sections of the interviews in which Village Health Workers spoke of their reasons for becoming involved, what they gained from participation (or why they remained involved), and the challenges they faced in their participation. In each of these broad areas, the academic partners created categories using in vivo coding and a constant comparison method to construct discrete subcategories (Charmaz, 1995; Zimmerman et al., 1995).

2. All names are pseudonyms.

References

Baker, E. A, Homan, S., Schonhoff, R., & Kreuter, M. W. (1999). Principles of practice for academic/practice/community research partnerships. *American Journal of Preventive Medicine, 16*(3), 86–93.

Charmaz, K. (1995). The grounded theory method: An explication and interpretation. In B. G. Glaser (Ed.), *More grounded theory methodology: A reader* (pp. 95–115). Mill Valley, CA: Sociology Press.

Collins, C., & Williams, D. R. (1999). Segregation and mortality: The deadly effects of racism? *Sociological Forum, 14,* 495–523.

Collins, P. H. (1990). *Black feminist thought and the politics of empowerment.* Boston: Unwin Hyman.

Collins, P. H. (1991). Learning from the outsider within: The social significance of black feminist thought. In M. Fonow & J. Cook (Eds.), *Beyond methodology* (pp. 35–59). Bloomington: Indiana University Press.

Crenshaw, K. W. (1995). Mapping the margins: Intersectionality, identity politics, and violence against women of color. In K. W. Crenshaw, N. Gotanda, G. Peller, & K. Thomas (Eds.), *Critical race theory: The key writings that formed the movement* (pp. 357–383). New York: New Press.

Dill, B. T., & Baca Zinn, M. (1997). Race and gender: Revisioning the social sciences. In M. Anderson, L. Fine, K. Geissler, & J. Ladenson (Eds.), *Doing feminism* (pp. 39–52). Lansing: Michigan State University, Women's Studies Program.

Eng, E., & Parker, E. A. (1994). Measuring community competence in the Mississippi Delta: The interface between program evaluation and empowerment. *Health Education Quarterly, 21,* 199–220.

Eng, E., & Parker, E. A. (2002). Natural helper models to enhance a community's health and competence. In R. De Clemente, R. Crosby, & M. Kegler (Eds.), *Emerging theories and models in health promotion research and practice* (pp. 126–156). San Francisco: Jossey-Bass.

Freudenberg, N. (1998). Community-based health education for urban populations: An overview. *Health Education and Behavior, 25,* 11–23.

Geronimus, A. T., Bound, J., & Waidmann, T. A. (1999). Poverty, time, and place: Variation in excess mortality across selected U.S. populations, 1980–1990. *Journal of Epidemiology and Community Health, 53,* 325–334.

Giddings, P. (1988). *In search of sisterhood: Delta Sigma Theta and the challenge of the black sorority movement.* New York: Morrow.

Gilkes, C. (1988). Building in many places: Multiple commitments and ideologies in black women's community work. In A. Bookman & S. Morgen (Eds.), *Women and the politics of empowerment* (pp. 53–76). Philadelphia: Temple University Press.

Green, L. W., George, M. A., Daniel, M., Frankish, C. J., Herbert, C. P., Bowie, W. R., & O'Neill, M. (1995). *Study of participatory research in health promotion: Review and recommendations for the development of participatory research in health promotion in Canada.* Vancouver, British Columbia: Royal Society of Canada.

Gutierrez, L. M., & Lewis, E. A. (1999). *Empowering women of color.* New York: Columbia University Press.

Hall, B. L. (1975). Participatory research: An approach to change. *Convergence, 11*(3), 25–27.

Hall, B. L. (1981). Participatory research, popular knowledge, and power: A personal reflection. *Convergence, 14*(3), 6–17.

Hall, B. L. (1992). From margins to center: The development and purpose of participatory research. *American Sociologist, 23*(4), 15–28.

Hatch, J., Moss, N., Saran, A., Presley-Cantrell, L., & Mallory, C. (1993). Community research: Partnership in black communities. *American Journal of Preventive Medicine, 9,* 27–31.

House, J. S., Lepkowski, J. M., Williams, D. R., Mero, R. P., Lantz, P. M., Robert, S. A. & Chen, J. M. (2000). Excess mortality among urban residents: How much, for whom, and why? *American Journal of Public Health, 90,* 1898–1904.

International Council for Adult Education. (1980). *Participatory research for adult education and literacy: Guidelines for practitioners.* Toronto: Author.

Israel, B. A, Checkoway, B., Schulz, A. J., & Zimmerman, M. A. (1994). Health education and community empowerment: Conceptualizing and measuring perceptions of individual, organizational, and community control. *Health Education Quarterly, 21,* 149–170.

Israel, B. A., Lichtenstein, R., Lantz, P. M., McGranaghan, R. J., Allen, A., Guzman, J. R., et al. (2001). The Detroit Community-Academic Urban Research Center: Lessons learned in the development, implementation, and evaluation of a community-based participatory research partnership. *Journal of Public Health Management and Practice, 7*(5), 1–19.

Israel, B. A., Schulz, A. J., Parker, E. A., & Becker, A. B. (1998). Review of community-based research: Assessing partnership approaches to improve public health. *Annual Review of Public Health, 19,* 173–202.

Jargowsky, P. A. (1999). The unknown city: Lives of poor and working-class young adults. *American Journal of Sociology, 105,* 549–551.

Johnson-Reagon, B. (1983). Coalition politics: Turning the century. In B. Smith (Ed.), *Home girls: A black feminist anthology* (pp. 356–369). New York: Kitchen Table/Women of Color Press.

Jones, J. H. (1981). *Bad blood: The Tuskegee syphilis experiment.* New York: Free Press.

Kieffer, C. H. (1984). Citizen empowerment: A developmental perspective. *Prevention in Human Services, 3,* 9–36.

Lantz, P. M., Viruell-Fuentes, E., Israel, B. A., Softley, D., & Guzman, J. R. (2001). Can communities and academia work together on public health research? Evaluation results from a community based participatory research partnership in Detroit. *Journal of Urban Health, 78,* 495–507.

Lugones, M., & Spelman, E. V. (1983). Have we got a theory for you! Feminist theory, cultural imperialism, and the demand for "the woman's voice." *Women's Studies International Forum, 6,* 573–581.

Maguire, P. (1990). *Doing participatory research: A feminist approach.* Amherst: University of Massachusetts, Center for International Education.

Maguire, P. (2001). Uneven ground: Feminisms and action research. In P. Reason & H. Bradbury (Eds.), *Handbook of action research: Participatory inquiry and practice* (pp. 59–69). Thousand Oaks, CA: Sage.

Massey, D., & Denton, N. (1993). *American apartheid: Segregation and the making of the underclass.* Cambridge, MA: Harvard University Press.

Morgen, S., & Bookman, A. (1988). Rethinking women and politics: An introductory essay. In A. Bookman & S. Morgen (Eds.), *Women and the politics of empowerment* (pp. 3–29). Philadelphia: Temple University Press.

Northridge, M. E., Vallone, D., Merzel, C., Greene, D., Shepard, P., Cohall, A. T., & Healton, C. G. (2000). The adolescent years: An academic-community partnership in Harlem comes of age. *Journal of Public Health Management and Practice, 6,* 53–60.

Park, P. (1993). What is participatory research? A theoretical and methodological perspective. In P. Park, M. Brydon-Miller, B. L. Hall, & T. Jackson (Eds.), *Voices of change: Participatory research in the United States and Canada* (pp. 1–20). Westport, CT: Bergin & Garvey.

Parker, E. A., Schulz, A. J., Israel, B. A., & Hollis, R. (1998). Detroit's East Side Village Health Worker Partnership: Community based lay health advisor intervention in an urban area. *Health Education and Behavior, 25,* 24–45.

Patton, M. Q. (1990). *Qualitative evaluation and research methods,* Newbury Park, CA: Sage.

Ramirez-Valles, J. (1999). Changing women: The narrative construction of personal change through community health work among women in Mexico. *Health Education and Behavior, 26,* 25–42.

Schulz, A. J., Israel, B. A., Parker, E. A., & Becker, A. B. (2002a). "I started knocking on doors in the community": Women's participation and influence in community based health initiatives. In S. Kar (Ed.), *Empowerment of women and mothers for health promotion.* New York: Russell Sage Foundation.

Schulz, A. J., Israel, B. A., Parker, E. A., Lockett, M., Hill, Y. R., & Wills, R. (2002b). Integrating research with action to address social determinants of health: The East Side Village Health Worker Partnership. *Public Health Reports, 117.*

Schulz, A. J., Parker, E. A., Israel, B. A., Allen, A., De Carlo, M., & Lockett, M. (2002c). Addressing social determinants of health through community based participatory research: The East Side Village Health Worker Partnership. *Health Education and Behavior, 29,* 326–341.

Schulz, A. J., Parker, E. A., Israel, B. A., Becker, A. B., Maciak, B. J., & Hollis, R. (1998). Conducting a participatory community based survey: Collecting and interpreting data for a community intervention on Detroit's east side. *Journal of Public Health Management and Practice, 4*(2), 10–24.

Schulz, A. J., Parker, E. A., Israel, B. A., & Fisher, T. (2001). Social context, stressors, and disparities in women's health. *Journal of the American Medical Women's Association, 56*(4), 143–149.

Service, C., Salber, E., & Jackson, J. (1979). *Community health education: The lay health advisor approach.* Durham, NC: Duke University Health Care Systems.

Stoecker, R., & Bonacich, E. (1992). Why participatory research? *American Sociologist, 23,* 5–15.

Wallerstein, N. (1992). Powerlessness, empowerment, and health: Implications for health promotion programs. *American Journal of Health Promotion, 6,* 197–205.

Zimmerman, M. A., Israel, B. A., Freudenberg, N., Becker, M. H., & Janz, N. (1995). Evaluating twelve AIDS prevention interventions: Methodology. In N. Freudenberg & M. A. Zimmerman (Eds.), *AIDS prevention in the community: Lessons from the first decade* (pp. 199–220). Washington, DC: American Public Health Association.

CHAPTER FIFTEEN

Community Based Participatory Research with Cambodian Girls in Long Beach, California

A Case Study

Ann Cheatham
Eveline Shen

Over the past two decades, there has been growing interest in working with youth in addressing public health issues such as homelessness, violence, HIV/AIDS, and substance abuse. With some notable exceptions, however (see Harper & Carver, 1999; Rogers, Feighery, Tancati, Butler, & Weiner, 1995; Wallerstein & Sanchez-Merki, 1994; Wang, Morrel-Samuels, Bell, Hutchison, & Powers, 2000), the youth involved in such projects have been informants whose roles at best have been advisory (McCormack et al., 2001). The Long Beach Community Based Participatory Research project on sexual harassment mounted by Asians and Pacific Islanders for Reproductive Health (APIRH) was an attempt to have research and organizing driven by young people themselves, with power to make important decisions and take action into their hands. The youth

Note: We would like to acknowledge and thank HOPE members Theary Chhay, Rotha Dom, Sothavy Meas, Ra Rok, Cheath Monica Ching, Mary Im, Molica Pov-Meas, Socheata Sun, Sophea Lun, Sothearith Chhay, and the many other HOPE members who contributed to this work. Thanks also go to Gina Acebo, Que Dang, Judy Han, Diep Tran, Betty Hung, Sopharn Lun, Rina Mehta, and Karen Chan. Many other individuals, groups, and organizations offered support that was essential to the success of this project, including the Cambodian Association of America, United Cambodian Community, Mount Carmel Cambodian Center, Cambodian Association of America, Student Leaders Against Sexual Harassment, Californians for Justice, California State University-Long Beach, Long Beach Sexual Assault and Crisis Agency, National Institute of Environmental Health Sciences, Khemara Buddhikaram Cambodian Buddhist Temple, Joanne O'Bryne, Doris Kagin, Francis Calpotura, Meredith Minkler, Leonard Syme, Dawn Phillips, Bobbie Smith Jenny Oropeza, Alan Lowenthal, and Betty Karnette.

were not helping the project but developing it themselves within a defined structure and theoretical framework.

This chapter will first describe APIRH and its Health, Opportunities, Problem-Solving, and Empowerment (HOPE) projects and then discuss the community based participatory research (CBPR) process that took place in Long Beach, California, as HOPE members worked to study and address the problem of sexual harassment. Following a look at the theory and principles that guided the project and the context in which it took place, the youth's identification of sexual harassment as an issue they wished to explore and address is described. The research and action components of the project then are discussed, including the policy changes that occurred as a result of this work. The chapter concludes with a discussion of some of the special challenges of working with youth, especially low-income youth of color, in CBPR; the approaches and strategies that worked best; and lessons for other such projects with and by youth.

ASIANS AND PACIFIC ISLANDERS FOR REPRODUCTIVE HEALTH AND THE HOPE PROJECTS

Asians and Pacific Islanders for Reproductive Health is a social, political, and economic justice organization fighting for Asian and Pacific Islander women's and girl's liberation through the lens of reproductive freedom. APIRH asserts that a woman has reproductive freedom when she has the power and resources to make healthy choices for herself and her family at home, at work, in school, and in all other areas of life. This means living in homes free from sexual and physical violence, living and working without fear of sexual harassment, and living without hatred due to sexual identity.

APIRH's expanded definition of reproductive freedom also extends to having all forms of work and labor valued and having the rights to earn equitable and livable wages, to eat safe and affordable food, and to determine and gain access to comprehensive health care for themselves and their families. Finally, it includes having the support and commitment of the government and private institutions for women to have or *not* have a child and to live in an environment that supports these choices (Asians and Pacific Islanders for Reproductive Health, 2001). To work toward a world in which women have reproductive freedom, APIRH strives to challenge the different ways in which racism, sexism, patriarchy, and poverty structurally and institutionally affect women's reproductive health and freedom.

Central to APIRH's work are two HOPE projects for Southeast Asian girls (aged fourteen to eighteen) in Long Beach and Oakland, California. These projects attempt to address the underlying causes of health, economic, social, and political disparities by building more collective power to hold institutions accountable for practices that affect community health and the quality of life of residents. The four core strategies in the HOPE approach are leadership development, popular education, community based participatory research, and community building.

The CBPR project described in this chapter was part of the Long Beach HOPE project, which works exclusively with Cambodian girls. APIRH decided to work with this population because Asian immigrant refugee communities have some of the nation's highest poverty and welfare rates. Cambodians in the United States are overwhelmingly concentrated in the lowest-paying jobs, and 43 percent are living in poverty (Yang, 2000). For organizing purposes, it is important to have large numbers (Staples, 1997), and Long Beach, with more than fifty thousand Cambodians—the largest number outside of Cambodia—more than meets this criterion. Because many Southeast Asian Americans have not yet gained U.S. citizenship and cannot vote, there is a general lack of involvement with mainstream political activity among them. Yet younger members of this population proved ripe for involvement in community organizing and CPBR around an issue of deep personal and collective concern. The CBPR project described in this chapter involved more than forty HOPE members in different capacities for over two years, with five involved through the entire process and fourteen participating for a year or more.

SETTING THE STAGE FOR PARTICIPATORY RESEARCH IN LONG BEACH

The CPBR process in this study was unique in that the "outside researchers," the APIRH staff, included experienced community organizers and popular educators, as well as an academically trained researcher, all of whom were working very closely with the Cambodian community in Long Beach. The staff's roles were to provide theory, political analysis, experience, and technical assistance with research, organizing skills, and perspectives on social movements. Staff provided guidance by asking challenging questions, facilitating training sessions, and employing popular education techniques (described later in this chapter) to help analyze issues. The responsibility and power that the staff had to make decisions and act to ultimately uphold the values and mission of APIRH and HOPE was openly acknowledged. As Margaret Le Compte (1995, p. 91) has argued, "Issues of power, agenda and voice are givens" in collaborative research but must be openly addressed and acknowledged. Dealing explicitly with issues of power in CBPR does not mean that power is always equally shared but rather that power dynamics are not hidden and that efforts at democratizing power take place to the extent possible.

Before beginning the project in Long Beach, APIRH staff developed a list of values and ideals capturing their vision of CBPR, which would help in providing direction for the process. These included using population education and the action-reflection cycle; continually revisiting the problem and tracking its changes; developing checkpoints for success; valuing and encompassing different ways of learning and using accessible language; having staff provide structure, process, and guidance, while knowing that their specific roles in relation to CBPR (initiator, consultant, collaborator, and so on; see Chapter Five) will continually change; and teaching the girls to navigate the outside community, academic, and professional realms.

As Barbara Israel and her colleagues note in Chapter Three, the core values and principles associated with CBPR should ideally be tailored to the particular group or project. Several values and guiding principles were thus established for this project, including these:

- Mutual learning
- Emphasis on the process, not just the outcome
- New definitions of success, making it not solely dependent on the outcome
- Youth ownership
- Integrity and faith that girls can make changes
- Shared authority, accountability, and ownership between HOPE members and APIRH
- Valuing every experience including disappointments
- Being explicit about the skills and experiences that staff and HOPE members bring
- Creating opportunities for HOPE members to be trainers

Consistent with these principles, HOPE members were given the support needed to develop a critical understanding of the issues they faced, based on an analysis of their own knowledge and experience. They then used this understanding to develop informal theory and a reproductive freedom analysis, to do research, and to take action to change structures that impinge on their reproductive freedom.

Providing Support for the Process

To undertake the CBPR process effectively, it was essential to have not only the HOPE members' understanding and full commitment but also the support of their parents, extended families, and communities. Several HOPE members found that their families were either apathetic about their participation or hesitant to allow it at all, making full participation impossible. In contrast, members who had the support of their families were much more likely to remain with the project throughout.

HOPE members often needed considerable personal support, beyond that provided by their families, in order to engage effectively in this work. APIRH staff offered such support, providing tutors, help in talking with teachers about schoolwork and grades, referrals to therapists, and help in getting to doctor's appointments to deal with possible pregnancies and other medical problems that they were uncomfortable dealing with through their families. In one instance, APIRH helped secure a loan for a member's mother so that she could pay the rent and her daughter could continue participating in the program.

The provision of a small stipend for each member helped demonstrate respect and appreciation of her time and work and allowed many to continue with the project at age sixteen, when they might otherwise have been obligated by financial necessity to stop to find employment.

One of the four key strategies of HOPE is community building, which, as Angela Blackwell and her colleagues (Blackwell, Tamir, Thompson, & Minkler, in press) point out, is a necessary precursor to effective CBPR. APIRH recognized that expecting the girls to come to numerous meetings and training sessions and to work on research, analysis, and organizing was realistic only if opportunities were also provided for having fun and building trust and relationships within their group. Providing time and space for team-building activities, including cultural events, informal discussions, and other social interaction opportunities (Walter, 1997), helped energize participants and build the motivation and interpersonal trust and support needed to engage effectively in CBPR.

Many different community-building activities occurred prior to and in conjunction with the CBPR project, including writing workshops, potlucks with Cambodian food, team-building games, sleepovers, and "rap sessions." These last proved particularly popular, and a safe environment, with structure and ground rules, was developed, within which the girls could share very openly about their personal lives.

Training for Participation in CBPR

To facilitate its CBPR work with HOPE, APIRH created training sessions designed to empower and develop grassroots organizing skills and political analysis and to foster leadership. As described later in this chapter, and consistent with the philosophy of Paulo Freire (1970), popular education lies at the heart of APIRH's trainings, and it continued throughout the entire participatory research process. Using a Freirian dialogic method, "teacher learners," in this case APIRH staff, posed questions to the HOPE participants, challenging the girls to draw on their own knowledge and experience to generate common themes, look at underlying causes and consequences, and come up with action plans for addressing shared concerns.

Emphasizing the feminist principle that "the personal is political" and using reproductive freedom as the core component of its training, APIRH staff helped HOPE participants see the structural and environmental causes of problems rather than internalizing these problems.

To help members become accustomed to the language and concepts of CBPR before they began their project, for example, staff led discussions of the different ways research is used by society and helped the girls differentiate between being exploited for research purposes and participating to make a contribution to their communities. Participants learned about marketing research and about academic and medical research that has hurt people, such as the Tuskegee study in which African American men were denied access to syphilis cures so that scientists could study the long-term consequences of the disease (Thomas & Crouse Quinn, 1991). The girls were engaged in dialogue about research in which they had already participated or with which they were familiar and how CBPR differed from more traditional approaches to research. Such dialogue helped the HOPE members develop a clear understanding of why a CBPR process was being employed and what they might gain by using CBPR to study and help bring about change in an area of concern to them.

Training sessions were also held to help HOPE members understand the differences between reproductive health and reproductive freedom. The impact of war and violence in Cambodia on their mothers and grandmothers; unsafe conditions in the garment industry, in which many of their mothers worked; racial profiling in the welfare-to-work system; and stereotypes of Asian women as exotic, passive, obedient, and quiet were discussed as social factors affecting Cambodian girls and women in Long Beach and their reproductive freedom.

Finally, the training sessions also helped place the CBPR work the members were going to begin in the context of community organizing and social movements and offered skill building in community organizing and in understanding power and power relationships. One particularly effective tool used was the "power flower" (see Figure 15.1). During this training session, each person colors in the outer petal of a flower for categories in which they are in the dominant group and the inner petal for categories in which they are not. Through a series of follow-up questions, participants are helped to understand the areas in which they do and do not have power both individually and as a group. They are asked to imagine how the world would be different if everyone had a chance

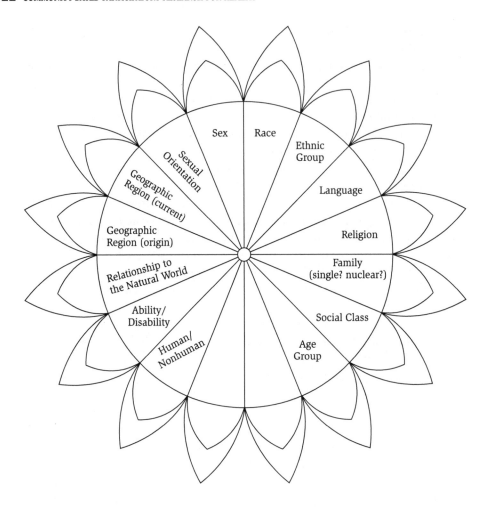

Figure 15.1 The Power Flower.

Source: From *Educating for a Change,* by R. Arnold, B. Burke, C. James, D. Martin, and B. Thomas, p. 13. Copyright © 1991 by Between the Lines Press. Reprinted with Permission.

to hold power and to discuss what happens when people who hold a lot of power abuse it (through racism or homophobic acts, for example).

The power flower proved a particularly valuable tool once the girls had selected and begun working on their issue (sexual harassment) and helped them avoid self-blame for situations that they now realized reflected broader power dynamics. This training also encouraged the viewing of various types of oppression as interlocking and introduced the important contributions of feminist and antiracist scholars (Collins, 2000; hooks, 1989) in furthering our understanding in this area.

IDENTIFYING SEXUAL HARASSMENT AS AN ISSUE

As noted earlier, the issue identification process employed by APIRH involves the use of popular education strategies to help members talk about their individual lives and then collectivize those experiences as they begin to see that many of their individual difficulties share the same societal roots. In addition, and consistent with Charlotte Bunch (1983) and Lee Staples (1997), who point out that a good issue is one that fits within a broader social agenda, APIRH staff facilitated the issue selection process with attention to the organization's explicit social justice agenda for reproductive freedom. Staff provided a structure of analysis, theory, coaching, facilitation, and resources so that members could consider potential issues they were concerned about in part in terms of whether and how they fit within this broader framework.

Numerous other criteria were used in issue selection. These included a potential issue's ability to challenge traditional gender (or racial or class or other) division of labor and societal roles, to stimulate leadership development among low-income Asian and Pacific Islanders (API) girls, to assert a new perspective on who gets defined as an expert and whose voices get heard, and to influence the understanding and approach to social change of API and progressive social movements and organizations.

The issue of sexual harassment, which became the central focus of the CBPR process, was an ideal one from APIRH's perspective: it came from the community, was clearly connected to the organization's broader reproductive freedom agenda, and lent itself to a careful analysis of the sociostructural roots of the problem.

Sexual harassment was first discussed when two of the HOPE members told the group of an incident that had occurred in their social studies class, when HOPE members had shared photos of their recent participation in a demonstration in the state capital. The teacher confiscated the pictures and went on to extensively criticize, to the class, the HOPE program and its activities in Sacramento. The teacher remarked to the two HOPE members, "If those gang-whores and sluts would only keep their jeans on, we would not need abortion programs like yours." Other members of the class who were friends of the girls were then told by the teacher to "write an essay about why bilingual education should not exist."

Critical learning comes from the scrutiny of everyday life (Sohng, 1996). Although the HOPE members did not initially identify this incident as sexual harassment, staff-led dialogue and training helped the girls identify the racism, sexism, classism, and sexual harassment embedded in this incident. The members were asked to go back to the power flower and think about which petals of the flower the teacher was drawing on when he made the statement about "sluts" and "gang-whores." Using Freirian problem posing, the staff also asked whether there were any equivalent terms to *sluts* and *whores* for men. They led a decoding of the word *gang* and how it is typically used in reference to young people of color who are poor, reflecting ageism, racism, and classism. Through this process, HOPE members developed a sophisticated analysis of the power dynamics involved in the incident experienced and further understood that the teacher's actions were indeed a potent example of sexual harassment.

As dialogue continued, HOPE members realized that they were being sexually harassed on a daily basis while often blaming themselves for the incidents that occurred. Staff again played a key role in initiating a process that Vio Grossi (1981) has termed "disindoctrination," or allowing people to detach themselves from myths imposed on them by the power structure that keep them from seeing their own oppression.

After additional popular education training sessions that helped the HOPE members understand internalized oppression, the social factors contributing to sexual harassment, and the consequences of such abuse, the girls were eager to move into action. They came up with recommendations for the prevention of further incidents of sexual harassment in the schools and arranged to meet with the school principals and separately with a district superintendent.

Although these meetings failed to get the desired results, subsequent debriefings provided excellent opportunities for the girls to use their critical reflection and analysis skills. For example, one of the principals had commented in the meeting, "I am just like you. I put on my pants the same way, but I am a man and you are a woman." This statement was considered in relation to the power flower, and it became clear that this individual was not just like the HOPE members. He held far more power than the girls on multiple dimensions (including gender, race, and class) in addition to holding a position that grants him final decision-making power for the school.

RESEARCHING THE PROBLEM

Both the critical reflection process and the failure of the initial meetings to achieve the desired outcomes reinforced for HOPE members the need for moving into the next phase of the CBPR process—studying the problem of sexual harassment in greater detail.

Staff posed questions to assist the members in brainstorming what they wanted to learn about sexual harassment, and forty different questions emerged. In addition to wishing to learn about the prevalence of such harassment and whether the perpetrators were teachers, staff, or students, HOPE members developed questions such as "How does sexual harassment affect students' ability to learn and participate in school?" "What do students and teachers already know about sexual harassment?" and "Is sexual harassment related to other health issues, such as sexually transmitted diseases (STDs), depression, pregnancy, drug and alcohol use, and smoking?" The members' earlier training through APIRH had made them familiar with a variety of research methods, including written surveys, interviews, photojournaling, document review, and observation. As Peter Reason (1994) notes, participatory research may use methods that look more "orthodox," making sense of them from the community perspective. In this instance, the HOPE members decided that written questions would be the most efficient means of getting the most questions answered about this sensitive and important topic.

The members then worked on writing the survey, with technical assistance from staff. An initial brainstorming session, in which members identified many potential ways in which sexual harassment at school could affect students, was particularly helpful in suggesting possible areas for questioning. These areas (for example, possible impacts on mental and physical health, self-esteem, grades, work habits, participation in class, and suicidal thoughts) were among the items explored through questions on the survey.

The HOPE members' insider knowledge of sexual harassment and related issues in their community also enabled them to come up with critical questions that outside researchers would not know to ask. For example, although having someone urinate in front of you is not a form of sexual harassment that is either common knowledge or cited in the literature, it was a critical issue for students in this community. The criteria used by the HOPE members in deciding whether or not to include a survey question were that the information gained from the question would help in the development of their organizing campaign, that it would not be repetitive, and that it could create new knowledge for future use.

To reduce possible error, the questions about physical and mental health were taken from the Behavioral Risk Factor Surveillance System, which has been in use since 1993. These questions have undergone several reliability and validity studies and been modified accordingly (Centers for Disease Control and Prevention, 2002). In addition to learning about standardized question items like these, the HOPE members learned about pretesting and did their own pretesting of the survey. Based on the pretesting, the final instrument was considerably shortened, and male students were eliminated from the target population.

The target population for the survey was female students at the high school the members attend in Long Beach. A nonprobability sample design was used and a quota sample taken. To obtain as large and diverse a group of participants as possible, the HOPE members placed themselves in strategic locations throughout the high school to distribute the survey. Completed surveys were returned by more than four hundred girls, or more than 25 percent of the target population.

Although APIRH staff had anticipated that the HOPE members themselves would be heavily involved in the subsequent data analysis stage of the project, the data collection had been so labor-intensive that the girls wanted a break. Indeed, an important staff role at this point and other points involved reminding the HOPE members how much they had accomplished through their work to date, having them think about what would be lost if they gave up, and engaging them in the kind of community-building activities that could help balance their task-oriented work with attention to their more social needs (Walter, 1997). By agreeing to analyze the data themselves, APIRH staff were both respecting the wishes of the HOPE members and providing the break they had desired.

The HOPE members did let staff know, however, the forms of data they wanted from the survey for use in the subsequent organizing phase of the project. The survey results provided strong evidence of the widespread nature and scope of the problem of sexual harassment that HOPE members had so often personally experienced. Some highlights of the survey include that over 87 percent of those surveyed had experienced sexual harassment. Sixteen percent had been harassed by a teacher or staff person. Fifty-four percent did not know that a grievance procedure existed or how to file a complaint about sexual harassment, and 35 percent talked less in class because of sexual harassment. Although there was a possibility of bias due to the nonprobability design of the survey, the analysis of findings suggested a possible association between sexual harassment and health, as well as the ability to learn and succeed in school.

MOVING INTO ACTION

With the survey work complete, the focus of the CBPR work turned to action for social change, within the conceptual framework of APIRH's unique organizing theory. In addition to its emphasis on the centrality of culture and identity and on political education as crucial to the support of strategic organizing and development, the theory stressed the importance of framing and reframing ideas as a main goal of the organizing and CBPR process. Sexual harassment was thus framed as an issue of school safety for girls, healthy sexuality, equitable education, environmental justice, and reproductive freedom.

The most effective direct action organized by HOPE to reduce sexual harassment was the Community Forum on School Safety. In preparation for this event, at which HOPE members would release their study results and their recommendations for action, visits to allies were made by HOPE members and staff to ask them to cosponsor the forum, sign on to the platform of recommendations, speak at the event, and contribute money. Actively building partners in this way enabled the forum to become a foundation for a large base of people to reframe the moral and practical dimensions of sexual harassment.

Families and friends of HOPE members, community members, and more than twenty representatives of community organizations attended the forum. In addition, attendees included two Long Beach school board members, the principals of the girls' high school, the Long Beach School District superintendent, a representative of the state legislature and of the city council, and reporters from the mass media.

As noted, HOPE members used the forum to release the dramatic results of their survey and, with support of APIRH staff, to present their tenets or recommendations for ensuring a safe learning environment for girls in Long Beach. These tenets were that all students have the right to a safe learning environment not compromised by gender discrimination, that eliminating sexual harassment should be a priority in order to ensure girls' right to learn in a safe school environment, that a more student-friendly grievance procedure should be adopted and publicized, and that training on sexual harassment should be instituted for teachers and students.

The forum was successful in shining a spotlight on and reframing the issue of student safety with a gender focus. In their media advocacy, HOPE members and their APIRH staff supporters were also able to link their issues with the heightened concern over school safety as a result of the Columbine, Colorado, school shootings in April 1999. Releases to the press therefore included such statements as "Students, parents, and community members want to see an effective response to sexual harassment, a threat just as real to girls' safety as guns, drugs, and gangs. This is a real danger to female students, and we want to see some accountability."

School officials adopted every one of the recommendations advocated by the HOPE members and their allies. The following fall, all 4,500 students at the high school were required to watch a video on sexual harassment during preregistration, and all were given educational materials about students' rights with respect to sexual harassment. Antiharassment posters designed and produced by HOPE members were displayed in almost every classroom and in many public spaces throughout the school, and a student-friendly version of the sexual harassment grievance procedure was provided to all students.

On a broader level, a community advisory board, including representatives of the school district and of local community groups, was formed to work on issues of sexual harassment in the Long Beach schools. As a result of the board's work, training on sexual harassment was provided to all tenth-grade health classes, teachers now receive in-service training on sexual harassment, peer counselors are getting training on how to counsel students who are sexually harassed, and a mechanism has been developed to monitor and address incidents of sexual harassment. Efforts to make these changes effective districtwide are indeed a major outcome of the project.

The forum and the careful work that preceded it also helped position APIRH as a progressive feminist voice in Long Beach rooted in the Cambodian community, raised awareness about school safety and the members' recommendations for addressing it, and helped develop the participants' political consciousness. The Cambodian community was also affected by the leadership presence of the HOPE members and saw its visibility and hence its power as a part of the broader community enhanced.

LESSONS LEARNED

Although the CBPR case study described in this chapter was clearly a success, a number of important lessons were learned along the way that in retrospect could have increased project effectiveness still further. Because of the dearth of social justice groups in Long Beach and the fact that the youth culture in that community doesn't include activism or social change work, for example, it might have been helpful to bring in earlier in the process other groups that do organizing with youth. Such groups from the Los Angeles area could have provided a much needed sense of support for the members. Forging such connections might also have given the members other people to turn to during hard times or when they just wanted more local advice, particularly from other youth engaged in this kind of work.

It would also have been more effective to have a senior organizer who was local, understood the community, and had experience running organizing campaigns, rather than having a consultant from APIRH's Northern California office fill that role. Although APIRH's position as an API-focused feminist organization was clearly important, this experience underscored the need for a larger pool of trained and culturally competent organizers, familiar with CBPR, who can undertake such work in their own locales.

Lessons were also learned about the need to plan for attrition, particularly in work with youth. This entire CBPR process took two years. Although five members were involved from beginning to end, many others played important roles for shorter time periods. It would have been helpful to plan for attrition from the beginning and to initially recruit more people to prevent loss of momentum when key individuals had to leave the project.

APIRH also learned from this process that youth need to feel that their work is connected to that of other youth and to see it moving forward. The importance of being shown and reminded of the results of one's work in order to foster continued engagement has been stressed in community organizing and CBPR in many venues (see, for example, Staples, 1997; El-Askari et al., 1998; Minkler, 2000). But as this case study suggests, it may be particularly important in work with youth. In addition, as noted earlier, young people, more than other community members in CBPR efforts, may need a great deal of one-on-one work and support in ensuring that their personal needs are met so that they can continue to participate in the project. Learning to maintain balance in the provision of such resources is a critical and ongoing challenge for adults engaged with youth in CBPR and related activities (Wallerstein & Sanchez-Merki, 1994).

In a conservative community like Long Beach in which organizing is not a part of the culture, the heightened importance of building allies and being well prepared in advance of meetings and events was also underscored. In this project, the conservative school administration was not prepared for an organizing effort involving important elements of the community and the mass media. They were caught off-guard, and this appeared to contribute to the HOPE members' and allies' successes in getting their recommendations for change accepted. Thinking ahead about the kind of culture that exists where CBPR is being attempted is critical, since this culture will affect the types of support needed for community based participatory research.

With some important exceptions, such as work done in the context of the National Black Women's Health Project (http://www.nationalblackwomenshealth project.org), the reproductive rights movement has been heavily white and middle-class (Rosen, 2000). An important lesson learned from this case study is that in order to have women of color, low-income women, or youth involved, it is necessary to discover people's self-interest and their community's interests. Done correctly, CBPR can be an ideal avenue for surfacing and acting on this information. Within the reproductive rights movement, CBPR that truly "starts where the people are" will mean working on a variety of issues beyond access to abortion.

A traditional approach to improving the reproductive health of Cambodian youth in Long Beach may have been to provide sex education, abstinence promotion, or free condoms. The CBPR process described in this case study involved going considerably deeper to enable youth in the community to identify, study, and address the root causes of reproductive health problems. At the same time, the CBPR process produced powerful new data on the prevalence of the problem of sexual harassment and its possible association with reproductive and mental health problems.

During the CBPR process, the research and its results moved HOPE participants and helped them see that far from being simply an individual problem, sexual harassment was affecting many people. They saw as well that by studying and addressing this issue, they could give something back to the community and make improvements for other students and female family members as well as for themselves. Because "the methods used to validate knowledge claims must also be acceptable to the group controlling the knowledge validation process" (Collins, 2000, p. 204), having the research gave the group considerable leverage. The survey captured the attention of the school authorities and the media in ways that individual accounts had not. The research also provided credibility and legitimacy to the organizing work.

A critical aspect of this process involved the youth's major role in designing the research and making all of the major decisions in this CBPR process, within the overarching framework provided by APIRH. The research gave the members facts and figures that they could in turn use in interesting other organizations to serve as powerful allies in their campaign. When members could say that 87 percent of the more than four hundred students surveyed had been harassed, the issue was raised to the community level, and more people got involved. If the community truly controls the CBPR process, its members may be better positioned to understand problems and make a difference.

References

Asians and Pacific Islanders for Reproductive Health. (2001). *HOPE project for girls: A reproductive freedom tour of Oakland.* Oakland, CA: Author.

Blackwell, A. G., Tamir, H., Thompson, M., & Minkler, M. (in press). Community based participatory research: Implications for funders. *Journal of General Internal Medicine.*

Bunch, C. (1983). The reform tool kit. In J. Friedman (Ed.), *First harvest: The Institute for Policy Studies, 1963–1983* (pp. 204–208). New York: Grove Press.

Centers for Disease Control and Prevention. (2002). *Health-related quality-of-life measure.* Atlanta: Health Care and Aging Studies Branch, Division of Adult and Community Health, National Center for Chronic Disease Prevention and Health Promotion.

Collins, P. H. (2000). *Black feminist thought: Knowledge, consciousness, and the politics of empowerment* (2nd ed.). New York: Routledge.

El-Askari, G., Freestone, J., Irizarry, C., Kraut, K., Mashiyama, S., Morgan, M. A., & Walton, S. (1998). The Healthy Neighborhoods project: A local health department's role in catalyzing community development. *Health Education and Behavior, 25,* 146–159.

Freire, P. (1970). *Pedagogy of the oppressed.* New York: Seabury Press.

Harper, G., & Carver, L. (1999). "Out of the mainstream" youth as partners in collaborative research: Exploring the benefits and challenges. *Health Education and Behavior, 26,* 250–256.

hooks, b. (1989). *Talking back: Thinking feminism, talking black.* Boston: South End Press.

Le Compte, M. (1995). Some notes on power, agenda, and voice: A researcher's personal evolution toward critical collaborative research. In P. McLaren & J. Giarelli (Eds.), *Critical theory and educational research* (pp. 91–112). Albany: State University of New York Press.

McCormack, K., Forthofer, M., Bryant, C., Eaton, D., Merritt, T., Landis, D., & McDermott, R. J. (2001). Developing youth capacity for community-based research: The Sarasota County demonstration project. *Journal of Public Health Management and Practice, 7*(2), 53–60.

Minkler, M. (2000). Participatory action research and healthy communities. *Public Health Reports, 115,* 191–197.

Reason, P. (1994). Three approaches to participative inquiry. In N. K. Denzin & Y. S. Lincoln (Eds.), *Handbook of qualitative research* (pp. 324–339). Thousand Oaks, CA: Sage.

Rogers, T., Feighery, E., Tancati, E., Butler, J., & Weiner, L. (1995). Community mobilization to reduce point-of-purchase advertising of tobacco products. *Health Education Quarterly, 22,* 427–442.

Rosen, R. (2000). The world split open: How the modern women's movement changed America. New York: Viking Penguin.

Sohng, S.S.L. (1996). Participatory research and community organizing. *Journal of Sociology and Social Welfare, 23*(4), 77–97.

Staples, L. (1997). Selecting and cutting the issue. In M. Minkler (Ed.), *Community organizing and community building for health* (pp. 175–194). New Brunswick, NJ: Rutgers University Press.

Thomas, S. B., & Crouse Quinn, S. C. (1991). The Tuskegee syphilis study, 1932–1972: Implications for HIV education and AIDS risk education programs in the black community. *American Journal of Public Health, 11,* 1498–1505.

Vio Grossi, F. (1981). The sociopolitical implications of participatory research: Yugoslavia International Forum on Participatory Research. *Convergence, 14*(3), 34–51.

Wallerstein, N., & Sanchez-Merki, V. (1994). Freirian praxis in health education: Research results from an adolescent prevention program. *Health Education Research, 9,* 105–118.

Walter, C. (1997). Community building practice: A conceptual framework. In M. Minkler, M. (Ed.), *Community organizing and community building for health* (pp. 68–87). New Brunswick, NJ: Rutgers University Press.

Wang, C. C., Morrel-Samuels, S., Bell, S., Hutchison, P., & Powers, L. S. (Eds.). (2000). *Strength to be: Community visions and voices.* Ann Arbor: University of Michigan.

Yang, K. (2000). *Status of southeast Asian Americans.* Paper presented to the Inter-Agency Working Group, White House Initiative on Asian Americans and Pacific Islanders, Washington, DC.

CHAPTER SIXTEEN

Community Based Participatory Research with a Hidden Population

The Transgender Community Health Project

Kristen Clements-Nolle
Ari Bachrach

Slowly and often painfully conventional researchers are coming to realize that working with the poor and voiceless is infinitely more rewarding than working on them.
—Cornwall & Jewkes, 1995

A
s several previous chapters in this book have demonstrated, community based participatory research (CBPR) is not a new research approach. With a few exceptions in environmental research, however, CBPR is rarely used in the field of epidemiology (Brown, 1992; Wing, 1998). According to Michael

Note: We would like to thank the research associates (Nikki Calma, Carla Clynes, Nashanta Stanley, Matt Rice, and Doan Thai), field coordinators (Vince Guilin, Scott Ikeda, Robert Guzman), and Transgender Community Advisory Board members (Connie Amarthitada, Nadia Cabezas, Crystal Catamco, Tamara Ching, Patrick Forte, Sage Foster, Liz Highleyman, Russell Hilkene, Carry Kissel, Jade Kwan, Yosenio Lewis, Lauren Michaels, Margaret Morvay, Major, Chenit Ong-Flaherty, Elise Shiver-Russell, Zak Sinclair, Claire Skiffington, Tammy Jean Spirithawk, Viny Tango, Gina Tucker, Adela Vasquez, Kiki Whitlock, and Willy Wilkinson) for all of their dedication and hard work.

We would also like to express our appreciation to the following community based organizations who assisted in recruitment and provided us space to conduct interviews and HIV testing: Asian and Pacific Islander Wellness Center, Center for Special Problems, Filipino Task Force on AIDS, FTM International, Glide-Goodlett HIV/AIDS Program, Instituto Familiar de la Raza, New Village, Proyecto Contra SIDA Por Vida, Southeast Asian Community Center, Tenderloin AIDS Resource Center, and Tom Waddell Clinic.

The Transgender Community Health Project was supported by the Centers for Disease Control and Prevention, Cooperative Agreement No. U62CCU902017-12, and the State of California, Department of Health Services, Office of AIDS Grant No. 97-10787. All study protocols and materials received approval from Committee on Human Research at the University of California, San Francisco.

Schwab and Leonard Syme (1997), community participation in the research process represents a new paradigm in epidemiology:

> It implies working across disciplines, and with the population itself, in defining variables, designing instruments, and collecting data (qualitative and quantitative) that reflect the ecological reality of life in that population, as people experience it. This collaboration is not easy. It calls for cross-disciplinary patience, as well as cultural sensitivity and competence, to overcome the differences of race, class, and age that generally exist between public health specialists and populations we are here to serve. Epidemiologists would not be required to surrender rigor, but they would be required to share power! [p. 2050].

This new paradigm is well suited for research with oppressed and marginalized populations who have historically been left out of the research process and may not trust outside investigators (Hall, 1981). Collaborating with local people in *all* aspects of the research process can build community confidence and trust, improve internal study validity, and facilitate the use of study results to improve community health. This chapter describes how CBPR was successfully used in an epidemiologic study with perhaps the most socially marginalized population in the United States: the transgender community. After a brief introduction to this hidden population and a summary of the study results, we will illustrate how CBPR guided the development and implementation of our research efforts.

We frame our case study within the CBPR principles originally outlined by Barbara Israel and her colleagues (Israel, Schurman, & Hugentobler, 1992) and further described in Chapter Three: community based participatory research is participatory, is cooperative, is a co-learning process, involves systems development, is an empowering process through which participants can increase control over their lives, and achieves a balance between research and action. We conclude with recommendations for other researchers who wish to use CBPR to conduct research with other marginalized and hidden populations.

THE TRANSGENDER COMMUNITY, THE STUDY, AND ITS RESULTS

Transgender is an inclusive term used to describe persons who do not conform to social gender norms associated with their physical sex (Gender Education and Advocacy, 2001). The transgender community is made up of a diverse group of individuals who may also self-identify as transsexual, transvestite, intersex, bigender, male (born female), or female (born male). Transgendered persons live their lives to varying degrees as their chosen gender, but in so doing, they endure severe social stigmatization as well as discrimination in housing, health care, and employment (Feinberg, 2001; Green, 1994; Lombardi, 2001).

A transgendered person may change his or her name and gender on all personal and legal identification, such as birth certificate, social security card, and driver's license. To enhance the secondary sex characteristics of their chosen gender, male-to-female (MTF) transgendered individuals often take estrogen, antiandrogens, and progesterone, and female-to-male (FTM) persons take testosterone. Some transgendered individuals also choose to have sex reassignment or gender confirmation surgeries. However, many lack the considerable financial resources to pay for such surgeries, which are rarely covered by health insurance.

The size of the transgender population in the United States is unknown because national and local data collection forms only include male and female gender categories. Similarly, we have little epidemiologic data to document the health of transgendered persons. Of particular concern in San Francisco, California, was the lack of information available on HIV infection in this hidden population. In the mid-1990s, anecdotal reports from members of the transgender community and health care providers suggested that HIV/AIDS may be a significant problem for transgendered persons. However, no large epidemiologic studies with the transgender community had been conducted in San Francisco or elsewhere to determine the prevalence of HIV and associated risk behaviors.

To address this limitation, researchers from the San Francisco Department of Public Health and members of the transgender community worked together to conduct the first large epidemiologic study with transgendered persons: the Transgender Community Health Project. Although the primary objective of the study was to obtain an estimate of HIV prevalence and risk behaviors among transgendered persons in San Francisco, the study also addressed access to health and prevention services and a range of psychosocial health issues.

From July 1 through December 31, 1997, a total of 392 MTF and 123 FTM transgendered persons were recruited, interviewed, and tested for HIV. Over one-third (35 percent) of MTF participants were found to be infected with HIV. African Americans and individuals with a history of injection drug use, multiple sex partners, and less education were significantly more likely to be HIV-positive. Among FTM participants, HIV prevalence (2 percent) and risk behaviors were much lower. However, FTMs who have sex with gay and bisexual men may be at risk due to low condom use. About two-thirds of MTF and over half of FTM participants were classified as depressed, and 32 percent of each population had attempted suicide (Clements-Nolle, Marx, Guzman, & Katz, 2001). As will be further described in the following case study, these alarming results greatly influenced policy, prevention, and health care for transgendered persons in San Francisco.

CBPR Is Participatory and Cooperative

The Transgender Community Health Project was initiated and driven by community concerns and priorities. Frustrated with data collection forms that only offered a binary (male/female) gender classification and keenly aware of the number of transgendered persons becoming infected with HIV, a group of transgendered individuals became vocal about the lack of epidemiologic data available on HIV for their community. This group of community members attended several San Francisco Health Commission and Health Department meetings and wrote letters stating the need to conduct a transgender HIV prevalence and risk behavior study. This persistent community organizing eventually resulted in the prioritization of such a study by the San Francisco HIV Prevention Planning Council.

In 1995, researchers from the health department asked the community members who played a role in getting the study prioritized to collaborate in the development of a transgender research grant application. This proposal was funded by the state of California Office of AIDS and the Centers for Disease Control and Prevention in 1996. At this time, ten more MTF and FTM transgendered volunteers were recruited to help plan and implement formative research for the proposed epidemiologic study.

The formative research consisted of thirty key informant interviews, eleven focus groups with one hundred transgendered persons, and four months of ethnographic community mapping. The transgender community collaborators played a particularly important role in developing the focus group questions, cofacilitating each focus group, and assisting in the analysis and publication of the focus group data (Clements-Nolle, Wilkinson, Kitano, & Marx, 2001). In addition, several community members worked very closely with health department researchers to conduct ethnographic mapping in neighborhoods thought to have high concentrations of transgendered persons. This helped determine the time of day and locations when recruitment should take place to ensure a diverse sample of MTF and FTM individuals for the epidemiologic study.

In 1997, a full community advisory board (CAB) was established to assist in the design and implementation of the quantitative study protocols. To ensure diversity and a range of experience among CAB members, some members were recruited through street outreach and others were recruited by writing letters to agencies that served the target population. This resulted in a twenty-four-member CAB that consisted almost entirely of MTFs and FTMs who were homeless, current sex workers, health care providers, and social service providers. The CAB members worked together to develop a mission statement and a set of agreements that were used to facilitate each meeting. The agreements outlined the need to respect one another's differences and helped create a safe space where people from various backgrounds could feel comfortable contributing to the research process.

The CAB initially met twice a month and then monthly to develop protocols, sampling plans, data collection instruments, and human subjects applications; pilot-test the instruments; interview and hire the research team; develop transgender-specific education and referral materials; and oversee participant recruitment and data collection activities. The expertise that the CAB members provided in developing the survey instrument was invaluable. Several CAB members met with health department researchers in between meetings to develop culturally appropriate ways to ask sexual behavior questions of MTFs and FTMs who may or may not have undergone sexual reassignment surgery. The resulting survey has served as a model for other jurisdictions conducting transgender studies.

The CAB also decided that interviewing and HIV testing should be conducted at seven different community based organizations located in the key neighborhoods identified by our ethnographic mapping. The CAB felt that a rotating presence in each neighborhood would help ensure recruitment of a diverse sample of participants and facilitate referrals to the very agencies where interviewing and HIV testing was conducted.

In May 1997, three MTFs (African American, Filipina, and Latina) and three FTMs (one Vietnamese and two whites) were hired as research associates. All of the research associates had strong ties with their respective communities, which helped the study gain access to different racial and ethnic, socioeconomic, and gender subpopulations within the transgender community. The research associates helped finalize the study instruments and were responsible for recruiting, interviewing, HIV-testing, providing referrals, and presenting the study results. The research associates quickly became aware that many of the agencies and clinics to which they referred study participants were not sensitive to the needs of transgendered people. To address this limitation, the research associates planned and conducted numerous transgender in-service training sessions at local agencies and clinics.

The research associates also believed that existing HIV prevention and referral materials did not reflect the reality of transgender identity and served to further alienate the community. Therefore, the research associates worked closely with CAB members to develop transgender-specific HIV education and referral materials. Created by and for members of the transgender community, these materials addressed issues specific to transgendered persons (for example, how to inject hormones safely) and used transgender-specific images (for example, a MTF transgendered person who had not undergone surgery was shown putting a condom on her penis). Such images validated transgender identity and expressed the importance of self-protection.

In December 1997, the research associates presented preliminary study results to participants, collaborating agencies, the HIV Prevention Planning Council, and the HIV Health Services Council. During the first six months of 1998, the CAB met every other month to develop the full analysis plan, review and interpret the results, and decide the content of reports, publications, and press releases. Community involvement began to drop off during this quantitative analysis phase. Some CAB members felt alienated by discussions of analysis, and others were simply not as interested in this phase of the research. The group decided that they trusted the health department researchers to clean, code, and analyze the data, and the CAB met only quarterly for the rest of the year to interpret results and guide data dissemination.

In 1999, the CAB resumed monthly meetings to plan a large community forum where the research associates presented the study results. The community forum was held at Glide Memorial Church in the Tenderloin (a low-income neighborhood from which a large number of study participants were recruited) and was attended by about two hundred people. The CAB asked that reporters not be invited to the forum because of the tendency of the media to sensationalize stories regarding the transgender community. An exception was made for a public radio station that presented a very objective summary of the study results.

After the community forum, the CAB membership changed. Several original CAB members had moved out of the area, and others felt that their work was completed. A front-line staff member and a program director from each agency serving the transgender community were asked to join the CAB to begin the process of translating the study results into action. The new eighteen-member CAB met bimonthly in 2000 and quarterly in 2001 to ensure that the research findings were widely distributed and used to secure funding for new HIV services, develop new categories for gender classification, and develop a transgender behavioral risk assessment instrument to be used by agencies providing HIV prevention for transgendered clients.

CBPR Is a Co-Learning Process

The health department researchers and transgender community members came to the table with different, but equally important, knowledge and skills. Throughout each phase of the research project, the two groups challenged and learned from each other, and this reciprocal transfer of knowledge was an especially valuable component of the Transgender Community Health Project.

The transgendered CAB members and research associates spent many hours educating the health department researchers about issues specific to the transgender community, such as the importance of self-identity and psychosocial reasons for risk taking that were crucial to appropriate study design, measurement, and data interpretation. Relying on local knowledge improved the quality of the research and, as will be seen later, helped facilitate the use of the results for program and policy development. The CAB members were trained in research methodology, and the research associates attended more than thirty-five training sessions on topics including HIV counseling, interviewing techniques, protection of human research subjects, research ethics, infection control, street outreach, suicide prevention, and referrals. In addition, the several research associates and CAB members acquired new skills by presenting the study results at local and national conferences and by coauthoring study publications.

Cross-training between MTF and FTM community members also occurred. Although both groups were part of the larger transgender community, it immediately became clear that their issues were very different. For example, MTFs were very concerned about employment discrimination and the high prevalence of sex work in their community, whereas for FTMs, the tendency to have unprotected sex as a way to feel sexually validated as male was a more pressing issue. MTF and FTM community members learned a great deal from each other, and the emerging differences profoundly informed the development of the sampling frame, questionnaire, and data analysis plan.

CBPR Involves System Development

According to Israel and her colleagues (1992), CBPR develops the competencies to diagnose and analyze problems and to plan, implement, and evaluate interventions aimed at meeting identified needs. Members of the CAB who worked at community based organizations were able to use the results from the Transgender Community Health Project to develop new or improve existing interventions at their agencies. For example, the finding that more unprotected sex occurred with main rather than casual or paying partners prompted several agencies to include the main partners of transgendered clients in their risk reduction interventions.

CAB members also decided to develop a simplified data collection instrument that could be used to evaluate interventions at the agency level. Health department researchers helped the CAB members develop a transgender-specific behavioral risk assessment and conducted several trainings on human subjects and survey administration. In this way, individuals at community based organizations were empowered to generate their own client-level data, rather than always relying on information that is gathered from outside researchers. As of this writing, the transgender behavioral risk assessment is still being used by community based organizations that serve transgendered persons in San Francisco.

CBPR Is an Empowering Process

The CAB members often refer to the Transgender Community Health Project as "the study we conducted." As one CAB member remarked, "This time we weren't the clowns, we were the researchers. We weren't asked to do a show or be in a float" (Vasquez, 2000). The CAB members were intimately involved in all phases of the research study, and their feelings of study "co-ownership" were evident from the outset. As CAB member Willy Wilkinson (2000) later wrote:

> I remember the feeling of excitement and commitment that permeated the room. For the first time ever, the responsibility to define and document our community's needs was in our hands, and we were going to do whatever it took to do it right, even if it meant frustration, struggle, and disagreement along the way. This process of community empowerment and self-determination cannot be forced or faked; it came because we were given the opportunity to meet as a community and grapple to define our lives and realities.

Feelings of community ownership were also apparent when the research associates presented the study findings to local agencies, boards, and planning councils. In addition, the research associates were guest lecturers for university courses and made presentations at local and national conferences. Through this process, the research associates emerged as positive role models in the transgender community and acquired valuable skills that they later used to pursue higher-level employment.

The Transgender Community Health Project also empowered the research associates to be themselves in a work environment. For some, this was the first opportunity they had been given to present themselves professionally as they expressed themselves personally. In addition, although many of the research associates had long histories of educating social service providers and the world around them about transgender issues, the study provided monetary and professional validation for this work. The research associates were considered experts in topics that are not typically valued in traditional work environments. Their collective knowledge of topics like sex work, hormones, and monolingual immigrant communities has been recognized by many as a key to the study's success.

CBPR Achieves a Balance Between Research and Action

The primary objective of the Transgender Community Health Project was to obtain a sound estimate of HIV prevalence and risk behaviors among transgendered persons in San Francisco. However, the research was not conducted in the absence of the kind of commitment to action that is a hallmark of participatory research (Cornwall & Jewkes, 1995; Hall, 1981).

As soon as the HIV prevalence data were confirmed, the results were returned to the community. First, a presentation was made to study participants, collaborating agencies, and local planning councils, and then a large forum was held where a community report was released. The research associates and CAB members participated in every presentation and offered programmatic and policy recommendations based on their review of the study data.

The release of findings from the Transgender Community Health Project occurred long before the intricate analyses necessary for publication were complete. Using these data, both the health department and local agencies were able to secure additional funds for HIV prevention and health services for transgendered persons. This resulted in the development and implementation of new programs for transgendered individuals in San Francisco more than two years before the first publication from the study went to press.

The study results have also been used by human rights groups to argue for improved health care and greater discrimination protection for transgendered persons. Recently, the San Francisco Health Services System Board asked for specific data from the Transgender Community Health Project on health issues and gender confirmation surgery, and these materials were used in their landmark decision to offer transgender health care (including sex reassignment surgery) to San Francisco city employees.

Other examples of the balance between research and action are evident when reviewing the accomplishments of the research associates and the CAB members. The in-service agency training sessions that were conducted by research associates throughout the study had a substantial impact on improving services for transgendered individuals in San Francisco. Although the training was originally developed for agencies to which we made frequent referrals, the research associates quickly began to receive requests for training from agencies throughout the Bay Area. Several of the research associates still do transgender in-service trainings.

CAB members attended several San Francisco HIV Prevention Planning Council meetings and successfully convinced the council to adopt new categories for classifying transgendered persons for data collection and service provision. Today, not only are such categories used by all community based organizations who contract with the San Francisco Health Department to provide HIV prevention, but many large HIV/AIDS data reporting systems in San Francisco now report data separately for transgendered persons. Efforts are currently under way to encourage federal agencies such as the Centers for Disease Control and Prevention to adopt similar data collection categories.

The Transgender Community Health Project represents a partnership between San Francisco Health Department researchers and transgendered community members, which was initiated in response to community concerns in 1996 and is still continuing today. This epidemiologic study provided valuable data on a hidden population with a complex array of social, physical, and mental health needs. Community collaborators worked closely with Health Department researchers to ensure that the study results were released in a timely manner and were used to effect social change and improve health outcomes for transgendered persons.

The Transgender Community Health Project helped secure funding for new health and prevention services, improve gender discrimination protection, change the gender categories on existing data collection forms, build agency capacity for data collection, and increase the transgender sensitivity of community based organizations. In addition, researchers from Los Angeles, New York, Boston, and Seattle have asked for assistance in conducting similar studies in their local jurisdictions. In time, the results of such studies may provide a broader understanding of HIV and other public health issues among transgendered individuals throughout the United States.

The overall success of the Transgender Community Health Project can likely be attributed to its effective engagement of CBPR. This research approach is very helpful for conducting epidemiologic research with marginalized and hidden populations who have historically been excluded from the research process and have little trust of outside researchers (see Chapter Four). By encouraging community participation in all phases of the research process, CBPR can demystify research, facilitate co-learning and capacity building, build community trust, improve study validity, and help ensure that the data generated will be used to influence program and policy change. However, researchers interested in using CBPR should realize that this approach requires flexibility, patience, and a long-term commitment.

A central tenant of CBPR is the need to address community-identified concerns (Cornwall & Jewkes, 1995). Outside researchers may find that they must abandon predetermined research objectives that are not congruent with community priorities. This may be difficult for a researcher who wants to respond a request for proposals from a funding agency that has already specified the research goals and objectives that it is willing to fund. In addition, CBPR's emphasis on returning data to the community and involving community collaborators as copresenters and coauthors may conflict with rules specified by academic or funding institutions. If the flexibility to negotiate research objectives and data dissemination rules is lacking, CBPR may not be an appropriate or feasible approach.

Funding agencies and researchers also need to be aware that using an equitable and collaborative research approach can be very time-consuming. If this process is rushed, important issues may be missed, and community members may become frustrated and disillusioned. As described in Chapter Three, CBPR involves a long-term commitment that typically extends beyond a given funding period. Many communities have had negative experiences with outside researchers, who typically seem to disappear as soon as they have obtained their data (Green & Mercer, 2001). Without making a commitment to stay involved until the data are used to effect change, outside researchers may have a difficult time obtaining the community trust necessary for CBPR.

Fortunately, support and funding opportunities for the use of participatory approaches in research that aims to decrease inequities in health status are increasing (Green & Mercer, 2001; Sclove, Scammell, & Holland, 1998). Such support may give researchers the flexibility and time needed to employ CBPR approaches with populations who are disproportionately affected by health and social problems but have had little opportunity to share their experience and knowledge. By recognizing the profound contribution that local experts can make to the research process, CBPR has the potential to contribute to improved community health and social well-being of marginalized and hidden populations.

References

Brown, P. (1992). Popular epidemiology and toxic waste contamination: Lay and professional ways of knowing. *Journal of Health and Social Behavior, 33,* 267–281.

Clements-Nolle, K., Marx, R., Guzman, R., & Katz, M. (2001). HIV prevalence, risk behaviors, health care use, and mental health status of transgender persons: Implications for public health intervention. *American Journal of Public Health, 91,* 915–921.

Clements-Nolle, K., Wilkinson, W., Kitano, K., & Marx, R. (2001). HIV prevention and health service needs of the transgender community in San Francisco. In W. Bockting & S. Kirk (Eds.), *Transgender and HIV: Risks, prevention, and care.* Binghamton, NY: Haworth Press.

Cornwall, A., & Jewkes, J. (1995). What is participatory action research? *Social Science and Medicine, 41,* 1667–1676.

Feinberg, L. (2001). Trans health crisis: For us it's life or death. *American Journal of Public Health, 91,* 897–900.

Gender Education and Advocacy. (2001). *Gender variance: A primer* [www.gender.org/resources/dge/gea01004.pdf].

Green, J. (1994). *Investigation into discrimination against transgendered people: A report by the Human Rights Commission.* San Francisco: City and County of San Francisco.

Green, L. W., & Mercer, S. (2001). Can public health researchers and agencies reconcile the push from funding bodies and the pull from communities? *American Journal of Public Health, 91,* 1926–1929.

Hall, B. L. (1981). Participatory research, poplar knowledge, and power: A personal reflection. *Convergence, 14*(3), 6–19.

Israel, B. A., Schurman, S. J., & Hugentobler, M. K. (1992). Conducting action research: Relationships between organization members and researchers. *Journal of Applied Behavioral Science, 28,* 74–101.

Lombardi, E. (2001). Enhancing transgender health care. *American Journal of Public Health, 91,* 869–872.

Schwab, M., & Syme, S. L. (1997). On paradigms, community participation, and the future of public health. *American Journal of Public Health, 87,* 2049–2051.

Sclove, R. E., Scammell, M., & Holland, B. (1998). *Community research in the U.S.: An introductory reconnaissance, including 12 organizational case studies and comparison with the Dutch Science Shops and the Mainstream American Research System.* Amherst, MA: Loka Institute.

Vasquez, A. (2001, March 7). Panel presentation, Transgender Community Health Project, PAR class, University of California, Berkeley, School of Public Health.

Wilkinson, W. (2000). *The Transgender Community Health Project: Participatory action research with a hidden population.* Unpublished manuscript, University of California, Berkeley, School of Public Health.

Wing, S. (1998). Whose epidemiology, whose health? *International Journal of Health Services, 28,* 241–252.

PART SIX

USING COMMUNITY BASED PARTICIPATORY RESEARCH TO PROMOTE SOCIAL CHANGE AND HEALTHY PUBLIC POLICY

In what is perhaps the most celebrated example of CBPR in the United States, Anne Anderson and her neighbors in Woburn, Massachusetts, worried about the high rates of childhood leukemia in their community, began two decades ago to gather data that led them to suspect a link with the community's water supply. Unsuccessful in their efforts to get local government authorities to test the water, they approached researchers at Harvard's School of Public Health, who worked collaboratively with community members, and also conducted their own analyses, to document what the community residents had long suspected. A subsequent civil suit against corporations that had for years dumped toxic chemicals into the town's water supply not only won a multimillion-dollar out-of-court settlement for victims and their families but is also credited with having been a major impetus for the reauthorization of federal Superfund legislation aimed at cleaning up the country's most hazardous toxic waste sites (Sclove, 1997).

The Woburn case study is a dramatic and admittedly atypical one in terms of the nature and magnitude of its policy-related outcome. Yet it is also a vivid reminder that CBPR's commitment to action need not shy away from action that takes the form of influencing public and private sector policy. In Part Six, we explore the important yet often neglected role that CBPR can play in influencing policy decisions on multiple levels. Makani Themba and Meredith Minkler begin in Chapter Seventeen by summarizing two conceptual frameworks for understanding the public policymaking process in the United States, as well as the steps or stages that tend to apply whether one thinks in terms of broad public policy or private sector policy arenas. They then highlight a complementary set of steps that CBPR partners should consider as they undertake research and use its findings to attempt to influence policy. Examples of the efforts of different CBPR partnerships and community coalitions around the country to influence diverse policies are presented, setting the stage for more detailed case examples in the remainder of Part Six.

In Chapter Eighteen, Juliana van Olphen and her colleagues provide an in-depth case study of the early steps taken in a CBPR project aimed at influencing policy to reduce substance abuse and HIV risk and in other ways facilitate the successful community reintegration of people leaving jail in New York City. They describe efforts by community partners and the Center for Urban Epidemiological Studies at the City University of New York to select and study the problem, narrow down the specific issue areas on which to focus, and move into next steps for research and action. The authors highlight the role of unfavorable public policies in widening health disparities and stress the potential of CBPR for building community capacity and ultimately affecting policy change.

As noted in Chapter Seventeen, although we tend to think of policy in terms of governmental decision making, CBPR can also play a critical role in influencing private sector policies at the workplace and in other nongovernmental arenas. We conclude Part Six with a powerful case study of a research partnership involving unionized low-wage hotel workers, most of them immigrant women, and their academic partners at the University of California in Berkeley and San Francisco. The project's aim was to carefully research and document the working conditions and health status of room cleaners and to use the findings, if appropriate, to influence subsequent workplace health and safety negotiations between union and management.

Pam Tau Lee and her colleagues' case study brings this book full circle: we learn how the topic for the research came from the community—low-wage room cleaners in San Francisco's tourist hotels—and how a core group of these women were involved in each stage of the research process. The case study emphasizes in particular, however, how the increasing individual and community empowerment experienced by room cleaners on the study team and the faith expressed in them by both their union and their academic partners enabled the women to play a key role in translating the study findings into action at the bargaining table. The policy changes they helped bring about, moreover, included not only a significant change in workload policy but also a commitment by the union to support additional participatory action research with hotel workers in diverse settings—research that is already under way.

In her examination of feminist research aimed at social change, Michelle Fine (1994) suggests that "the raison d'être for such research is to unsettle questions, texts, and collective struggles; to challenge what is, incite what could be, and help imagine a world that is not yet imagined." In these final chapters, as in those that preceded them, we hope to demonstrate again the particular potency of CBPR for helping us imagine and realize a more just and equitable society in which individuals and communities have a genuine voice in influencing the factors that determine their health.

References

Fine, M. (1994). Dis-stance and other stances: Negotiations of power inside feminist research. In A. Gitlin (Ed.), *Power and method: Political activism and educational research* (pp. 13–35). New York: Routledge.

Sclove, R. E. (1997). Research by people, for people. *Futures, 29,* 541–549.

CHAPTER SEVENTEEN

Influencing Policy Through Community Based Participatory Research

Makani N. Themba
Meredith Minkler

One of the critical differences between community based participatory research (CBPR) and more traditional approaches to inquiry lies in the former's commitment to action and helping to foster social change as an integral part of the research process (Cornwall & Jewkes, 1995; Gaventa, 1981; Hall, 1992; Israel, Schulz, Parker, & Becker, 1998). As the case studies in this book have illustrated, action may take many forms, including increasing community dialogue about a difficult or taboo topic or securing changed practices at a local school or health care institution, while bringing broader public attention to bear on a previously ignored problem or issue. Such outcomes are important. Yet to influence the lives of large numbers of people, action aimed at changing policy is often critical.

As Toby Citrin (2000, p. 84) has noted, "For grassroots community-based organizations, the term 'policy' is an abstract concept not clearly related to the quality of life of the community, even though many community residents do, in fact, engage in activities to address 'policy issues.'" Similarly, academics engaged in CBPR, like those involved in more traditional research approaches,

Note: The authors gratefully acknowledge the helpful comments provided by Sonja Herbert and Nick Freudenberg on an earlier version of this manuscript. We are grateful as well to Allan Stecker and to Ron Nixon for his work and helpful information on the environmental justice protocol. Thanks also are due Lawrence Wallack and the Berkeley Media Studies Group for their immense contributions to our thinking about the ability of community residents and their academic and professional partners to harness the power of the media to promote healthy public policy.

have often shied away from policy level activity, partly because they tend to think of policy and policy processes as occurring on the national and state levels. These levels are often perceived as being far removed from the local contexts of a CBPR project. As Rist (1994) has argued, although research may influence policy at this level, it tends to be a very minor player amid the many often competing and contradictory forces at work.

Of more immediate relevance to many who engage in CBPR is the possibility of affecting policy on the local level. Much of the best work in local policy development translates existing community concerns into concrete action. As CBPR begins with community selection of an issue, the bridge to policy advocacy should be a logical one. Yet although people, particularly in low-income communities, may be used to having outsiders come in to "mobilize" them around predetermined issues (Minkler & Pies, 1997), they have often had little experience in getting a hearing for their own issues in the corridors of power—and having power listen. Done well, as the examples here suggest, such local involvement can make a critical difference in the local policy environment and can sometimes also help build momentum for related policy changes on the state or national levels.

Nancy Milio (1998, p.15) has defined public policy as "a guide to government action at any jurisdictional level to alter what would otherwise occur. The intent is to achieve a more acceptable state of affairs and, from a public health perspective, a more health-promoting society." She goes on to suggest that organizational policy typically involves a single agency or type of organization (for example, the health department or public schools) while broader policies tend to operate across multiple organizations and affect large populations. In addition to regulatory, legislative, or other formal actions, policy can also be the informal norms or expectations that govern people's actions.

Although government policy on the local level is the primary focus of this chapter, the potential for changing the policies of local businesses and other organizations through alternative means should also be considered. A "policy initiative" is therefore defined broadly here as a planned set of activities, with clear goals and objectives, to change informal or formal mechanisms that affect people's lives.

Many models of policy processes exist with relevance for CBPR in public health and related fields (see, for example, Brownson, Newschaffer, & Ali-Abarghoul, 1997; Longest, 1998; Milio, 1998; Steckler, Dawson, Goodman, & Epstein, 1987). Such models tend to have in common an emphasis on the various stages of policy development, from initiation through adoption, implementation, evaluation or assessment, and reformulation or repeal (Milio, 1998). They also frequently place a heavy emphasis on the sociopolitical environments in which policymaking takes place, recognizing that developing good policy requires a careful examination of the larger context in which the issue is embedded. Finally, models of the policy process typically stress the often circuitous processes involved in policy development. In Milio's words, policy processes "are not linear, and are often punctuated by legal and social challenges, retrenchment or rescissions. They are always embedded in historical and current social contexts. Policy making processes shape content as interested parties attempt to direct the course and pace of policy development to their own needs and priorities" (1998, p. 17).

In this chapter, we briefly review two conceptual frameworks for understanding the public policy process and the steps involved in policy formulation and enactment. Most of the chapter then examines a third framework developed by one of us, Makani Themba, which is more heavily focused on policy advocacy and has relevance for influencing both public policy and policies made outside the public policy arena. Examples and illustrations of opportunities for CBPR involvement at each stage of the policy process are provided. As this chapter demonstrates, although not all CBPR lends itself to the seeking of change on the policy level, CBPR practitioners are increasingly finding the opportunities for policy-level action a potent component and outcome of collaborative inquiry processes.

THE POLICY MAKING PROCESS: TWO CONCEPTUAL MODELS

Longest's (2001) model of the public policymaking process in the United States (see Figure 17.1) is helpful to anyone engaged in CBPR because it stresses the fact that the "window of opportunity" for influencing this process opens whenever there is "a favorable confluence of problems, possible solutions, and political circumstances" (p. 110). Features of the model include the following facts:

- It is a "distinctly cyclical" process, with a circular flow of interactions and influences between the various stages.

- It is an open system, defined as "one in which the process interacts with and is affected by events and circumstances in its external environment."

- It emphasizes several distinct process components but stresses their intimate interdependence.

- It is a highly political process, reflecting a mix of influences on both public and individual interests and rarely proceeding on the basis of rational or empirical decision making.

The three interconnected phases of the public policymaking process identified in Longest's model are as follows:

- *Policy formulation,* encompassing activities involved in setting the policy agenda and later in the actual development of legislation

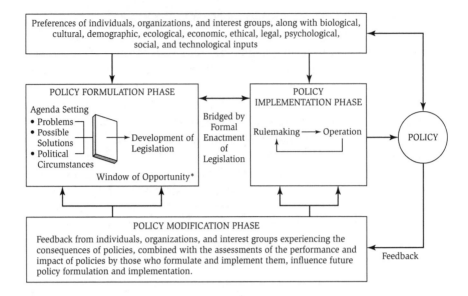

Figure 17.1 A Model of the Public Policymaking Process in the United States.

*The window of opportunity opens when there is a favorable confluence of problems, possible solutions, and political circumstances.

Source: From "The Process of Public Policy Making: A Conceptual Model," by B. B. Longest Jr., Fig. 1, P. 110, in *The Nation's Health* (6th Ed.), Edited by P. R. Lee and C. L. Estes. Copyright © 2001 by Jones and Bartlett Publishers. Reprinted with Permission of Jones and Bartlett Publishers.

- *Policy implementation,* involving all those activities connected with rule making to guide the actual implementing and operationalizing of a policy
- *Policy modification,* including the revisiting and possible alteration of all previous decisions and compromises made during the policymaking process

As Longest's model suggests, the formal enactment of legislation serves as a bridge between the policy formulation process and the subsequent implementation phase (see Figure 17.1). The third or policy modification phase in turn comes into play as a feedback loop through which minor tweaking of the legislation or a major revisiting of the agenda-setting process may take place. Both the political nature of policymaking and the dynamic nature of the external environment in which policymaking occurs underscore the likelihood of policy modification—and in extreme cases, even repeal—during this phase.

The policymaking process just described is expanded upon by Steckler and Dawson (1982) and their colleagues (Steckler et al., 1987), who offer a conceptual model consisting of seven stages. We shall briefly describe each of these, along with its relevance for CBPR.

Problem Awareness and Identification

In this first phase, a particular health or social problem is "brought to the public agenda and recognized as an important and legitimate problem which should be addressed by policy" (Steckler & Dawson, 1982, p. 279). Competition among interest groups and the sheer number of complex health and social problems that cannot be solved by individual or micro-level intervention suggest how formidable this first stage actually is. The commitment of CBPR to community, rather than outside-expert-driven issue selection, however, underscores the importance of having the voices of CBPR community partners heard and critically inform agenda setting at this early problem identification stage.

Problem Refinement

Problem refinement involves the movement from a broad formulation of the policy issue to a more specific problem statement including concrete policy objectives. As Steckler et al. (1987) note, although this stage typically involves investigation and analysis of the extent of the problems and the populations affected, it is also inherently political. Particularly in the case of controversial issues (for example, a proposal to allow needle exchange to prevent HIV/AIDS), interest groups on opposite sides of the issue are likely to present vastly different data and data interpretations. CBPR that can help illuminate and bring forward authentic community voices at this stage can play a critical role in framing (or reframing) the problem.

Setting Policy Objectives

Although attempts at setting policy objectives often occur as part of the problem refinement process, the formulation of objectives for the long haul is likely to occur only after a working consensus has been reached about the nature and extent of the problem being addressed. Typically stated in broad terms in order to address the concerns of many competing interest groups, policy goals and objectives may in fact contain internal contradictions as a result of the many political compromises involved in their adoption (Steckler & Dawson, 1982). Once again, CBPR can play a critical role in this stage of the process by helping ensure that the real interests of community members are not forgotten in the process of compromise and negotiation.

Designing Alternative Courses of Action

The intentionally broad nature of policy objectives and the fact that they not infrequently contradict one another suggest the likelihood of a number of alternative courses of action being put forward. Participants in a CBPR project may be among the many competing interest groups to offer suggested programs or other courses of action at this stage, in the hopes that at least some of their recommendations for action will be mirrored in the final policy or program adopted.

Estimating the Consequences of Alternative Actions

Once alternative programs or other policy strategies have been proposed, an evaluative stage ensues during which CBPR partners also may wish to weigh in. Policy analysis during this stage typically involves assessing who benefits and who pays for the various actions being proposed, which health or social problems are being addressed and with what likely effectiveness, potential interaction effects between the proposed action and a variety of societal factors, and what other alternative actions might be developed to achieve the same or different policy objectives (Milio, 1998; Steckler et al., 1987; Themba, 1999). Opportunities for public comment at this stage may provide an excellent chance for CBPR partners to re-present the merits of the particular actions they advocate, within a framework that addresses the analytical questions being asked at this stage. To enhance their impact, the partners should estimate the logistics, costs, and potential savings of the various options under consideration, demonstrating that they've "done their homework."

Assigning Implementation Responsibility

The often neglected implementation phase of the policy process involves both ensuring that an agency or other entity within the bureaucracy has clear responsibility for carrying out a new program or policy and undertaking local program development (Steckler et al., 1987). A variety of barriers frequently get in the way of effective program implementation. Key among these are failure to assign adequate fiscal and personnel resources; lack of enthusiasm (or actual opposition) among those changed with overseeing policy implementation; and the inertia that often characterizes bureaucracies (Longest, 1998; Milio, 1998; Themba, 1999). By offering relevant technical assistance and working, often with other program supporters, to press for overcoming structural barriers (rather than simply assuming that things are moving forward), CBPR partners may again have a key role to play in this phase of the policy process.

Evaluation

Although health researchers, practitioners, and other CBPR partners are often engaged in program evaluation, there is frequently a disconnect between local program evaluation and evaluation of the larger policy process. Yet practitioners of CBPR may have valuable roles to play in this stage as well, particularly if the principles of participatory evaluation can be introduced early on in the evaluative process (see Chapter Thirteen). Such evaluation would include an examination of such outcomes as how well a resultant program resembled what the policy had intended and the relative efficacy of different aspects of the program. But it also would include ongoing, collaborative inquiry into whether and how well the CBPR partners were staying "on track" in their own process (Fetterman, Kaftarian, & Wandersman, 1996) and in achieving their policy-related goals and objectives.

In sum, and whether we think in terms of broad stages (for example, policy formulation, implementation, and modification) or more discrete phases within these stages, understanding the policymaking process is critical to CBPR partners interested in attempting to influence this process. Moreover, for most of the stages in the policymaking process, there are corresponding advocacy steps through which CBPR partners may seek to influence policymaking efforts. We turn now to some key considerations and advocacy steps relevant for those interested in attempting to influence either public policy or policies in the private sector through CBPR.

DEFINING AND FRAMING A POLICY GOAL

As Citrin (2000, p. 84) has pointed out, "While academics and practitioners are inclined to look first at policymaking and then at its impacts on constituent groups, community residents usually reverse this process, looking first at their daily needs and then at the way these are affected by policy decisions." The general policy goal for a CBPR project flows, by definition, from the community's identification of the problem and outcomes of the dialogical processes in which it has engaged in order to better explore this issue or problem. Yet as just suggested, policy goals must also take into account a wide variety of additional factors, and a key part of getting to action in CBPR involves ensuring that those other contextual factors are considered in formulating a policy goal. A good policy goal requires cutting or shaping the issue into effective or doable action that engages broader community interest and support. Framing the problem or issue in ways that will attract a wide constituency whose members care enough about the issue to become actively involved is critical at this stage. In addition, and consistent with the principles of CBPR delineated in Chapter Three, the policy goal adopted should incorporate features that help a community or community based organization or coalition achieve such goals as the following:

- *Building community and organizational capacity* by expanding the leadership base and creating more involved community members
- *Solving real problems,* ideally through policy impacts that can be concisely stated in twenty-five words or less
- *Contributing to a sense of community,* bringing more people together and giving them a sense of their own power and leadership
- *Laying the foundation for more good policy,* serving as an incremental step on the path toward the community partners' larger goals and placing this specific policy goal within a longer-term community strategic action plan
- *Bringing the community closer to its vision* of a healthy community and a better world

An additional frequently cited feature of a good policy goal in this era of cost containment is that it pays for itself. CBPR efforts to reduce the plethora of alcohol and tobacco outlets in low-income communities of color might thus craft a policy goal of establishing local permit fees for the selling of these products or conditional use permits for such environmental land uses as billboards (Themba, 1999). Whatever the ultimate goal selected, however, CBPR partners should be guided in their thinking by a coherent set of guiding considerations so that the selected goal has good likelihood for success and for contributing to subsequent community building in the process.

SELECTING A POLICY APPROACH

After selecting a policy goal, CBPR partners will need to determine who has the power to make the change, whether that be an elected official, a planning commission, or a locally headquartered business. As noted earlier, although the focus of this chapter is primarily on efforts to influence local public policy (for example, through initiatives and ordinances), efforts to similarly bring about policy changes in relevant private sector arenas and other complementary strategies for change also should be considered. Let us look at a range of possible policy-related strategies.

Voluntary Agreements

Voluntary agreements are "pacts between a community and one or more institutions that outline conditions, expectations, or obligations without the force of law" (Themba, 1999, p. 91). Such agreements provide a useful alternative when there isn't enough support to enact more formal regulations. Ideally, written memorandums of understanding should be developed that clearly spell out the conditions of the agreement, and care must be taken to ensure that the terms of the agreement are being honored.

Some voluntary agreements are forged as legislation that offers incentives for parties who would be regulated to consent to regulation or oversight. One such agreement, the Louisiana Green Scorecard, was administered by the state—although it was the Louisiana Coalition for Tax Justice that worked with a university based research partner to design and disseminate it. Backed by a broad coalition of civil rights groups, labor unions, teachers, tenants groups, and environmental organizations, the Scorecard was a voluntary regulatory process that companies seeking or receiving state tax incentives could go through if they were interested in receiving these subsidies. The tool evaluated companies' environmental performance and tied their performance to the amount of tax breaks they received. Although the legislation was difficult to enforce due to its voluntary nature, and although it was ultimately dropped when a new administration was elected a year later, it succeeded in pressuring companies to invest in new pollution prevention equipment. As a result, more jobs were created, and air pollution and toxic emissions were reduced by 177 million pounds (Themba, 1999).

Legal Actions

Well-framed legal actions, such as lawsuits and other court actions, can also accomplish significant long- and short-term goals, even if they simply involve getting the other party to the table. Yet such actions can be tedious and expensive, as well as a major distraction if not integrated into a broader community agenda (Themba, 1999). Further, failure to identify the right defendants (for example, the parent company of a major local polluter) can lead to embarrassing and demoralizing defeats. In lieu of (or in addition to) bringing a lawsuit, simply filing complaints about bad or illegal practices with the appropriate regulatory agency can be an effective policy approach.

In Idaho, organizations working in low-income communities were reasonably confident that the state's low number of enrollees in the Child Health Insurance Program (CHIP)—a program that provided low-cost health insurance to low-income families—was due to poor administration practices. They needed evidence, however, to use in confronting the state Department of Health and Welfare (DHW) and pressure for change.

The Idaho Community Action Network (ICAN), a coalition of both organizations and more than one thousand local residents of six mostly low-income communities, took on this charge, working in partnership with academic partners at Virginia Tech. Through door-to-door canvassing and other means, the ICAN members began by identifying twenty-five families they believed to be eligible for CHIP or Medicaid coverage. Borrowing a methodology used to test for housing discrimination, they then examined whether the CHIP program was practicing discrimination. ICAN helped the families apply for the program and recorded their experiences as they worked their way through the labyrinthine process over several weeks. In addition to providing informal advising on this early stage of the process, ICAN's academic partners then helped analyze the data. The results clearly showed that applicants of color were treated differently from white applicants—although all applicants were treated poorly—and spelled out the nature of this discriminatory treatment in a report to the DHW (Idaho Community Action Network, 1999).

ICAN then filed an administrative complaint with this state agency as well as the U.S. Department of Health and Human Services, outlining findings from the report. At the federal level, ICAN highlighted the ways in which the Idaho CHIP policies were markedly different from national norms. For example, the CHIP application was seventeen pages long in Idaho, whereas many other states had shorter and less intimidating applications. ICAN was able to win new policies guiding the implementation of CHIP, including a new four-page application and added safeguards for the treatment of Spanish-speaking applicants (Themba, Delgado, Vribe, & Calpotura, 2000).

Studies and Moratoriums

Mandated studies and moratoriums pending data collection can be helpful under certain circumstances. Although CBPR can uncover valuable information about an unhealthy or unlawful institutional practice, far more extensive study may be necessary to provide the hard data needed to support a policy change. In such instances, CBPR partners may identify a policy goal of getting a mandated study or other data collection performed (or protecting what is currently being collected, such as data on racial/ethnic disparities in health). When a Los Angeles coalition's preliminary investigation led it to fight for and get a mandated city study on wage levels, the resulting information was so disconcerting that it laid an important basis for subsequent work toward a living-wage law (Themba, 1999).

Another useful policy approach may involve calling for a moratorium on continued policy enactment until more data are available. A moratorium on the conversion of low-income housing into tourist units in downtown San Francisco in the early 1980s provided valuable time for a neighborhood planning coalition to study and demonstrate the impacts of such conversions on the city's growing homeless population. The "breathing time" allowed by a moratorium also can enable CBPR partners to help organize neighborhood hearings or town hall meetings and forums with legislators in attendance. Such events, particularly if well publicized and offering a blend of the numbers and stories needed to help influence pubic opinion (Wallack, Woodruff, Dorfman, & Diaz, 1999), can help mobilize support for a policy change.

Electoral Strategies

Electoral strategies, like legal approaches to policy change, tend to be extremely time-consuming and labor-intensive. Yet such approaches, including ballot initiatives, referendums, or even support of candidates can have considerable payoff over the longer term. As Steckler and Dawson (1982, p. 289) suggest, "States which offer the possibility of a referendum or initiative enable citizens themselves to become policy makers." There are short-term payoffs as well. Electoral campaigns can help raise the profile of an issue, attract volunteers, and pull an issue out of the purview of nonsupportive policymakers and place it directly before a more supportive public. Whether helping to craft an initiative or becoming involved in an effort to react to an existing policy through a referendum, CBPR partners can facilitate bringing an issue to public attention.

Electoral strategies were among a range of approaches used as part of the California Wellness Foundation's Violence Prevention Initiative, a $60 million grantmaking program that began in 1993 with the goal of reducing youth violence in the state. An important component of the initiative—the effort to curb the sale and wide availability of handguns—included efforts by the Pacific Center for Violence Prevention at San Francisco General Hospital's Trauma Foundation to coordinate data gathering, policy, and media advocacy training and other activities in collaboration with community based organizations, grassroots advocates, business representatives, health professionals, law enforcement and education groups, and local and state political figures and organizations (Wallack, 1999).

The efforts were tailored to the issues of specific communities. In suburban Livermore, for example, widespread concern over "junk guns" or "Saturday night specials"—poor-quality, low-cost, and easily concealed handguns popular among youth—led to the passage of a referendum that effectively banned the sale of junk guns in that city (Wallack, 1999). This measure, which ratified the 3–2 decision of the city council to ban the weapons, was the first such public vote in the state. By the fall of 1998, fully sixty-seven cities and half a dozen counties had enacted local ordinances placing limits on handguns (Legal Community Against Violence, 1998). A bill banning the manufacture and sale of such weapons statewide was also passed. Although quickly vetoed by then Governor Pete Wilson, a similar bill was signed by his successor, Governor Gray Davis, and became effective in January 2000.

As Lawrence Wallack (1997, p. 49) has noted, "The public health approach to violence prevention" involves not only epidemiological methods and the application of social and behavioral sciences research but also "[mobilizing] communities to participate in the definition and solution of violence problems" through multiple means. Although CBPR was just one of many components of the fight against gun violence in California, the collaborative study and mounting of electoral campaigns by multiple partners was a crucial part of the picture and provides a potent example of the power of such partnerships.

Each of these policy-related approaches—voluntary agreements, legal actions, mandated studies and moratoriums, and electoral strategies—has both advantages and disadvantages that must be carefully weighed by CBPR partners in their efforts to select the alternative most likely to succeed. Next we describe some of the key considerations and advocacy steps that are relevant in the use of a variety of alternative approaches to policy change and that complement and expand on the policy process stages in the conceptual models just described.

IDENTIFYING A TARGET

As noted earlier, decisions about the particular policy approach best suited to a given CBPR effort should be driven in part by a careful analysis of the most appropriate change target or decision-making body with the power to bring about the changes sought. Several key questions may be helpful to community members and their outside research partners as they choose an appropriate target, including these (Themba, 1999):

- Who or what institutions have the power to solve or ameliorate the problem and grant the community's demands?
- Are there key actors who must be approached first as gatekeepers to the people with real power?
- What would motivate key actors to take the actions you want to see (for example, would a politician who is up for reelection be aided by your cause)?
- Which targets are appointed? Which are elected?
- Are their relevant bodies (such as commissions or subcommittees) that are open to community participation and that one or more of your members might join?
- What are the most strategic sources of power for influencing the targets (for example, voters, consumers, faith-based organizations, taxpayers, investors, neighborhood organizations)?
- What are the target's self-interests where this issue is concerned?
- Who would have jurisdiction if you redefined the issue (for example, if you turned a tobacco advertising issue into a question of fair business practices)? Would this increase your likelihood of success?

As suggested by some of these questions, each potential decision-making body or target will require different organizing strategies to move the target to action. A critical part of the CBPR process will therefore include strategic analysis in narrowing down potential targets and research into each target's self-interests, strengths, and vulnerabilities. Not infrequently, such research will reveal the existence of a more vulnerable target with whom the possibility of success is greater. This target is often referred to as the *primary* target on whom pressure is focused. Recent community organizing and CBPR around billboard advertising of alcohol and tobacco provides a good case in point. Participants have found it more effective, for example, to target local and in some cases state governments to restrict the placement and content of ads than to pressure the billboard industry itself to give up a sizable portion of its revenue from such advertisements (Themba, 1999). In other instances, there may need to be additional, secondary targets to bring about the desired change.

SUPPORT, POWER, AND OPPOSITION

Building support for a CBPR policy goal or approach often requires building a coalition of organizations that come together temporarily for a specific reason (Berkowitz & Wolff, 2000; Wandersman, Goodman, & Butterfoss, 1997). As Shoshanna Sofaer (2001, p. 9) has pointed out, "Policy-oriented coalitions can be relevant on several jurisdictional levels, depending on which level of government or private policy-making group is responsible for the target policies." In deciding whether to put together such a coalition, CBPR partners should consider the kinds of support needed to win, which groups are most likely to support the policy goal or initiative, and which can influence the target or decision maker. Community members of the CBPR team can be particularly helpful at this stage in sharing their knowledge of key community players and the potential interests of each. Both informal groups (for example, parents of children with asthma) and formal community organizations should be considered as potential allies. Each potential ally's commitment to the issue and self-interests, as well as both the resources and the possible risks and liabilities their involvement might entail, need to be considered in building a base of support for the policy action being proposed.

At the same time that CBPR partners work to build their own power base, they need to think strategically about the interests and potential power base of the opposition. Community interests in lead abatement, improved air quality, and the like may thus translate into policy initiatives whose implementation would hurt a powerful industry or a local employer's bottom line. Since these likely opponents may also have powerful lobbies or make substantial contributions to the coffers of elected decision makers, the importance of their opposition should not be minimized. CBPR partners need to consider such matters as whose interests may be adversely affected by a policy initiative, in what ways they may be affected, and whether the proposed initiative will cost money or raise fees or taxes. As in other forms of community based research and organizing, the need for "doing your homework," to understand in detail who pays for a proposed policy, and to be able to justify it to the decision makers being targeted is critical to success.

STAGES IN DEVELOPING AND IMPLEMENTING A POLICY INITIATIVE: OPPORTUNITIES FOR CBPR INVOLVEMENT

Regardless of the form a policy change effort may take, several key stages should take place (see Table 17.1), each of which offers unique opportunities for CBPR involvement. Let us examine each of these stages from a policy advocacy perspective.

Table 17.1. Stages in the Policy Process and Corresponding Steps in Policy Advocacy.

Policy Change (Steckler and Dawson)	Policy Advocacy (Themba)
Problem awareness and identification: Advocates and policymakers identify problems or issues to be addressed in future legislation	*Testing the Waters:* Advocates gather information by listening to constituents, research and other means to identify a policy approach to shared problems or actualizing a vision
Problem refinement: Work is done to refine identified problems and issues; choose priorities	*Defining the Initiative:* Advocates define the policy initiative based on community input and organizing opportunities.
Setting policy objectives: Clear objectives for the policy are identified based on problem refinement process.	*Strategy and Analysis/Direct Issue Organizing:* Outreach, media and organizing to build support for the policy; identify and neutralize opponents.
Designing alternative courses of action: In the policy arena, identifying alternatives is an important part of the process as it often operates as a "market" with competing interests. *Estimating the consequences of alternative actions:*	*In the Belly of "The Beast":* Advocates tend to identify alternatives only if they assess that they do not have the clout to win their original proposal. Still, the time engaged with officials often requires compromise and caution. Here's where advocates negotiate and push around what the content of the policy will be, implementation processes, funding levels, etc. *Victory and Defense:* Celebrating victories amongst constituents and in the media is important to organizing goals. But time for celebration is often short, as progressive policy initiatives must anticipate legal and other challenges.
Assigning implementation responsibility: Decisionmakers identify what agency will have responsibility (and often resources) for implementation.	*Enforcement and Evaluation:* Community groups work to ensure that their hard won legislation is enforced and that there are mechanisms for oversight.
Evaluation: Formal mechanisms for assessing policy impact and outcomes.	Participatory evaluation ideally is employed throughout the process, with CBPR partners actively engaged.

Assessing the Policy Environment and Testing the Waters

As Milio (1998, p. 20) suggests, "Organized activity surrounding the policy making process in any given issue is set in a historical context derived from past experience with similar issues and current constraining circumstances that affect all interested parties." Thus demographic, epidemiological, political and other factors all are likely to influence the reception a given policy initiative will receive and its chances for success. Monitoring the policy environment must therefore begin as a key component of the data gathering that will inform what a potential policy initiative might look like.

At the same time that they are assessing the environment, CBPR partners may "try on" or test a number of potential approaches to addressing their issue. Broad community support, legality, and the likelihood of success are key among the criteria that should be considered at this early stage. The importance of monitoring the policy environment and testing the waters was demonstrated in San Diego, California, when a community coalition, organized in the wake of a juvenile shooting, mobilized to study and take action to prevent such violence. The group's first goal was broad gun control. However, research on the legislative remedies available and consideration of the policy environment—an environment dominated by powerful gun lobbies—indicated that they should consider regulatory initiatives with a narrower scope. These were the banning of "junk guns" and local regulation of bullet sales. Although regulating bullet sales was felt to be too tough a fight for the coalition at that time, targeting junk guns proved effective. As noted earlier, coalitions nationwide have taken on junk gun bans and won them at the local and state levels. As with many of these other coalitions, the key in San Diego was identifying a narrower focus in ways that divided their opposition and made a win more likely (Staples, 1997; Themba, 1999; Wallack et al., 1999).

Reframing the Issue and Defining the Initiative

A critical step in the action phase of CBPR for policy change involves helping community partners refine the issue they have collectively identified and collaboratively examined so that it becomes a clear policy initiative. In the context of CBPR, the best policy initiatives often come from having community partners articulate their ideal policy and then looking for the best mechanism to bring that vision to reality (Themba, 1999). Reframing the issue may be needed at this point so that the policy initiative that is crafted clearly reflects the community's interests while also showing sensitivity to broader environmental issues (Milio, 1998) and the concerns of real or potential allies and other stakeholders. A CBPR project focused on preventing youth violence, for example, and targeting a local city council with the goal of limiting handgun availability and increasing youth employment opportunities may reframe its initial initiative to emphasize the social and economic aspects of youth violence (Wallack, 1994). By tapping into the aspects of the issue of greatest concern to local council members and reframing the issue to reflect these concerns, the CBPR partners may substantially increase their chances for success.

Part of reframing may also involve defining issues nationally and internationally, as well as locally. Many environmental groups, for example, have researched the practices of companies seeking to build a new plant in order to assess their record on environmental issues in other states or countries. Where unethical or dubious practices are uncovered, this information can be used in legal or educational campaigns. Similarly, local CBPR groups attempting to mobilize against the tobacco industry have sometimes studied and publicized its increased targeting of people of color in Third World countries and the nations of the former USSR (World Health Organization, 1996). Revealing such practices overseas may have value at home in delegitimizing the image of multinational parent companies that allow or encourage such practices.

Strategic Power Analysis

Once the initiative has been identified, the CBPR partners conduct a strategic "power analysis" to identify the targets, allies, opponents, and other factors that will be important in the campaign. Kurt Lewin's (1947) classic "force field analysis" may be used at this stage, as participants lay out the driving forces in support of the initiative and the likely resisting or restraining forces that may work against its success. Methods for removing or weakening the resisting forces and both adding new driving forces and strengthening the power of those already operative are then considered. A "SWOT analysis" may be conducted at this stage, through which participants lay out the *strengths* and *weaknesses* internal to their case and the *opportunities* and *threats* in the external environment that may influence their chances of success (Barry, 1997). As in force field analysis, participants in a SWOT strategic planning exercise also consider steps that may be taken to build their strengths, minimize weaknesses, capitalize on external opportunities, and respond to potential outside threats (Barry, 1997). Often the initiative is refined further in the light of this new information.

A SWOT analysis figured prominently in the decision by tobacco control organizations working in African American communities to mount a campaign to shut down "X Brand" cigarettes. Typically, the focus in tobacco control is on further regulation because the industry is both very powerful and well funded. However, Duffy Distributors, the "inventor" of X Brand, was a small, family-operated business in predominantly white Charlestown, Massachusetts, not far from Boston.

Activists were angry because the brand appeared to use symbolism associated with a then-popular Spike Lee movie on Malcolm X. Talks with the company about withdrawing the brand were not making headway. The power analysis and strategic planning process revealed that concerted media pressure would likely force the small company to discontinue the brand. They were right. In just two weeks, the company could not withstand the barrage of media coverage, protests, and bad publicity and decided to drop the brand altogether. Without research and power analysis to guide the group's strategy, it might have settled for far less (Themba, 1996).

Although the X Brand action was a clear success story, strategic analysis and related processes can also be helpful when victory may be less likely or incomplete. As Rochefort and Cobb (1993) suggest, the feasibility analysis conducted during this stage of the policy process may well suggest possible compromise positions, which can in turn be explored in advance but held in reserve as backup positions to be used if a compromise appears necessary.

Organizing Support for the Initiative

Informed by the power analysis and strategic planning, organizing for the proposed policy change begins. A variety of strategies may be useful at this stage, including town hall meetings, door-to-door canvassing, outreach to additional organizational partners, and media advocacy. Defined as the strategic use of mass media to advance a social or public policy initiative (U.S. Department of Health and Human Services, 1989), media advocacy has increasingly been used by local community groups and CBPR partners to deliver their message and create pressure for change (Wallack, 1994; Wallack et al., 1999).

Media advocacy is critical to policy advocacy. Important political debates are carried out in fifteen-second sound bites, and a single news story can be the catalyst for new legislation. For better or worse, the media are clearly central to setting the public agenda, with news media playing a particularly important role as the public's "official story." It is now nearly axiomatic that what story is chosen for coverage and how it is covered largely determines public sentiment—especially among public officials.

Given the importance of the media's agenda-setting and legitimizing functions, data and research play critical roles in establishing the credibility of community policy initiatives with policymakers and the public at large. CBPR findings have been particularly important to efforts that were unpopular or focused on communities with few resources. For example, welfare rights groups partnered with Virginia Polytechnic University researcher Susan Gooden to disseminate research on discrimination in workfare programs. Gooden's work documented what many organizers knew anecdotally—that women of color did not receive equal access to training, placement, and employment services. Groups leveraged the data in an intensive media campaign to pressure the federal government to enact civil rights protections for program participants. The media campaign helped raise awareness about problems with the administration of workfare programs and put pressure on state and federal agencies to make changes (Themba et al., 2000).

In the Belly of the Beast

Once the initiative is on the table and support is made clear, groups will work closely with decision makers to ensure that the policy is actually enacted. Often further research and expertise are needed as community groups and researchers make their case. It is at this stage that CBPR partnerships are at greatest risk, as decision makers will often look to researchers and other traditional "experts" for input and sometimes act to exclude community based groups that they perceive are less "professional." These classic "divide and conquer" tactics have hurt a wide variety of movements.

To address this problem, environmental justice advocates (groups working to address dimensions of racism in environmental policy) used part of their national meeting in 1994 to hammer out protocols for community work with researchers in order to avoid further conflicts. Representatives of more than two dozen groups were involved in this effort, including national coalitions and regional networks representing smaller community based groups like the Asian Pacific Environmental Network in California, the Southern Organizing Committee, and South Carolina CLEAN. Similar protocols have been developed by other groups working to foster more effective community-researcher partnerships (see Chapter Three and Appendix A), and sample memorandums of understanding have been published and widely disseminated (Fawcett, Francisco, Paine-Andrews, & Schultz, 2000).

Victory and Defense

In the case of progressive policies, winning enactment can mean that a corporate court challenge is soon to follow (Themba, 1999). CBPR practitioners in their roles as advocates must prepare for the possibility of litigation at the beginning of the initiative and be ready to play an active role in any legal action even if the local government (and not their group) is the defendant. CBPR partners have played an important role in this stage of the policy process by working with communities to craft public testimony with an eye toward building a strong public record as a defense against any future litigation. Research on alcohol outlets and increased homicide rates helped Los Angeles' Community Coalition defend against a challenge to an ordinance regulating liquor stores. The coalition partnered with researchers and attorneys to intervene in an alcohol industry lawsuit against the city in a process in which a community group steps into a lawsuit on the side of a public agency defendant to ensure that community interests are well defended (Mosher & Works, 1994). Similarly, Baltimore's Citywide Liquor Coalition made sure that its attorney worked closely with the city attorney throughout an initiative process. Their objective was to carefully craft testimony that would be part of a strong public record in preparation for the litigation that would follow passage of the policy they were supporting (Themba, 1999). In sum, and although celebrating a victory is always in order

(Staples, 1997), preparing for challenges to a controversial new policy is also a critical part of the action in which CBPR partners may usefully engage.

Enforcement and Evaluation

After the policy is enacted and has cleared any legal challenges, the work to get the new law enforced begins. For initiatives with powerful opposition, negotiation continues around issues like the timeline for implementing the policy, interpretation of particular clauses, and fitting the new policy in with other staffing priorities. Researchers and community based groups working together have helped agencies identify existing enforcement models and propose new enforcement procedures that meet community needs. In addition, research partners have helped community groups design processes for evaluating new policies with an eye toward strengthening these policies and their enforcement. One example of such a partnership was the work of South Carolina Fair Share with University of South Carolina researchers on enforcement and effectiveness of new child health insurance policies. Research partners were able to develop a participatory evaluation process that provided accessible information on how well the program was working and why. Armed with good data, community groups could take an active part in the implementation process in an informed, ongoing way (Themba et al., 2000).

CBPR has been an important asset in community based policy development. It has helped identify, make visible, and legitimize issues so that they are placed on the public's agenda. It has also helped community advocates attract media attention for long-standing but long ignored issues when there are newsworthy findings. The best initiatives use research as a way of documenting and elucidating problems that are already of concern to communities, in ways that help build confidence in community based knowledge and ways of knowing (Ansley & Gaventa, 1997).

In policy arenas, CBPR can be an agent for the democratization of information through active involvement of communities in data gathering by giving community based groups equal access to the kinds of data that help drive policymaking. It can help them influence the policy process in ways that can benefit the groups of which communities are a part. As noted at the beginning of this chapter, research is of course only one of the many factors that influence policy and is indeed a minor player when compared to political realties and funding considerations (Rist, 1994). Yet as the examples in this and several other chapters illustrate, community groups and their research partners who are intentional about policy outcomes from the beginning can help build CBPR projects that result in lasting, formal community change for the better.

References

Ansley, F., & Gaventa, J. (1997, January-February). Researching for democracy and democratizing research. *Change,* pp. 46–53.

Barry, B. W. (1997). *Strategic planning workbook for nonprofit organizations.* St. Paul, MN: Amherst H. Wilder Foundation.

Berkowitz, B., & Wolff, T. (2000). *The spirit of the coalition.* Washington, CD: American Public Health Association.

Brownson, R. C., Newschaffer, C. J., & Ali-Abarghoul, F. (1997). Policy research for disease prevention: Challenges and practical recommendations. *American Journal of Public Health, 87,* 735–739.

Citrin, T. (2000). Policy issues in a community-based approach. In T. A. Bruce & S. Uranga McKane (Eds.), *Community-based public health: A partnership model* (pp. 83–90). Washington, DC: American Public Health Association, 2000.

Cornwall, A., & Jewkes, R. (1995). What is participatory research? *Social Science and Medicine, 41,* 1667–1676.

Fawcett, S. B., Francisco, V. T., Paine-Andrews, A., & Schultz, J. A. (2000). A model memorandum of collaboration: A proposal. *Public Health Reports, 115,* 174–179.

Fetterman, D., Kaftarian, S. J., & Wandersman, A. (Eds.). (1996). *Empowerment evaluation: Knowledge and tools for self-assessment and accountability.* Thousand Oaks, CA: Sage.

Gaventa, J. (1981). Participatory research in North America. *Convergence, 14,* 30–42.

Hall, B. L. (1992). From margins to center: The development and purpose of participatory research. *American Sociologist, 23*(4), 15–28.

Idaho Community Action Network. (1999). *All kids need a healthy start: DHW doesn't play fair with children's health.* Boise: Author.

Israel, B. A., Schulz, A. J., Parker, E. A., & Becker, A. B. (1998). Review of community-based research: Assessing partnership approaches to improve public health. *Annual Review of Public Health, 19,* 173–202.

Legal Community Against Violence. (1998). *Communities on the move.* San Francisco: Author.

Lewin, K. (1947). Quasi-stationary and social equilibria and the problem of social change. In T. Newcomb & E. Hartley (Eds.), *Readings in social psychology* (pp. 340–344). New York: Holt, Rinehart and Winston.

Longest, B. B., Jr. (1998). *Health policymaking in the United States* (2nd ed.). Chicago: Health Administration Press.

Longest, B. B., Jr. (2001). The process of public policy making: A conceptual model. In P. R. Lee & C. L. Estes, *The nation's health* (6th ed., pp. 109–115). Sudbury, MA: Jones & Bartlett.

Milio, N. (1998). Priorities and strategies for promoting community-based prevention policies. *Journal of Public Health Management and Practice, 4*(3), 14–28.

Minkler, M., & Pies, C. (1997). Ethical issues in community organizing and participation. In M. Minkler (Ed.), *Community organizing and community building for health* (pp. 120–138). New Brunswick, NJ: Rutgers University Press.

Mosher, J., & Works, R. (1994). *Confronting Sacramento: State preemption, community control, and alcohol-outlet blight in two inner-city communities.* San Rafael, CA: Marin Institute.

Rist, C. (1994). Influencing the policy process with qualitative research. In N. K. Denzin & Y. S. Lincoln (Eds.), *Handbook of qualitative research* (pp. 545–557). Thousand Oaks, CA: Sage.

Rochefort, D., & Cobb, R. (1993). Definition, agenda, access, and policy choice. *Policy Studies Journal, 21,* 56–71.

Sofaer, S. (2001). *Working together, moving ahead: A manual to support effective community health coalitions.* New York: Baruch College, School of Public Affairs.

Staples, L. (1997). Selecting and "cutting" the issue. In M. Minkler (Ed.), *Community organizing and community building for health* (pp. 175–194). New Brunswick, NJ: Rutgers University Press.

Steckler, A., & Dawson, L. (1982). The role of health education in public policy development. *Health Educational Quarterly, 9,* 275–292.

Steckler, A., Dawson, L., Goodman, R. M., & Epstein, N. (1987). Policy advocacy: Three emerging roles for health education. *Advances in Health Education and Promotion, 2,* 5–27.

Themba, M. N. (1996). *Chalk one up for David: The African American Tobacco Education Network and the fight to stop X Brand.* Sacramento, CA: African American Tobacco Education Network.

Themba, M. N. (1999). *Making policy, making change: How communities are taking law into their own hands.* San Francisco: Jossey-Bass.

Themba, M. N., Delgado, G., Vribe, J., & Calpotura, F. (2000). *Grassroots innovative policy program.* Oakland, CA: Applied Research Center.

U.S. Department of Health and Human Services. (1989). *Media strategies for smoking control: Guidelines.* Washington, DC: U.S. Government Printing Office.

Wallack, L. (1994). Media advocacy: A strategy for empowering people and communities. *Journal of Public Health Policy, 15,* 420–436.

Wallack, L. (1997). Strategies for reducing youth violence: Media, community, and policy. In California Wellness Foundation, *1997 Wellness Lectures* (pp. 41–69). Berkeley: University of California Press.

Wallack, L. (1999). The California Violence Prevention Initiative: Advancing policy to ban Saturday night specials. *Health Education and Behavior, 26,* 841–858.

Wallack, L., Woodruff, K., Dorfman, L., & Diaz, I. (1999). *News for a change: An advocate's guide to working with the media.* Thousand Oaks, CA: Sage.

Wandersman, A., Goodman, R. M., & Butterfoss, F. D. (1997). Understanding coalitions and how they operate: An "open systems" organizational framework. In M. Minkler (Ed.), *Community organizing and community building for health* (pp. 261–277). New Brunswick, NJ: Rutgers University Press.

World Health Organization. (1996). The tobacco epidemic: A global public health emergency. In *Tobacco alert: Special issue: World No Tobacco Day.* Geneva, Switzerland: Author.

CHAPTER EIGHTEEN

Advocating Policies to Promote Community Reintegration of Drug Users Leaving Jail

A Case Study of First Steps in a Policy Change Campaign Guided by Community Based Participatory Research

Juliana van Olphen
Nicholas Freudenberg
Sandro Galea
Ann-Gel S. Palermo
Cassandra Ritas

Public health professionals increasingly recognize policy analysis and advocacy as a crucial intervention strategy for improving the health of communities and populations. In the past two decades, many observers have advocated for health educators and other public health professionals to become more involved in policy analysis and advocacy (see, for example, Holtgrave, Doll, & Harrison, 1997; Krieger & Lashof, 1988; Steckler & Dawson, 1982; Steckler, Dawson, Goodman, & Epstein, 1987). A growing body of scientific literature provides evidence for the role that policies play in determining adverse health outcomes (Brownson, Newschaffer, & Ali-Abarghoui, 1997; Geronimus, 2000; McKinlay, 1993) and in increasing social and racial inequalities in health (James, 1993; Kawachi, Kennedy, Lochner, & Prothrow-Stith, 1997; Krieger, 1993; Krieger, Rowley, Herman, Avery, & Phillips, 1993; Williams &

Note: The New York Urban Research Center is supported by the U.S. Centers for Disease Control and Prevention. The Robert Wood Johnson Foundation and the New York City Department of Health supported additional work described in this chapter. All views expressed herein are those of the authors and do not necessarily represent the positions of the funders or other institutions. The work described here would not have been possible without the active participation of the Center for Urban Epidemiological Studies Community Action Board.

Collins, 1995). This evidence provides further impetus for political action aimed at improving health.

Despite these advances, there remains a significant gap between our understanding of the social, political, and economic determinants of health and the application of that knowledge. Only recently has the public health literature begun to more regularly include policy recommendations (Boufford & Lee, 2001; Kates, Sorian, Crowley, & Summers, 2002), and others still grapple with the question of whether public health professionals should be policy advocates (Krieger & Lashof, 1988). Although most authors have argued that public health professionals have a responsibility to participate in public health policymaking, there is little consensus on strategies for participation in this process (Holtgrave et al., 1997; Krieger & Lashof, 1988; Steckler & Dawson, 1982; Steckler et al., 1987).

Public health professionals may make use of several avenues to influence policies. They can, for example, act as policymakers themselves, assume administrative positions, effectively communicate research to policymakers, and empower communities to influence policymaking themselves (Holtgrave et al., 1997; Krieger & Lashof, 1988; Steckler et al., 1987). It is this last strategy—the political empowerment of communities—that will be the focus of this chapter. In particular, we will present a case illustration of how public health professionals have been involved in the early stages of policymaking in a community based participatory research framework.

The growth of research about the role of social determinants and structural processes in public health has been accompanied by a broader understanding of political factors as determinants of health and disease (Diez-Roux, 1998; McMichael & Powles, 1999). The recognition that these processes and structures are important health determinants has led to a search for better ways to study community-level influences on health (Israel, Schulz, Parker, & Becker, 1998). Public health professionals have increasingly embraced a community based participatory research approach because it recognizes that socially and economically marginalized communities often lack the power to tackle many of the problems they face. Moreover, such an approach can empower communities to become more involved politically in order to bring resources and decision-making power into communities. At the same time, communities with few resources to alter the fundamental socioeconomic or political causes of morbidity and mortality may have modest potential to bring about this scale of change.

Therefore, while it is important to both mobilize and strengthen the assets, resources, and relationships within communities, it is equally important to attend to the power differentials between communities that produce and maintain social inequalities in health (James, Schulz, & van Olphen, 2001). A significant challenge in integrating policy analysis and advocacy in community based participatory research is to find an appropriate balance between taking action to improve health in the short run and building partnerships that will in the longer run change the resource allocation policies that harm poor communities.

Finally, community based participatory research recognizes the importance of local knowledge in designing and implementing interventions to create and sustain healthy policies. This ensures that community experience informs the policy analysis and design phases and that a community's interests drive the policy development process. Communities can create, reinforce, or undermine policies, and people are less likely to comply with policies if the process that created them is perceived as unfair (Tyler, 1990). When communities are centrally involved in policy design and implementation, participatory decision making becomes an integral part of the policy process. Public health researchers engaged in CBPR are both independent stakeholders and liaisons between policymakers and community members. In these newly defined roles, researchers and community members collaborate to develop the necessary tools, information, and language to influence policymakers and mobilize communities to improve health.

In this chapter, we describe the first stages of a campaign to change local policies that contribute to the adverse health consequences of illegal drug use in two New York City neighborhoods: Central and East Harlem. We describe the evolution of the community based participatory research center that initiated this project, with attention to how diverse stakeholders came together and selected drug use as a priority focus. We then show how the complex nature of the drug problem in Central and East Harlem called for an ecological approach to inform a multilevel model of the determinants of substance use. This facilitated the development of various interventions targeting different pathways through which substance use affects health.

In describing our process, we adopt the stages of policy development described by Steckler and Dawson (1982) and reviewed in Chapter Seventeen. Because we are still in the early phase of the intervention, we will focus in particular on the first three stages: problem awareness and identification, problem refinement, and setting policy objectives. Finally, we explore the strengths and challenges involved in developing and implementing a policy intervention in a CBPR framework. Throughout the chapter, we pay close attention to the tension between maintaining a community based and participatory focus and also addressing the broader external forces that shape health and disease.

THE CENTER FOR URBAN EPIDEMIOLOGICAL STUDIES

As discussed in Chapter Three, the U.S. Centers for Disease Control and Prevention initiated in 1995 a new program, the Urban Research Centers (URC), designed to develop innovative strategies to improve the health and well-being of urban low-income populations (Higgins, Maciak, & Metzler, 2001). Centers were established in Detroit, Seattle, and New York City, the site described in this case history.

The New York URC, founded in 1996 as part of the Center for Urban Epidemiological Studies (CUES), is located at the New York Academy of Medicine, a 150-year-old organization dedicated to improving health and health care in New York City (Freudenberg, 2001a). Its original goals were to bolster the research capacity of several New York City medical institutions to carry out epidemiological studies of urban health problems.

Over the next four years, CUES was transformed from a traditional academic research organization, whose investigators chose projects based primarily on their own interests and the availability of funding, into a more community-oriented, participatory institution committed to bringing some direct benefits to the neighborhoods in which it worked. Some manifestations of these changes include decisions to focus on the geographic communities of Harlem and East Harlem in which CUES was located; to concentrate on a few health problems regularly identified as community priorities—HIV, hepatitis C, and related infectious diseases, substance abuse, and asthma; to join and work with several neighborhood coalitions and networks on these local health problems; and to establish a community action board to provide ongoing guidance to all CUES projects.

The CUES Community Action Board (CAB) includes community service providers, representatives of citywide health organizations (such as the department of health and several medical and academic centers), representatives of advocacy groups, and neighborhood residents. Diverse stakeholders were invited to participate on the CAB, based on their perceived interest and expertise in local health problems, and these stakeholders in turn identified other community partners. The CAB meets monthly to review CUES projects and to plan new initiatives. In 1998, the CAB planned a citywide conference on childhood asthma that included researchers, service providers, and parents of children with asthma. In 2000, it sponsored a community forum on substance use called "Breaking the Barriers," in which service providers, policymakers, and current and former drug users met to identify needs, critique policy, and suggest new directions for city, state, and federal policies. These forums helped bring greater visibility to the URC and to bring together a wide range of diverse stakeholders. Although both meetings were marked by disagreements and controversy on the underlying causes of the high rates of asthma and substance use in these communities and on appropriate solutions, most participants welcomed the opportunity to exchange views. Both conferences helped characterize CUES as a place that could bring together diverse stakeholders to consider practical, scientific, and policy dimensions of community health issues.

In 1999, when CUES decided to focus on substance use as one of its priorities, the CAB articulated the goal of "making it easier to get help for a drug problem in Harlem than to get drugs." This aim explicitly recognized the perception that the easy availability of drugs and the limited access to both formal and informal substance abuse services contributed to the harm that drugs and alcohol imposed on these communities.

Based on its analysis of the substance use problem in Central and East Harlem, on the scientific staff's interpretation of previous epidemiological and social science research on this issue, and on the life and work experience of CAB members, URC participants developed a multilevel model of the determinants of substance use. This ecological model (Sumartojo, 2000; Waldo & Coates, 2000) identified factors that contributed to substance use at the individual, family, neighborhood, service provider, and policy levels. It was designed for use in developing interventions that could operate at one or more levels to reduce the harm associated with illicit drugs and alcohol (Galea et al., in press).

SUBSTANCE ABUSE IN HARLEM

In East and Central Harlem, substance abuse has long been a significant problem and an important contributor to the high rates of other conditions such as HIV, homicide, and violence (McCord & Freeman, 1990). The Harlem Household Survey, conducted from 1992 to 1994, found that 10 to 35 percent of respondents had used either heroin, cocaine, or crack cocaine in their lifetime—a rate four to ten times the average for New York City or for the United States (Fullilove et al., 1999). It has been estimated that in the early 1990s, some 11,050 people in East Harlem and 13,100 people in Central Harlem were injection drug users, constituting 18.8 and 11.9 percent of the respective communities' populations, the highest rates in New York City (New York City Health Systems Agency, 1991; Rose, 1992).

Previous research suggests that substance use is both a direct precursor to poor health and a contextual factor that contributes to a breakdown in the social environment that in turn affects health (Currie, 1993; Fullilove et al., 1999; Rose, 1992; Wallace, Fullilove, & Wallace, 1992). Specifically, poverty and lack of employment opportunities can make the illegal drug market more attractive, and the wide availability of drugs both makes use easier and contributes to health-damaging community norms and values (Anderson, 1999). The crack epidemic beginning in the 1980s has been linked to increases in STDs, violence, and community disorganization (Bourgois, 1995; Cohen et al., 2000). Substance abuse is also thought to be a consequence of the harsh socioeconomic conditions of a neighborhood (Bachman, O'Malley, & Johnston, 1984; Currie, 1993; Wallace et al., 1992), as well as a problem that is exacerbated by unhealthy public policies. Drug policies that impede access to sterile syringes (Coffin, 2000) and housing policies that evict families from public housing when a household member is convicted of a drug crime (Vera Institute of Justice, 2000) are among these unhealthy policies. In sum, substance use both shapes and is shaped by the social environment.

As noted, based on a model depicting the multiple pathways through which substance use affects health (Galea et al., in press), CUES developed a variety of interventions. Several community research studies had documented widespread agreement among service providers and substance users concerning the lack of available information about, and barriers to access to, job training, job opportunities, housing services, and services for people who have been in jail (Galea et al., in press). The experience of CAB members also suggested the need to improve job training and placement, housing, and other services for drug users with complex problems. To address these problems, CUES, in partnership with current and former drug users, is developing a "survival guide" designed to help drug users and their families find the information and resources needed to meet their needs (Factor et al., 2002). CUES also created a Web based resource guide to help community service providers make more appropriate referrals for drug users.

The survival guide and the resource guide are designed to help drug users and service providers to find more readily and efficiently the information, services, and ongoing social support they need. The guides seek to break down the isolation that both users and providers often experience and to relieve the frustration involved in searching for help at the moment a user is ready to seek assistance. The guides also aim to contribute indirectly to a more integrated network of formal and informal services. The guides have the advantage of being relatively easy to produce and distribute, of being visible products that bolster the self-confidence of CUES participants, and of equally involving researchers and CAB members. Their primary drawbacks are their limited potential for impact and their inability to address the deeper underlying social determinants of drug use. The CUES Policy Work Group set out to address these more fundamental issues.

Beginning in 1999, the CUES CAB began to discuss how to develop a policy-level intervention to reduce substance use in Central and East Harlem. The goal was to develop and then evaluate an intervention designed to support and be supported by the other levels of intervention (for example, the survival guide, the community forums, and the resource guide for providers). In 2000, the CAB formed the Policy Work Group, which included both members and CUES staff, to develop a plan for the policy initiative. Over the next two years, five to ten individuals participated actively in this group.

Early in the development of the intervention, the Policy Work Group recognized the need to collect more information in order to better understand the problem of substance use at the policy level. The Policy Work Group launched a set of activities to investigate the issue in more depth. In the early phase of this stage, identified as stage 1, problem awareness and identification, in Steckler and Dawson's framework, researchers from Hunter College at the City University of New York, a partner collaborating with CUES, carried out a survey of seventy-nine counselors, social workers, and managers in drug treatment and social service agencies to assess their perceptions of policy obstacles to meeting the need for drug users in Central and East Harlem (McKnight, 2000). Interviews with CAB members and policy experts identified eight policy arenas for investigation: drug treatment; public assistance; child protective services; housing; Medicaid and managed care; mental health; police; and corrections, probation and parole. Survey participants were asked to rate thirty specific policies in terms of how harmful or helpful they were to their clients and how the policies served as barriers to getting services and reducing drug use. In addition, study participants were asked to identify the three policies that served as the biggest obstacles for their clients. Eleven policies were rated as harmful to their clients by more than 50 percent of the study participants. Of these, three addressed drug treatment policies, three addressed correctional policies, and two addressed Medicaid regulations. Fewer than 20 percent of those participating in the study said these eleven policies did not affect their clients, and fewer than 15 percent (and in most cases, fewer than 5 percent) said these eleven policies were helpful to their clients. Two policies were rated as helpful by more than half of those participating: mandatory drug treatment for people on welfare was rated as helpful by more than 60 percent of service providers, and an aggressive police response to domestic violence reports was rated as helpful by about half of the participants. Finally, the study documented that many service providers were unaware of various policies and their impact on clients, with more than 30 percent reporting that they were unaware of eight of the thirty policies investigated.

CUES staff also organized two facilitated discussions with local service providers on policy obstacles, one at the Community Forum on Substance Use and the other at a conference sponsored by a major Harlem service provider. About twenty people attended each session. Using the previous survey findings as a starting point, these groups discussed and refined the problem list and then ranked policy issues on their importance as deterrents to their clients' receiving services.

As a third source of information, Policy Work Group members reviewed published papers and previous reports on policy issues related to substance abuse in New York City and Central and East Harlem and identified policies that other groups had suggested for action (for example, Davis and Johnson, 2000; Nelson & Trone, 2000; Office of the Comptroller, 2000; Vera Institute of Justice, 2000).

Based on these sources of information and their own experience working with drug users in Harlem, the group identified several possible policy issues. These included lack of housing for drug users, insufficient quantity and quality of drug treatment services, welfare policies that put unrealistic demands on users in recovery, and jail discharge planning and aftercare policies. The Policy Work Group asked several questions to assess which of these policies to target for action, including these:

1. How important is this policy to getting needed and appropriate services for drug users in Central and East Harlem?

2. How likely is it that the CAB members and the Policy Work Group can make a difference on this issue with the resources, previous experience, and time frame available?

3. Can a community based intervention make a difference on this issue, or would we need to work on a city, state, or national level to effect change?

4. What other organizations are working on this issue? Are some willing to work with us? Is there a need for another organization to become involved?

5. To what extent will work on this issue support and be reinforced by other CUES projects?

In the summer of 2001, based on a discussion of these questions, the CUES Policy Work Group selected the topic of jail based discharge planning and community reintegration of released inmates as its focus for action. Several factors led to this decision. First, the survey and discussions with community service providers had consistently identified jail policies related to discharge and aftercare as one of the top three problems affecting their drug-using clients. Second, previous policy reports had identified several dimensions of jail policies that contributed to drug problems (for example, lack of drug treatment in jail and lack of discharge planning), making it easier to consider options for action than in more uncharted areas. Moreover, substantial evidence suggested that community reintegration from jail constituted a critical moment in the natural history of several public health problems—substance abuse, infectious disease, mental health, lack of health care—and provided an opportunity for intervention to promote health and prevent disease (Freudenberg, 2001b; Hammett, 2001; Hammett, Gaiter, & Crawford, 1998; Hammett, Roberts, & Kennedy, 2001).

Third, a few members of the Policy Work Group had already been working in the New York City jails on community reintegration and discharge planning for almost a decade, giving them an intimate knowledge of the relevant barriers and facilitators to action, possible partners, and the existing policy climate. Choosing this issue would give the CUES policy focus the benefit of this experience. Fourth, the selection of this issue would provide CUES with an opportunity to begin a dialogue between the community and stakeholders in other areas such as criminal justice, health care, law enforcement, and public safety, all issues of concern to many Harlem residents. We believed that an open discussion of community reintegration of people leaving jail could pave the way for addressing other important policies in the future and help reframe the issue of drug use from primarily an individual law enforcement issue to a more social community problem. Moreover, we believed that the combination of a long period of declining crime rates in New York City and a new mayoral administration and city council could create a window of opportunity for policy change (Longest, 2001) on the issue of community reintegration. Finally, the links among jail policy, substance abuse, and community health seemed clear (Freudenberg, 2001b), making action squarely within the mission of CUES.

JAIL DISCHARGE POLICIES IN NEW YORK CITY AND THEIR IMPACT ON DRUG USE

Critical to making the case for policy change is "doing your homework" and demonstrating that current approaches and programs are seriously inadequate (see Chapter Seventeen). Such data gathering is also an important precursor of and adjunct to the second and third steps in the policy process, problem refinement and setting policy objectives (Steckler et al., 1987). In their review of data and statistics on jail discharge policies, CUES members learned that in 2000, a total of 124,501 people were admitted to New York City jails. The annual budget for the New York City Department of Correction was $834 million. Although complete data on home addresses of arrestees are incomplete and inaccurate, it was estimated that about 16,000 inmates (13 percent) had an Upper Manhattan (Harlem and adjacent neighborhoods) address at the time of their arrest. Four-fifths were released directly back to their community, meaning that about 12,800 people returned from jail to Harlem communities in that year. The average length of incarceration was forty-five days. The remaining 20 percent were sentenced to state prison. The annual readmission rate was 50 percent; that is, half of those released from jail were reincarcerated within the year. The average annual direct cost for incarceration in a New York City jail was about $56,000, or about $6,904 for the average forty-five-day stay (New York City Department of Correction, 2001; Office of the Mayor, 2001).

Surveys of drug users arrested in New York City suggested that about 80 percent had used illicit drugs in the days prior to their arrest (Arrestee Drug Abuse

Monitoring Program, 2000). Between a quarter and a half of inmates had a drug charge as their highest offense (New York City Department of Correction, 2001). The New York City Health and Hospitals Corporation estimated in 1997 that 25 percent of detainees made use of mental health services while in jail. Despite receiving services while incarcerated, however, there was no routine discharge planning for inmates to ensure that upon release, they would have ongoing access to treatment and services or assistance in obtaining Medicaid or other benefits (Vera Institute of Justice, 2000; Office of the Mayor, 2001).

Partners in this CBPR effort also learned that previous reports (Lynch & Sabol, 2001; Mead, 1996; Nelson, Deess, & Allen, 1999; Nelson & Trone, 2000; Travis, Solomon, & Waul, 2001) had identified several policies that harm community reintegration, including the following six:

- *Correctional policies* such as the release of inmates in the middle of the night without a specific discharge plan, limited availability of substance abuse treatment services within the jail, and inadequate procedures to provide inmates with the identification papers needed to gain access to services after release. The consequences of these policies are the release of inmates who are not ready to get help for the problems that had sent them to jail or are unable to find the help they want. As a result, they are more likely to return to drug use or crime, damaging their own health as well as the well-being of their families and communities.

- *Health care policies* such as a waiting period for Medicaid eligibility after release and inadequate systems for sharing medical information from jail health services (such as lab tests and prescriptions) with community based health providers. These policies make it difficult for ex-offenders to comply with prescribed treatments for HIV, tuberculosis, or psychiatric illness or to get help for health problems before they require hospitalization.

- *Substance abuse service policies* such as having to wait for Medicaid eligibility to pay for drug treatment; for women, requiring postponing reunification with children if they want to enter a residential drug treatment program; and funding shortfalls that limit the intensity and quality of available treatment services. These problems make it more difficult for drug-using ex-offenders to find or complete drug treatment services after release.

- *Housing policies* such as the requirement that public housing projects evict people convicted of drug crimes and their families, the refusal of city homeless shelters to accept people coming out of jail, and the lack of programs that allow inmates to enter the rental housing market. Without adequate housing, many newly released inmates return to street life, crime, and drug use.

- *Employment policies* that allow discrimination against former inmates, and the lack of sufficient job training or educational programs for sectors of the economy where jobs are available. These policies make it more difficult for inmates to avoid the illegal economy, with its pull to continuing drug use.

• *Broader city policies* that do not provide a mechanism for coordinated planning of services and policies among the many city, state, and federal agencies and nonprofit organizations that serve inmates leaving jail. Thus, despite the fact that many city, state, and federal agencies spend significant public money on services for newly released inmates, the lack of coordination results in limited accountability, gaps in and duplication of services, and high rates of recidivism.

Having developed the list of policy barriers to community reintegration, the CUES Policy Work Group faced the daunting task of focusing on a few issues and setting objectives that were achievable yet capable of having some public health impact on Central and East Harlem. As described by Steckler and Dawson (1982), the process of investigating the nature and extent of the problem is key to problem refinement (stage 2 of the policy process) and to achieving some agreement among stakeholders about the nature and extent of the problem. It is only then that stakeholders can begin to formulate policy objectives (stage 3 of the policy process). Problem refinement involved in-depth discussions among the work group members about the common causes of several of the problems identified, such as the lack of coordination among various city agencies charged with providing services for people returning from jail to their communities. For example, inmates are often discharged from jail without referrals to mental health treatment, social services, shelter or affordable housing, or employment services. The Policy Work Group thus faced the dilemma of, on the one hand, understanding that all the problems newly released inmates faced were connected and required action (for example, without mental health care, some inmates would have difficulty getting housing) and, on the other hand, acknowledging that CUES needed to choose one or two issues if it wanted to succeed. In addition, the Policy Work Group was, as always, mindful of selecting issues that reflected community concerns. Policy initiatives that are community-driven build community capacity and increase the likelihood of community participation in the implementation phase (Themba, 1999).

By the end of 2001, the group had begun stage 3, setting out general areas within which specific objectives could be developed and narrowing its list of possible policy objectives to four: (1) obtaining identification for inmates prior to their release from jail, (2) improving coordination among city agencies serving inmates, (3) improving access to substance use treatment for newly released inmates, and (4) obtaining a waiver for the waiting period for Medicaid eligibility after release from jail. Because this phase of the policy process is interactive and complex, it is crucial to go back to key players for their input, however.

To make its decision on which of these options to pursue, the group decided to carry out the following activities:

- Organize several focus groups with recently released inmates to elicit their perceptions and priorities for action

- Interview local and city officials to assess the political and financial barriers to change in the proposed areas

- Meet with local and citywide advocacy groups to learn both their prior experiences on these four issues and their willingness to join a campaign to change policy (In addition, these consultations will help the group decide whether to begin a communitywide versus a citywide effort.)

- Develop detailed policy briefs analyzing policy history, current status, and opportunities for change

After these tasks are completed, the information will be used to refine the specific policy objectives in order to ensure that these objectives are feasible and likely to meet with success. As we move into this next phase, we will proceed through the subsequent stages of the policy process as outlined out by Steckler and Dawson (1982): designing alternative actions, estimating consequences of alternative actions, selecting a specific course of action, assigning implementation responsibility, and evaluation. Investigating and designing different courses of action for achieving our policy objectives will require the involvement and buy-in of stakeholders from many different areas, including criminal justice, health care, and public safety. A significant challenge in the action phase concerns the mobilization of support among constituencies with differing political ideologies. This will require framing the policy issues and their solutions realistically but also creatively in order to suggest significant payoff in the long run.

IMPLICATIONS FOR POLICY ANALYSIS AND ADVOCACY WITHIN A COMMUNITY BASED PARTICIPATORY FRAMEWORK

Integrating policy analysis and advocacy in a CBPR framework recognizes that disparities in health are, in part, consequences of policies that are unfriendly and unhealthy to communities with fewer resources. Although this case study describes only the first stages of our policy-level work to reduce the harm associated with substance use in Central and East Harlem, the intervention as a whole addresses the multiple and interacting factors that contribute to the substance use problem at the individual, service provider, and community levels. Framing the problem of substance use in this way recognizes the complexity of the problem.

The CBPR approach calls for a process that is inclusive and comprehensive in defining health problems and their solution. In this project, academics, service providers, community groups, drug users, and community residents have played active roles throughout the process. Since many community partners live and work in the communities of East and Central Harlem, they are intimately familiar with their neighborhood's history and concerns, enabling them to see connections among various problems (such as the connection between substance use and the lack of affordable housing and jobs that pay a living wage) and to assist in identifying the sources of these problems. Moreover, community leaders' linkages to social networks and community institutions serve as the basis for building community partnerships and mobilizing communities for social change. These linkages are essential in identifying those in the community already working to address similar issues and in recruiting resources and expertise. The Policy Work Group benefited from community input in identifying policy priorities, which reflected local understanding of the community context, and in mobilizing resources for change.

In this case history, we have focused on the first phase of the policy process, what Longest (2001) calls policy formulation and what Steckler and Dawson (1982; Steckler et al., 1987) define as the first three of seven stages. Participatory strategies can make unique contributions in each stage (see Chapter Seventeen). It should also be noted that participatory approaches have their disadvantages. In this case, it took almost two years for a working group to emerge, define a problem, and achieve a common plan of action. Others have noted that CBPR can be a slow and time-consuming process (Higgins et al., 2001). The time and energy required for this process can be especially burdensome to community partners who have limited time, financial, and human resources and few personnel to devote to the process. Since coming together, CAB members have collaborated on many efforts to secure additional funding to support community partners. These have included working with investigators on research proposals to study community reintegration from jail as a social process that affects HIV infection and seeking public funds to open a drop-in center for returning inmates. Though not always successful, these activities have been crucial to building trust and commitment between CAB members. In addition, the investments of time and energy by community partners and other institutions have immediate benefits, such as sharing of resources and creating social ties across organizations. These investments, properly nurtured, can become social capital to invest in later projects.

In the long run, using a community based participatory research approach to influence policy is important not only for mobilizing community resources and expertise but also for building the capacities of politically disadvantaged communities to advocate for change. This presents a dilemma if we consider that community members control limited resources because of the long-term social, political, and economic exclusion they have experienced (Geronimus, 2000). As Halpern (1995, p. 5) notes, "Those who have the least role in making and the largest role in bearing the brunt of society's economic and societal choices [are left] to deal with the effects of those choices." How do we thus avoid unrealistic expectations of what community based participatory approaches can be expected to achieve? In this project, we have attempted both to set achievable goals and to link our efforts to other community struggles (horizontal integration) and broader citywide, state, and national efforts (vertical integration). We have also sought to engage advocacy organizations, service providers, and elected officials, demonstrating our desire to develop linkages among diverse stakeholders and to try new options should one strategy fail. This approach follows Green and Mercer's (2001) recent proposal for a model of community research that includes all relevant constituencies, not just the residents of a specific geographic neighborhood. Broner, Franczak, Dye, and McAllister (2001) describe a similar process, emphasizing the benefits of working to achieve consensus among diverse participants. Whether we will be successful in connecting our modest goals to the larger social movement seeking more basic reforms of the criminal justice system remains to be seen (Rodriguez & Stoller, 2000).

Approaching policy change through a community based participatory framework is critical to widening the base of advocacy for achieving directed social change. This framework emphasizes an ecological approach that views any given problem (in this case, substance use) as a complex interaction of biological, social, economic, cultural, historical, and political factors. Framing the question in this way creates the potential for addressing more fundamental causes of the problem but also increases the risk of biting off more than we can chew and ultimately failing.

The Policy Work Group, through addressing policies focusing on jail based discharge planning and community reintegration, recognizes that substance use is a social problem exacerbated by the lack of affordable housing, educational, and economic opportunities. Through CBPR, we identified policy barriers in the areas of housing, employment, corrections, and health. We then engaged in an in-depth discussion and investigative process devoted to more fully understanding each policy area and identifying the barriers to intervention. Achieving success in addressing and changing policies will require joining forces with new partners, such as correctional facilities, housing agencies, and advocacy organizations. In order to mobilize support among these partners, the Policy Work Group will need to frame the issues in ways that are meaningful to systems with vastly different missions and cultures.

An unanticipated challenge in this effort has been finding the right balance between defining specific policy objectives and acknowledging the multiple policy determinants of inmates' vulnerability. On the one hand, political success requires choosing a few achievable targets for policy change. On the other hand, our analysis of the problem has taught us that multiple policy changes (more discharge planning, improved drug treatment, more low-income housing, and better access to health care) will be needed if we are to improve the health of people leaving jail. Like other community advocates, the Policy Work Group engages in an ongoing struggle to define realistic goals while continuing to articulate our broader vision.

Our optimism that we can make progress on this issue is based on the consensus among many stakeholders that the harm caused by substance abuse in Central and East Harlem requires urgent action and that traditional approaches to addiction, public safety, criminal justice, and community health have not proved adequate to solve the problem. Most important, both Central and East Harlem have a long history of mobilization to confront and reduce the harm that externally shaped policies imposed on these communities (see Bascom, 1999; Meier, 1996; Smith & Sinclair, 1994; Young Lords Party, 1971). Our success in achieving our policy goals will depend in large part on our ability to become part of this tradition. CBPR approaches provide a vehicle by which public health professionals can link their efforts with the broader aims of improving living conditions, reducing inequality, and promoting social justice.

References

Anderson, E. (1999). *The code of the street: Decency, violence, and the moral life of the inner city.* New York: Norton.

Arrestee Drug Abuse Monitoring Program (ADAM). (2000, June). "1999 Annual Report on Drug Use Among Adult and Juvenile Arrestees." A Program of the National Institute of Justice. Research Report.

Bachman, J. G., O'Malley, P. M., & Johnston, L. D. (1984). Drug use among young adults: The impacts of role status and social environment. *Journal of Peers and Social Psychology, 47,* 629–645.

Bascom, L. (1999). *Renaissance in Harlem: Lost voices of an American community.* New York: Bard Books.

Boufford, J. I., & Lee, P. R. (2001). *Health policies for the 21st century: Challenges and recommendations for the U.S. Department of Health and Human Services.* New York: Milbank Memorial Fund.

Bourgois, P. (1995). *In search of respect: Selling crack in El Barrio.* New York: Cambridge University Press.

Broner, N., Franczak, M., Dye, C., & McAllister, W. (2001). Knowledge transfer, policymaking and community empowerment: A consensus model approach for providing public mental health and substance abuse services. *Psychiatric Quarterly, 72,* 79–102.

Brownson, R. C., Newschaffer, C. J., & Ali-Abarghoui, F. (1997). Policy research for disease prevention: Challenges and practical recommendations. *American Journal of Public Health, 87,* 735–739.

Coffin, P. O. (2000). Syringe availability as HIV prevention: A review of the modalities. *Journal of Urban Health, 77,* 302–326.

Cohen, D., Spear, S., Scribner, R, Kissinger, P., Mason, K., & Wildgen, J. (2000). "Broken windows" and the risk of gonorrhea. *American Journal of Public Health, 90,* 230–236.

Currie, E. (1993). *Reckoning: Drugs, the cities, and the American future.* New York: Hill & Wang.

Davis, W. R., & Johnson, B. D. (2000). Criminal justice contacts of users and sellers of hard drugs in Harlem. *Albany Law Review, 63,* 877–922.

Diez-Roux, A. V. (1998). Bringing context back into epidemiology: Variables and fallacies in multilevel analysis. *American Journal of Public Health, 88,* 216–222.

Factor, S. H., Galea, S., Garcia de Dueñas, L., Saynisch, M., Blumenthal, S., Canales, E., et al. (2002). Development of a "survival" guide for substance users in Harlem, New York City. *Health Education and Behavior, 29,* 312–325.

Freudenberg, N. (2001a). Case history of the Center for Urban Epidemiologic Studies in New York City. *Journal of Urban Health, 78,* 510–520.

Freudenberg, N. (2001b). Jails, prisons, and the health of urban populations: Review of the impact of the correctional system on community health. *Journal of Urban Health, 78,* 214–235.

Fullilove, R. E., Fullilove, M. T., Northridge, M. E., Ganz, M. L., Bassett, M. T., McLean, D. E., et al. (1999). Risk factors for excess mortality in Harlem: Findings from the Harlem Household Survey. *American Journal of Preventive Medicine, 16*(3S), 22–28.

Galea, S., Factor, S. H., Bonner, S., Foley, M., Freudenberg, N., Latka, M., et al. (in press). An Urban Research Center in Harlem, New York City: A case study in collaboration between the community, service providers, and academics. *Public Health Reports.*

Geronimus, A. T. (2000). To mitigate, resist, or undo: Addressing structural influences on the health of urban populations. *American Journal of Public Health, 90,* 867–872.

Green, L. W., & Mercer, S. L. (2001). Can public health researchers and agencies reconcile the push from funding bodies and the pull from communities? *American Journal of Public Health, 91,* 1926–1929.

Halpern, R. (1995). *Rebuilding the inner city: A history of neighborhood initiatives to address poverty in the United States.* New York: Columbia University Press.

Hammett, T. M. (2001). Making the case for health interventions in correctional facilities. *Journal of Urban Health, 78,* 236–240.

Hammett, T. M., Gaiter, J., & Crawford, C. (1998). Reaching seriously at-risk populations: Health interventions in criminal justice settings. *Health Education and Behavior, 25,* 99–120.

Hammett, T. M, Roberts, C., & Kennedy, S. (2001). Health-related issues in prisoner reentry. *Crime and Delinquency, 47,* 390–409.

Higgins, D. L., Maciak, B., & Metzler, M. (2001). CDC Urban Research Centers: Community-based participatory research to improve the health of urban communities." *Journal of Women's Health, 10,* 9–15.

Holtgrave, D. R., Doll, L. S., & Harrison, J. (1997). Influence of behavioral and social science on public health policymaking. *American Psychologist, 52,* 167–173.

Israel, B. A., Schulz, A. J., Parker, E. A., & Becker, A. B. (1998). Review of community-based research: Assessing partnership approaches to improve public health. *Annual Review of Public Health, 19,* 173–202.

James, S. A. (1993). Racial and ethnic differences in infant mortality and low birth weight: A psychosocial critique. *Annals of Epidemiology, 3,* 130–136.

James, S. A., Schulz, A. J., & van Olphen, J. (2001). Social capital, poverty, and community health: An exploration of linkages. In S. Saegert, J. P. Thompson, & M. R. Warren (Eds.), *Social capital and poor communities* (pp. 165–188). New York: Russell Sage Foundation.

Kates, J., Sorian, R., Crowley, J. S., & Summers, T. A. (2002). Critical policy challenges in the third decade of the HIV/AIDS epidemic. *American Journal of Public Health, 92,* 1061–1063.

Kawachi, I., Kennedy, B. P., Lochner, K., & Prothrow-Stith, D. (1997). Social capital, income inequality, and mortality. *American Journal of Public Health, 87,* 1491–1498.

Krieger, N. (1993). Epidemiology and the web of causation: Has anyone seen the spider? *Social Science and Medicine, 39,* 887–903.

Krieger, N., & Lashof, J. C. (1988). AIDS, policy analysis, and the electorate: The role of schools of public health. *American Journal of Public Health, 78,* 411–415.

Krieger, N., Rowley, D. L., Herman, A. A., Avery, B., & Phillips, M. T. (1993). Racism, sexism, and social class: Implications for studies of health, disease, and well-being. *American Journal of Preventive Medicine, 9*(Suppl.), 82–122.

Longest, B. B., Jr. (2001). The process of public policy making: A conceptual model. In P. R. Lee & C. L. Estes, *The nation's health* (6th ed., pp. 109–115). Sudbury, MA: Jones & Bartlett.

Lynch, J. P., & Sabol, W. J. (2001). Prisoner reentry in perspective. *Crime Policy Report, 3,* 1–26.

McCord, C., & Freeman, H. (1990). Excess mortality in Harlem. *New England Journal of Medicine, 322,* 173–178.

McKinlay, J. B.(1993). The promotion of health through planned sociopolitical change: Challenges for research and policy. *Social Science and Medicine, 36,* 109–117.

McKnight, C. (2000). *A survey of perceptions of Harlem and East Harlem service providers on policies affecting drug users.* Unpublished master's thesis, Hunter College, New York.

McMichael, A. J., & Powles, J. W. (1999). Human numbers, environment, sustainability and health. *British Medical Journal, 319,* 977–980.

Mead, D. M. (1996). *A profile of the Citizens' Budget Commission.* New York: Citizens' Budget Commission.

Meier, D. (1996). *The power of their Ideas: Lessons for America from a small school in Harlem.* Boston: Beacon Press.

Nelson, M., Deess, P., & Allen, C. (1999). *The first month out: Post-incarceration experiences in New York City.* New York: Vera Institute of Justice.

Nelson, M., & Trone, J. (2000, October). Why planning for release matters. *Issues in Brief,* pp. 1–8.

New York City Department of Correction. (2001). *Summary statistics, FY 2000.* New York: Author.

New York City Health Systems Agency. (1991). *Data book.* New York: Author.

Office of the Comptroller, Office of Policy Management. (2000). *Quitting drugs, quitting crime: Reducing probationers' recidivism through drug treatment programs.* New York: Author.

Office of the Mayor. (2001). *Mayor's management report, 2001.* New York: Author.

Rodriguez, D., & Stoller, N. (2000). Reflections on critical resistance. *Social Justice, 27,* 180–194.

Rose, D. (1992). The epidemiology of HIV infection and AIDS in East and Central Harlem, New York. *Mount Sinai Journal of Medicine, 59,* 493–497.

Smith, K., & Sinclair, A. (1994). *The Harlem cultural/political movements, 1960–1970.* New York: Gumbs & Thomas.

Steckler, A., & Dawson, L. (1982). The role of health education in public policy development. *Health Education Quarterly, 9,* 275–292.

Steckler, A., Dawson, L., Goodman, R. M., & Epstein, N. (1987). Policy advocacy: Three emerging roles for health education. *Health Education and Promotion, 2,* 5–27.

Sumartojo, E. (2000). Structural factors in HIV prevention: Concepts, examples, and implications for research. *AIDS, 14*(Suppl. 2), S3–S10.

Themba, M. N. (1999). *Making policy, making change: How communities are taking law into their own hands.* San Francisco: Jossey-Bass.

Travis, J., Solomon, A. L., & Waul, M. (2001). *From prison to home: The dimensions and consequences of prisoner reentry.* Washington, DC: Urban Institute.

Tyler, T. R. (1990). *Why people obey the law.* New Haven, CT: Yale University Press.

Vera Institute of Justice. (2000). *Why planning for release matters.* New York: Author.

Waldo, C. R., & Coates, T. J. (2000). Multiple levels of analysis and intervention in HIV prevention science: Exemplars and directions for new research. *AIDS, 14*(Suppl. 2), S18–S26.

Wallace, R., Fullilove, M. T., & Wallace, D. (1992). Family systems and deurbanization: Implications for substance abuse. In J. H. Lowinson, P. Ruiz, & R. B. Millman (Eds.), *Substance abuse: A comprehensive textbook* (2nd ed., pp. 944–955). Baltimore: Williams & Wilkins.

Williams, D. R., & Collins, C. (1995). U.S. socioeconomic and racial differences in health: Patterns and explanations. *Annual Review of Sociology, 21*, 349–386.

Young Lords Party. (1971). *Palante: Young Lords Party.* New York: McGraw-Hill.

CHAPTER NINETEEN

Participatory Action Research with Hotel Room Cleaners

From Collaborative Study to the Bargaining Table

Pam Tau Lee
Niklas Krause
Charles Goetchius

The hospitality industry, with approximately forty-three thousand tourist hotels nationwide, is a major employer of low-wage service workers in metropolitan areas of the United States. Yet despite high rates of injury and disability experienced by these workers, very little health research has been conducted on this population (American Hotel and Lodging Association, 1999; U.S. Department of Labor, 1998).

The study described in this chapter grew out of concerns by low-wage hotel room cleaners and their union, the San Francisco–based Hotel Employees and Restaurant Employees Union (HERE) Local 2. For many years, these workers, 99 percent of whom are female and 95 percent of whom are immigrants, had complained of high rates of injuries and musculoskeletal disorders. The union was aware that many had undergone surgery and several had become permanently disabled. Believing that these injuries could be job-related, the union leadership contacted the University of California (UC) Labor Occupational Health Program (LOHP) in Berkeley to assess its interest in helping to conduct original research that would look at workload, health, and employee-employer relationships. The union envisioned a study that would involve participatory

Note: Portions of this chapter are adapted from "The Impact of a Worker Health Study on Working Conditions," by P. T. Lee, N. Krause, C. Goetchius, & M. Casey, to be published in the *Journal of Public Health Policy.* Copyright © 2002 by the *Journal of Public Health Policy.* Adapted with permission.

action research (PAR) with hotel room cleaners themselves in the role of study collaborators. LOHP was to serve as an intermediary with university based researchers at UC's School of Public Health in conducting original research that would look at workload, health, and employee-employer relationship issues.

As Randy Stoecker (in Chapter Five) and others (Reason, 1994) have suggested, collaborations between universities and community organizations such as unions often arise from the interests and priorities of the academic partners rather than the community organizations or groups. Similarly, the selection of research methods and the design of the study are usually considered within the domain of the academics. This study took a nontraditional path with the union initiating the partnership and defining the research priorities and methods, which included having hotel room cleaners play an active role in many aspects of the research. Because of LOHP's strong track record in facilitating joint labor-management initiatives around issues of health and safety, the union—which had no prior experience in working with academic based researchers—was comfortable having this organization direct the project.

THEORETICAL FRAMEWORK

For the purposes of this study, participatory action research was defined as "systematic investigation, with the collaboration of those affected by the issue being studied, for the purpose of education and taking action or effecting social change" (Green et al., 1995, p. 4). As discussed in earlier chapters, this community-driven approach to research begins with the goals and questions of the community, is participatory at every level, is culturally sensitive, and uses a diversity of communication tools and languages. It involves sharing of power and resources with the community and attempts to build a common language among partners (Northridge et al., 2000). In Hagey's words, "Participatory research is a means of putting research capabilities in the hands of deprived and disenfranchised people so that they can transform their lives for themselves" (1997, p. 1).

A participatory study assembles an appropriate team of research partners, which in this case included health educators and medical researchers, to work in genuine collaboration with the community. It ensures that ownership of data and methods of dissemination are considered collaboratively, and it includes a participatory evaluation process that examines the potential and actual impact of the intervention (National Institute of Environmental Health Sciences, 1997). Other objectives include education and empowerment of the community by making resources available for the study of community-defined issues, facilitation of activism, and involvement of both the researchers and the community in improving conditions and quality of life (Hagey, 1997). Although a participatory research approach is particularly appealing to institutions such as labor unions, however, applying its principles can be challenging. As Hagey (1997, p. 4) has pointed out, "Participatory action research, accepting the politics of research, requires a good emotional quotient (EQ), a high tolerance for conflict and excellent group process skills. By definition [it] employs group process to generate and utilize research." Willingness to share power and build trust is key (Cornwall & Jewkes, 1995; Northridge et al., 2000). In this chapter, we describe the partners involved in this participatory research effort, examine the challenges and dilemmas faced at different stages of the research, and give a brief overview of the study findings. We then examine how the findings were used to influence policy and practice and the role of the room cleaners and their academic partners at the bargaining table.

RESEARCH PARTNERS AND THEIR ROLES AND CONCERNS

HERE Local 2, which represents approximately 75 percent of all nonmanagerial hotel employees in San Francisco, was the lead community organization in this research. The union membership consists of more than 8,500 workers, the majority of whom are employed in the twenty-three major hotels that have contracts with the union local.

In addition to donating considerable amounts of their own time, the union leaders allocated staff and substantial funding. The union thus supplemented an initial grant of $30,000 from the Rockefeller Foundation with most of the additional $100,000 needed to see the project through to completion.

The room cleaners themselves, who typically make up 27 percent of the workforce in the hotel industry (U.S. Department of Labor, 1998), were another key partner in the study. Ninety-nine percent of San Francisco room cleaners are female, with Filipinas accounting for 31 percent, other Asians 35 percent, and Latinas 28 percent. For approximately 95 percent of the room cleaners, English is a second language (Center for Occupational and Environmental Health, 1999). Through Local 2, this diverse membership has frequently participated in activities such as picket actions, organizing drives, and workplace committees. Although none had previously been involved as research partners, these earlier activities may have contributed to individual and community capacity building and laid important groundwork for the women's active participation in the present study.

As noted, LOHP was responsible for direction of the project, coordination between the union and School of Public Health researchers, and facilitation and training of room cleaner groups involved in the project. Established in 1974, LOHP is a public service arm of the Center for Occupational and Environmental Health at the School of Public Health. Its primary purpose is to serve working people and their unions, particularly in Northern California, and to assist them in taking an active role in identifying and controlling occupational hazards.

Known for its innovative, action-oriented training methods, LOHP is also recognized for work at the policy level to advance prevention strategies and its strong record of successful collaborations with community based organizations.

To facilitate a true community based participatory research (CBPR) study, LOHP identified as potential collaborators public health researchers who were knowledgeable about and comfortable with the use of this approach. Physician and epidemiologist Niklas Krause, a faculty member in Occupational and Environmental Medicine at the University of California, San Francisco, with extensive experience in collaborating with both unions and management, was the lead public health researcher suggested by LOHP and joined the project after a meeting with union representatives. Pam Tau Lee, LOHP's labor services program coordinator, served as codirector and brought with her professional background her own personal experience years earlier as a room cleaner.

By agreeing to collaborate on this project, both HERE and the academic researchers were entering uncharted waters. HERE knew the workers were getting hurt and sick from the job, but would the data provide this evidence? How could the union mobilize members for action without compromising the scientific protocols? And for the academic partners, how could the needs of the union be respected while the methodological rigor and scientific integrity of the study was also maintained? The union puts it this way: "This was like a marriage with no chance of getting a divorce in case things didn't work out." The academic partners realized they could collaborate with HERE when, after a series of exploratory discussions, the union representative made it known that he felt comfortable with the process and would abide by the findings, even if they turned out to be negative for the union. That statement set a tone of mutual trust.

LOHP's work to facilitate the relationship helped build a foundation for the sharing of power. Assuming the role of a third party, LOHP helped build bridges between the union and the academic researchers. According to one union spokesperson, "We needed a third party to keep us [the union] in line. We had to be disciplined and learn how to participate but not taint the process. A third party helped us sort through our concerns and helped us present these in a way the researchers could understand. We didn't know anything about the world of the academics, and we wouldn't have been able to figure out what to do without the help of people who understood us and understood the researchers as well."

LOHP sometimes held separate discussions with the union and the researchers to hear concerns and brief each party on the interests, needs, constraints, and culture of the other. LOHP also played an important role in keeping the project on track, keeping the parties informed, and arranging check-in conference calls before moving the project to the next phase.

As Barbara Israel and her colleagues discuss in Chapter Three, partners in a CBPR project may be differentially involved in different stages of the research. In the present study, for example, Niklas Krause and the academic partners took primary responsibility for study design. Consistent with CPBR principles, however, they were respectful of and attentive to community partner concerns. So even though these researchers would have preferred a joint labor-management setting for the study, they understood the union's expressed need to focus its limited resources on researching specific room cleaner health and workload issues. Since these topics were unlikely to generate interest or involvement from the employers in this period just prior to contract negotiations, the union's preference for a study design that was more limited in scope was given close attention by the academic partners and guided their development of the research design.

DEFINING RESEARCH TOPICS AND ENHANCING COMMUNITY PARTICIPATION

Over the years, room cleaners had complained that their workload had increased. Here was an opportunity to cut through the rumors to find out if a significant number of new duties had been added and if so, with what, if any, impacts on worker health.

The team agreed to an approach that would combine the knowledge of the workers and the best available science. A core group of twenty-five room cleaners was identified, whose racial and ethnic composition reflected that of the workforce: all but two (one African American and one Caucasian) were Latina, Filipina, and Chinese. All core group members were women, and they were chosen on the basis of the high regard in which peers held them and their tendency to seek out union representatives on job-related concerns. An effort was also made to include women with varying lengths of seniority, including new hires (under two years), midterm (seven to ten years), and senior employees (fifteen to twenty years).

The core group members attended six focus group sessions, held every two weeks for three hours after work. LOHP facilitated group discussions to look at workload, physical strain, relationship with management, and worker disability. The information that emerged in these discussions provided the study team with several specific issues that could then form the basis of more in-depth collaborative research.

Several steps were taken to enhance participation in the focus groups. Since English was not the first language for the great majority of participants, simultaneous interpretation into Spanish and Chinese and translated written materials were made available at each session. Dinner and a stipend of $15 per hour were provided to each participant to communicate appreciation for their expertise and recognition of the hardship of meeting for three hours after work, particularly since many of the women lived outside San Francisco and had a long commute by bus after dark to get home.

In keeping with CBPR's emphasis on local capacity building and empowerment (Green et al., 1995; Hagey, 1997; Israel, Schulz, Parker, & Becker, 1998) and to inform the focus group discussions, LOHP integrated training on ergonomics and control measures into the sessions. Each session utilized adult education techniques and interactive activities such as illness and injury reports, body charting for workplace pain, brainstorming, and risk mapping. As part of this last activity, participants drew visual maps of their workplaces on which they then identified the various physical, chemical, ergonomic, and other stressors to which they were routinely exposed (Brown, 1995; see Appendix G) as a basis for subsequent discussion.

Using as a prop a mock hotel room, which was set up with two beds, a bathtub, a sink, furniture, and equipment, the participants were given a short introduction to ergonomic risk factors. The focus group facilitator then asked for volunteers to go through the motions of cleaning a room while the rest of the participants called out "freeze" when they spotted a risk factor for injury. Through this process, the study team found that factors like the weight and awkwardness of linen carts and vacuum cleaners and ineffective cleaning products that required repeated scrubbing were all sources of ergonomic and other forms of stress.

To facilitate the academic partners' understanding of what questions to pose regarding workload and tasks, the room cleaners listed on index cards every task required to get their job done. The LOHP facilitator then asked the group to identify the tasks that generated time pressures or other stresses for the room cleaner. Finally, participants were asked to identify when these particular duties were introduced as part of a room cleaner's job. Participants explained, for example, that linen carts used to be fully stocked during the evening by utility personnel, but over time, that crew was gradually eliminated and its duties turned over to the room cleaners.

DESIGNING AND PILOT-TESTING THE SURVEY

Once the outside researchers and the core group members had identified the specific data needed, a questionnaire was developed to be distributed to larger numbers of room cleaners. This stage began with the academic partners combing through standardized questionnaires in order to select appropriate psychosocial questions. They also selected and developed other items that would capture accurate information about workload, job pressure, and employer relations. A draft questionnaire was produced and shared with the union, which expressed concern that a long and difficult questionnaire could discourage the room cleaners from completing the entire survey. The researchers in turn explained their view that completeness was necessary to maintain the scientific integrity of standardized scales and to provide valid points of comparison. They further suggested that this was important for meeting the union's objective of being able to compare the health conditions of room cleaners with those of other working populations. The core group of room clearers played a key role at this point. After piloting the draft questionnaire, they shared their perception that the instrument was indeed too long and included some questions that were difficult to understand as a result of having been written in English and then translated into Spanish and Chinese. They helped reword a number of items, recommended that others be deleted, and further suggested that survey "helpers" fluent in different languages be available at each survey site to assist the room cleaners in understanding the intent of the questions and the complex directions for filling out the form.

Through this collaborative process, the academic partners were helped to refine the questionnaire while LOHP and the union came away with concrete ideas for how to design the implementation phase, including the training and use of survey helpers.

SELECTING THE SAMPLE POPULATION

The academic partners asked the union to select hotels that differed by business category, by type of customer, or by quality of labor-management relations. Variation in such hotel characteristics, they explained, would allow for statistical comparisons that identify the effects of the different work environments on the health and well-being of room cleaners. Only if differences in working conditions were related to differences in health status could changes in working conditions be proposed to improve the health of hotel workers.

The union explained that San Francisco hotels generally fall into four categories: luxury/business, convention/business, tour group/business, and family/tour group. The union selected four hotels, one from each business category. Two of these hotels had a relatively positive labor-management relationship and two had a more adversarial one. The union provided the latest scheduling and seniority lists from the four selected hotels, and LOHP and the academic partners then worked with a subcommittee of workers from these hotels to update the lists.

OUTREACH PLAN AND SURVEY LOGISTICS

To ensure a high participation in the survey component of the study, an outreach effort was developed that was in effect a "minicampaign" waged by the union and its rank-and-file. The union appointed and trained leaders from each of the four hotels to be active members of an outreach team, with one leader selected for each approximately twelve workers on the basis of language and other sociocultural factors. Armed with copies of seniority lists, outreach team members followed up with individual workers, explaining the importance of their involvement.

The union supplemented this activity with letters sent to each worker's home, and union staff and workers also distributed leaflets at the various work sites. Announcements were made by union staff at union committee meetings, stressing the importance of this study and encouraging members to contact their friends at these hotels to participate.

Three survey sites—two at churches and one in a union hall—were set up within walking distance of the hotels and staffed by five to twelve people who were available at times convenient for the workers. To maintain confidentiality, rooms were selected that had their own separate entrances and were also strictly off limits to union staff and employers.

In addition to the room cleaners who agreed to serve as survey helpers, LOHP hired several UC graduate students and community social service workers who spoke and understood Spanish, Chinese, or Tagalog and could serve in this role as well. LOHP conducted a special training session for the helpers, covering the protocol for administration of the survey, their role as interpreters and explainers, and the importance of not influencing participants' answers.

On the day of the survey, the outreach leaders stationed themselves at the time clocks at the various hotels, where workers punched out at the end of the day, or just outside the employee entrances. When the room cleaners finished their shifts, those who agreed to participate walked to their survey site together and were greeted by a welcome person and survey helpers. To further ensure the neutrality and confidentiality of the process, completed questionnaires were collected only by the university partners, not union members. Finally, and because many of the room cleaners lived in areas that had poor evening transportation, arrangements were made to take these workers home, thus making it less burdensome for them to participate.

The detailed planning that went into the outreach and logistics of survey administration proved very successful: a total of 258 women took part in the survey, resulting in a participation rate of 69.2 percent of all eligible room cleaners.

ANALYZING THE DATA

Once the questionnaires were collected, the information was entered into a database program by a graduate student researcher. The academic partners then prepared and provided simple frequency tables for all answers to the questions, stratified by hotel. In keeping with the CBPR principle stressing community ownership of data (Brown & Vega, 1996; Hagey, 1997; see also Appendix A), the LOHP focus group facilitator then brought together the original core group of twenty-five room cleaners and two UC researchers to review the information. The room cleaners, academic partners, union president, and union staff broke into several small groups to discuss the data. Each small group was assigned a different set of data. They were asked to review the information and come back to the whole group with their analysis. After the small groups reported on their findings, others attending were free to provide additional information or other perspectives. Although this discussion was originally scheduled for three hours, it proved so fruitful that participants voluntarily met for an additional hour.

Because the academic partners did not have firsthand knowledge of how rooms are cleaned, they had many questions and looked to the room cleaners for clarification. For example, when the academic partners questioned why "lots of garbage in the room" surfaced as a big workload problem, core group members explained that there is now far more garbage because convention and meeting participants collect bags of brochures and trinkets. Convention catalogues and brochures left in a room can weigh ten pounds or more. Guests eat on the run and bring in take-out food, leaving paper containers, cans, and bags on tables or in wastebaskets. More garbage translates into more trips to pick up trash and heavier wastebaskets.

Core group members also explained that "linen" had emerged as a major problem in the study because many hotels now use three sheets per bed and more pillows. A king-size bed can require up to six pillows, requiring more travel to and from the linen closet.

Informed by insights like these, the academic partners spent another four months doing more analysis and cross-checking the data before writing their final report and submitting it to the union.

SELECTED FINDINGS AND STUDY CONCLUSIONS

The preliminary report prepared for the union based on this study (Krause, Lee, Thompson, Rugulies, & Baker, 1999) suggested that the overall health status of room cleaners appeared to be worse than that of the general U.S. population. More than three-quarters of the room cleaners reported work-related pain or discomfort. In 73 percent of all cases, this was severe enough to result in a visit a doctor, and in 53 percent of all cases, it required taking time off from work. Yet only 50 percent had reported this pain to their supervisors or management, and only 23 percent had a formally reported work-related injury during the last year. The relatively high frequency of work-related musculoskeletal symptoms could not be explained by the aging of the workforce, as was suggested by management in discussions with the union. The study indeed found equally high rates of musculoskeletal symptoms among younger and older employees.

Significant differences in health status and work days lost due to work-related pain were found among the four types of hotels, with employees of one hotel reporting consistently better than average health on nearly all health measures. Further analyses were planned to determine to what extent these differences were caused by variations in physical workload and psychosocial working conditions, both of which appear to be more favorable at the hotel showing better health status (Krause et al., 1999).

Prior research has documented that heavy manual labor may lead to overuse and injury of the musculoskeletal system (Bernard, 1997; Institute of Medicine, 2001). Although no longitudinal data were available, the results of this study suggested that the physical workload of the room cleaners had increased over the last five years. The extent of the increase, the particular tasks involved, and the reasons for the increase differed among the four hotels studied.

In addition to physical job demands, 83 percent of room cleaners reported constant time pressure. Poor job security, limited opportunities for mobility, and high levels of job strain (measured as the combination of high job demands and little job control) (Theorell et al., 1988) were also frequently reported. Together, the findings suggested that more than a third of the room cleaners experienced high levels of job stress. Although the study team concluded that the effects of these combined stressors on the well-being, health, and productivity of hotel room cleaners merited further study, it was also able to draw some important conclusions. The findings of an association between poor working conditions and reduced health in hotel room cleaners, high levels of job stress, and work-related pain and disability could in turn serve as a basis for action.

TRANSLATING RESEARCH FINDINGS INTO ACTION

As noted earlier, the study findings were first presented to the union, which would use them as a critical empirical basis for its negotiations at the bargaining table.

Prior to getting to the table, however, other actions were taken in which the women played a key role. The participatory research in which they had been partners indeed helped uncover information that helped them and their union gain a deeper appreciation of their issues and add legitimacy to their fight. That legitimacy, and in some cases the women's excitement over being part of the research process, helped spur their readiness to act.

Many of the women took part in lobby actions at their hotels—four of the largest and best-known tourist hotels in San Francisco. The union called meetings in hotel lobbies during work hours to report on the status of their campaign for a contract. Many room cleaners took the bold step of stopping work to come down to take part in these meetings. At several hotels, focus group participants spoke about their involvement in the study, the issues they had personally raised, and what they had learned through their participation, as a means of educating their fellow workers.

Core group members and study participants also took part in the strike vote, which authorized the union and workers to stop work if the contract bargaining was stalled or not progressing well. A focus group participant was also one of the primary speakers at the strike vote.

During a picket line action in front of one of the hotels, a focus group member and the union representative invited other room cleaners to have their hands photographed to show their employers as a symbol of the toll in terms of wear and tear that the job was taking on room cleaners' bodies. Two dozen women volunteered, and the photographs were later presented, along with the women's names, to their employers at the bargaining table.

On Labor Day, a union action and sit-down civil discipline action took place on the cable car tracks outside one of the hotels. Approximately ten room cleaners demonstrated their commitment to the fight by participating in the sit-in and getting arrested. For the majority of these women, this was the first time they had participated in this kind of action.

Finally, and throughout this process, core group members and focus group participants played a leadership role in their hotels, keeping the workforce informed and mobilizing room cleaners for involvement in both preliminary actions and the bargaining session itself.

Thirty bargaining sessions took place, and the focus group and survey results were two of the main vehicles used to help influence the desired changes in hotel policy. Approximately twenty room cleaners attended these daylong bargaining sessions, forfeiting their wages to do so.

Both academic partners and room cleaners themselves played a vital role at the bargaining table. At the union's request, the lead UC researcher presented the study findings at a joint contract negotiation session between union and management. A forty-five-minute presentation was made to the entire negotiating committee of over one hundred people, including the union leadership along with many rank-and-file negotiators, the twenty-three hotel general managers, their lawyers, and human resource personnel. Well over two hundred room cleaners came to hear the presentation and signify their support.

The presentation was followed by an hourlong closed-door session with the employer group and three union representatives. The commitment by the academic partner to present the report in person and to undergo questioning by the employer group lent credibility to the research and allowed the employers to ask questions and discuss the findings.

Equally important, however, was the active involvement of the room cleaners themselves at the bargaining table. In the afternoon negotiating session, a panel of six room cleaners spoke, including several who had been leaders in the focus group and other aspects of the study. Prior to their presentations, the women selected for the panel met at the union and outlined their talks, received help in writing a simple script, and practiced several times.

When the panel began, each woman told her life story, including the kinds of jobs she had held in her native country and in the United States, the injuries she had incurred as a room cleaner, and the results of these injuries, including severe pain, operations on wrists and shoulders, daily medications, and the wearing of braces. The women also talked about the physical and psychological demands of the job and explained the hardship their injuries caused for them and their families (for example, leaving them with no energy for playing with their children or helping them with homework). Each of the speakers added that room cleaning involved by far the most difficult work she had ever done, and two cried openly during their testimony. In part because of their involvement in the research, the women could speak with great passion and clarity about their situation, the increase in workload they had experienced, and the proposals the union was making to protect their health.

The data from the study enabled the union and the room cleaners to make and justify a contract proposal calling for a significant reduction in housekeeping workload. The union was successful in negotiating a contract that reduced the maximum required assignment from fifteen rooms to fourteen rooms per day. In some hotels, special cleaning requirements could drop the maximum assignment to thirteen rooms. By lowering the maximum work assignment, these workers set a new standard that could then potentially be used in efforts to protect the health of room cleaners across the country. The union also won agreements for future health and safety studies covering other categories of hotel workers, including food servers, telephone operators, and kitchen workers. Finally, they successfully negotiated to have all housekeeping meetings interpreted and to have any materials provided translated as needed as well.

Although the primary use of study findings was in influencing policy, successful efforts were also made to bring about changes in practice through less formal means. Some of the hotels, for example, agreed to revise their health and safety programs, some of which inadvertently discouraged workers from reporting work-related injuries.

Finally, presentations of the methods and the outcomes were shared with other groups in the hopes of encouraging further use of participatory methods in occupational health research. Presentations at national and statewide academic meetings, conferences of health and safety educators, and a popular education workshop, sponsored by UCLA, for Labor Occupational Safety and Health Program (LOSH) personnel were among the venues in which this research project was shared. In several of these, room cleaners served as cop-resenters. Partly as a result, there is growing interest in using this study as a template for further participatory research with workers, and the study is cur-rently being replicated in several hotels in Las Vegas.

The study also contributed to individual and community capacity building. One of the Latina focus group members was subsequently elected to the union's executive board. Two Chinese women who had been active in the study were hired as staff and are now union organizers working in a campaign involving a large nonunion hotel. Several other women active in the study and not previ-ously shop stewards took on that role. One of the focus group members spoke at a national convention of the Hotel Employees and Restaurant Employees Union, where she introduced the newly elected secretary-treasurer of the union to employees—a very high honor.

Core group members and others who played leadership roles in the study have also participated in formal presentations about the research, with several flying to other cities (Toronto, Las Vegas, and Los Angeles) to talk about the study and their own roles in the research.

Finally, all of the core group members and many of the other study partici-pants now take part in hotel joint labor and management problem-solving com-mittees, and for many, such activity was a direct outgrowth of their active involvement in the study and the sense of empowerment it had engendered.

The hotel room cleaners study presented in this chapter is an example of a CBPR project that succeeded in "balancing research and action" (Israel et al., 1998) in part by influencing policy. The study findings constituted the primary data used by the union in its contract negotiation sessions, and the active par-ticipation of hotel workers at the bargaining table, and in many of the steps leading to the table, was crucial to the negotiations' success.

This case study also demonstrated the effectiveness of a unique partnership among a major union, its university research collaborators, and women from an often invisible sector of the economy for the purposes of community based participatory research. The vital role of the university-based Labor Occu-pational Health Program as an organization that could serve as a bridge between the various partners and facilitate the research process was also demonstrated.

Although a hoped-for goal of this participatory research project was to provide data that could be used in subsequent contract negotiations, an empha-sis on maintaining high research standards and ensuring that the study findings were not influenced by the union's agenda was adhered to throughout. As noted earlier, it was indeed the union's openness to supporting the study regard-less of the findings it might produce that enabled a relationship based on trust between the academic and union partners to blossom. Finally, reflected throughout the project was its commitment to living up to CBPR's emphasis on community capacity building and empowerment. As illustrated here, a heavy accent was placed throughout on building on the strengths of the room cleaner partners, increasing their problem-solving abilities, and providing opportunities for them to articulate their own concerns and issues in their own voices.

As the San Francisco hotel room cleaners study is used as the basis of subsequent projects in Las Vegas and other settings, it is hoped that the potential for new collaborations among unions, workers, and academic partners will emerge as a major new vista for community based participatory research. It is also hoped that this study will serve as an example of how the application of research findings can be used to promote policy change—in this case, to improve working conditions for low-wage immigrant workers.

References

American Hotel and Lodging Association. (1999). *1998 lodging survey: Lodging services, facilities, and trends.* New York: Author.

Bernard, B. P. (Ed.). (1997). *Musculoskeletal disorders and workplace factors.* DHHS (NIOSH) Publication No. 97-141. Cincinnati, OH: U.S. Department of Health and Human Services, National Institute for Occupational Safety and Health.

Brown, L., & Vega, W. (1996). A protocol for community-based research. *American Journal of Preventive Medicine, 12*(4), 4–5.

Brown, M. P. (1995). Worker risk mapping: An education-for-action approach. *New Solutions, 5*(2), 22–30.

Center for Occupational and Environmental Health. (1999, December). UC Berkeley pioneering hotel workers study gets results. *Bridges,* pp. 4–5.

Cornwall, A., & Jewkes, R. (1995). What is participatory research? *Social Science and Medicine, 41,* 1667–1676.

Green, L. W., George, M. A., Daniel, M., Frankish, C. J., Herbert, C. P., Bowie, W. R., & O'Neill, M. (1995). *Study of participatory research in health promotion: Review and recommendations for the development of participatory research in health promotion in Canada.* Vancouver, British Columbia: Royal Society of Canada.

Hagey, R. (1997). Guest editorial: The use and abuse of participatory action research. *Chronic Diseases in Canada, 18*(1), 1–4.

Institute of Medicine. (2001). *Musculoskeletal disorders and the workplace: Low back and upper extremities.* Washington, DC: National Academy Press.

Israel, B. A., Schulz, A. J., Parker, E. A., & Becker, A. B. (1998). Review of community-based research: Assessing partnership approaches to improve public health. *Annual Review of Public Health, 19,* 173–202.

Krause, N., Lee, P. T., Thompson, P. J., Rugulies, R, & Baker, R. L. (1999). *Health and working conditions of San Francisco hotel room cleaners: Preliminary report to the Hotel Employees and Restaurant Employees International Union.* Unpublished report, University of California, Berkeley, School of Public Health.

National Institute of Environmental Health Sciences. (1997). *Advancing the community-driven research agenda.* Research Triangle Park: University of North Carolina.

Northridge, M. E., Vallone, D., Merzel, C., Greene, D., Shephard, P., Cohall, A. T., & Healton, C. G. (2000). The adolescent years: An academic-community partnership in Harlem comes of age. *Journal of Public Health Management Practice, 6,* 53–60.

Reason, P. (1994). Three approaches to participative inquiry. In N. K. Denzin & Y. S. Lincoln (Eds.), *Handbook of qualitative research* (pp. 324–339). Thousand Oaks, CA: Sage.

Theorell, T. A., Perski, T., Akerstedt, F., Sigala, G., Ahlberg-Hulten, A., Svensson, J., & Eneroth, P. (1988). Changes in job strain in relation to changes in physiological state. *Scandinavian Journal of Work, Environment, and Health, 14,*189–196.

U.S. Department of Labor, Bureau of Labor Statistics. (1998). *Occupational outlook handbook* (1998–99 ed.). Washington, DC: U.S. Government Printing Office.

APPENDIXES

A PROTOCOL FOR COMMUNITY BASED RESEARCH

Leland Brown
William A. Vega

This protocol is a starting point for a wider dialogue around the nature of academic research—specifically, who it serves, who it benefits, and who reports it. In essence, the question is, "How relevant is academic research to the specific health needs of our community?"

The protocol was developed in 1994 by a committee of the Oakland Community Based Public Health Initiative (CBPHI), a collaboration of community based organizations, the University of California, Berkeley, School of Public Health, and the Alameda County Department of Public Health. The CBPHI in turn was part of the nationwide W. K. Kellogg Foundation funded Community Based Public Health Initiative (CBPHI) designed to promote long-term change in institutions of public health research and public health practice. As Dr. Thomas Bruce (1995, p. 11) formerly of the W. K. Kellogg Foundation, has pointed out, "If an informed and involved community works in active collaboration with a responsive and knowledgeable health agency, enormous progress can be made against many resistant health problems." The aim of this protocol was to establish ground rules on how research institutions and communities in Oakland might best work together. Of special concern was moving from models focusing on community deficits and professional-client relationships to

Note: Adapted with permission of Elsevier Science from "A Protocol for Community Based Research," by L. Brown and W. A. Vega, *American Journal of Preventive Medicine, 12*(4), 4–5. Copyright © 1996 by *American Journal of Preventive Medicine.*

models that empower communities by building on local assets and professional-community partnerships (Kretzman & McKnight, 1993). The CBPHI community based research protocol reinforces the type of dialogue that must occur between communities and research institutions in order for legitimate community based solutions to local public health problems to emerge. The protocol ensures that rigorous, academically sound community based research can and should involve communities at every step.

The protocol was developed as a series of questions around which the community-researcher dialogue can take place. It is by no means exhaustive. The questions can be viewed from at least two perspectives: (1) questions that communities should ask every researcher and (2) questions every researcher should ask himself or herself.

1. How will research processes and outcomes serve the community?

   Will community people be hired?

   Will community people be trained?

   Will the research build on community assets and enhance them?

   Will there be continuity over time?

2. How will the community be involved in defining the objectives of the research?

3. Are researchers committed to doing the follow-up necessary to implement larger applications?

4. How will the community be involved in the analysis of the data?

   What are the hypotheses?

   What are the biases?

5. What perceptions about the community are likely to be created or persist as a result of analysis and publication of the results? Will the spirit of confidentiality be violated as a result of making public the research findings?

6. How, when, and by whom should findings be released?

7. What is the focus of the research vis-à-vis addressing long-term community needs?

8. Are the research methods sufficiently rigorous yet true to community based principles that incorporate perspectives and beliefs of community residents?

Perhaps one of the most germane and elusive questions for university based researchers is who really represents their community. This question is not static, as time and circumstances create new landscapes and landscape architects within the community. It is sometimes impossible to know who can represent the true spirit of the community. Nevertheless, the questions on our list cannot be answered without the benefit of community participation involving those who will be the subjects of research and the potential beneficiaries of that research. If answers to the questions can be mutually agreed on, the results and the effects of collaborative research will be worth far more than time and money invested in the conduct of this research. This should be a lesson for federal, state, and private funding sources as well. Such research takes time, enormous goodwill, and infinite patience.

References

Bruce, T. A. (1995). Community health science: A discipline whose time has already come. Research linkages between academia and public health practice. *American Journal of Preventive Medicine, 11* (suppl.): 1–7.

Kretzman, J. P., & McKnight, J. L. (1993). *Building communities from the inside out: A path toward finding and mobilizing a community's assets.* Evanston, IL: Center for Urban Affairs and Policy Research. Northwestern University.

Tracing Federal Support for Participatory Research in Public Health

Lawrence W. Green

In the international history of health education and public health, among other fields of social development and technical assistance, much has been made of the need for people's participation. Health promotion has emerged as a field spanning health education and other aspects of public health and social policy development, with participation, expressed as enabling people to control the determinants of their health, written into the very definition of this emerging field (World Health Organization, 1986).

At first, the emphasis on participation in the health field was on the need for people's participation in the adoption or endorsement of programs or services delivered by science to their localities. Later emphasis shifted to the need for people's cooperation in the implementation of such programs; later still, in advocating and planning programs and policies; and most recently, in the research itself. These gradual shifts from downstream to upstream involvement of people in the continuum from research to policy and practice have resulted from various converging strands of theory, practice, politics, and policy (Green, 1986). Many of these strands are reflected in the chapters of this book. The purpose of this appendix is to reflect on the corresponding trends and current efforts in U.S. federal support for participatory research.

EARLY FEDERAL INTEREST IN PARTICIPATORY
HEALTH RESEARCH

Without attempting to retrace the history of federal attempts to encourage the ideals of participatory democracy in a society governed by representative democracy, we can at least note the paradox of centralized government attempting to safeguard and ensure decentralized "states' rights" and even local autonomy and self-determination. The Revolutionary War was fought ostensibly to free the colonies from distant governance. That and the Civil War, and the subsequent era of reconstruction of the South, must have set in the American psyche a need to use federal powers to protect victims of local tyranny while honoring the need for local self-governance.

C.-E. A. Winslow wrote about "the great sanitary awakening" coming to full flower in 1850 in Europe and following the Civil War in the United States. He viewed "the new public health" in the early twentieth century as an extension of the "golden age of bacteriology," based on, "Above all, . . . a campaign of popular education to acquaint the public with the good tidings" (Winslow, 1923/1984, p. 52). He defined public health as "organized community efforts" to complement and mobilize the sciences of sanitation, epidemiology, hygiene, medicine, and nursing (Winslow, 1920). These early stirrings of a popular public health viewed participation of the public not as an end in itself, not as a social philosophy, but as a very pragmatic, instrumental extension of science.

Harry Mustard wrote in 1948 that "the pace toward a stronger Federal Government has been greatly accelerated. . . . Large units of government tend in general to press upon smaller ones, to help them, to guide them, to give them money, to anesthetize them, to circumscribe their respective local autonomies" (p. 19). But the Tenth Amendment to the U.S. Constitution set limits on this accretion of centralized power: "The powers not granted to the United States by the Constitution nor prohibited to it by the states are reserved to the states respectively, or to the people." This was especially decentralizing in health, where the Constitution accorded very little specifically to the federal government.

Many of the federal laws passed during the 1960s under Kennedy's New Frontier and Johnson's New Society initiatives in health and other antipoverty efforts carried the phrase "maximum feasible participation." The main provision for participation was a 51 percent requirement for lay membership on local health planning boards and other bodies receiving federal funds. The Vietnam War, however, siphoned away most of the resources that the legislation intended to flow to these groups, so that the lay board members found themselves having to volunteer their time and skills to perform managerial functions just to keep the neighborhood health centers and other local entities operating. This undermined the purpose of lay board membership and participatory planning, making the citizen participant planners into managers rather than independent critics or overseers of management. Washington became dependent on this volunteer labor to maintain its programs while also maintaining the war effort, even imagining this to be a value apart from cost savings. In his retrospective on community action in the War on Poverty, Daniel Patrick Moynihan referred to this as "maximum feasible misunderstanding" (1969). The disenchantment spread rapidly to the youth volunteer movement (Moffett, 1971) and continues to haunt latter-day initiatives to revive participatory approaches in health planning and research.

Participatory approaches had another incarnation of federal life in the environmental health field, independent of the personal health services that most neighborhood health centers and other community health planning boards were attempting to address during the 1960s and 1970s. A series of monographs on "community organization techniques for community environmental management," published by the Bureau of Community Environmental Management in the Public Health Service, grew originally out of the training experience of the Office of Urban Environmental Health Planning. "The trainees returning to their home communities did not know how to go about getting support for doing needed interjurisdictional surveys of their areas, preliminary to professional plans" (Nix, 1970, p. iii).

This identified gap fueled a growing interest in participatory research approaches to community development work in various federal agencies in the United States and Canada in the 1980s, following on this early domestic effort. Several reviews have chronicled the explosion of literature in the 1980s in education, social work, agriculture, and health, particularly from projects sponsored by American and Canadian federal agencies and foundations engaged in and drawing from experience in developing countries (Park, Brydon-Miller, Hall, & Jackson, 1993). The Royal Society of Canada, with funding from various Canadian federal sources, sponsored a review of the North American extension and adaptation of these efforts in health promotion in the early to mid-1990s (Green et al., 1995).

The Health Resources and Services Administration and the Indian Health Service pursued a model of "community-oriented primary care" in the 1980s that had many of the markings of community based participatory research, though it was not always participatory. Staff of migrant health centers, community health centers, and Indian Health facilities were trained to practice "denominator medicine" by conducting community assessments of the population served by the practice and to engage the community collaboratively in doing so (Nutting, 1987).

This was also a period of growing insistence by Congress and federal agencies on accountability by state and local grantees for their expenditure of federal funds, requiring in each grant a partnered evaluation between the agencies receiving the funds and the local stakeholders. The Anti-Drug Abuse Act of 1988, for example, authorized the Community Partnership Demonstration Grant Program, administered by the Office for Substance Abuse Prevention (later renamed the Center for Substance Abuse Prevention). The initial 251 grantees were required to plan and conduct process and outcome evaluations of their projects, with sole authority to select and contract with local evaluators. The systematic efforts to study the struggles and successes of these and other local evaluation partnerships led to the recognition that one of the notable successes was the learning and building of local capacity for research, evaluation, and ultimately greater control of program planning and management (Yin, Kaftarian, & Jacobs, 1996). This led to, or in retrospect was the consequence of, the formulation or adaptation of a subspecies of participatory research approaches that came to be called "empowerment evaluation" (Fetterman, 1994) and "participatory and empowerment evaluation" (Dugan, 1996).

THE CURRENT EFFORTS OF FEDERAL HEALTH AGENCIES IN PARTICIPATORY RESEARCH

The National Institute of Environmental Health Sciences (NIEHS) was the first of the National Institutes of Health (NIH) to undertake, in 1995, a sustained effort in community based participatory research (CBPR). Among the NIH research institutes, this one has been under the greatest pressure to undertake participatory research because the public has expressed greater skepticism about the science of environmental health than about medical science. This skepticism arose from and has endured the decades of industrial pollution during which manufacturing and mining companies, in particular, quoted science of dubious validity to reassure employees or residents that their toxins were not toxic to people or were neutralized before being dumped into soil or streams. The pressure mounted for something like community based participatory research following Love Canal and other residential pollution disasters in which residents perceived the government scientists as protecting industry or failing to represent community knowledge, concerns, and perspectives in their environmental research.

The Division of Extramural Research and Training of the NIEHS (2002) defines CBPR as "a methodology that promotes active community involvement in the processes that shape research and intervention strategies, as well as in the conduct of research studies." NIEHS has funded fifteen CBPR projects at about $6.1 million per year and in March 2000 hosted a conference on successful models of CBPR, seeking "to expand the acceptance, use, and applicability of CBPR as a valuable tool in improving the public health of the nation" (O'Fallon, Tyson, & Dearry, 2000, p. 5). It also initiated in February 2002 a federal interagency working group for CBPR. The purpose of this group is to strengthen communication among federal agencies with an interest in supporting CBPR methodologies in the conduct of biomedical research, education, health care delivery, or policy.

The Agency for Healthcare Research and Quality (AHRQ) sponsored and hosted a conference on CBPR in November 2001, well attended by staff of many federal agencies and an array of others, mostly proponents of CBPR but some skeptics as well. AHRQ also sponsors its EXCEDE program with ninety leaders from across the country looking for ways to advance CBPR. It is also sponsoring a special issue of the *Journal of General Internal Medicine* that will be devoted to CBPR. This would be the first major foray of the subject into the mainstream medical literature. Like the Royal Society auspices of the report in Canada, this could have a legitimizing effect for the subject.

At the Centers for Disease Control and Prevention (CDC), a long tradition of "bootstrap epidemiology" and strong ties to state and local health departments have provided a sympathetic environment for the promotion of participatory concepts in the development and fielding of surveillance systems, planning, training, evaluation, and research. Without reaching too far into that history, the Health Education and Risk Reduction grants of the 1970s, the Planned Approach to Community Health (PATCH) relationships between CDC and the states and communities in the 1980s, and the REACH initiative for minority health issues in the 1990s have all had a participatory research mandate at their core. The university based Centers for Health Promotion and Disease Prevention Research funded through CDC by Congress after authorizing legislation in 1984 and continuing to this date have had a clear mandate for greater collaboration between academic researchers and state or community public health practitioners and citizen groups. A committee of the Institute of Medicine, National Academy of Sciences, commissioned by CDC to assess the prevention research centers in the mid-1990s concluded that the centers still needed to "adopt a community-based approach to their research and demonstration efforts" (Stoto, Green, & Bailey, 1997).

The Prevention Research Centers (PRCs) represent a nationwide network of academic, public health, and community partners linking science and practice. Three centers were first funded in 1986. The program currently has twenty-six centers. The PRCs now compete for approximately $40 million per year by submitting proposals for peer-reviewed cooperative agreements. Responding to the IOM recommendation, CDC has placed considerably more emphasis on building collaborative community partnerships through the PRCs and other programs. For example, since 1998, community advisory groups are required, representing community members, volunteers, health and education professionals, and representatives of the local and state service organizations. The community advisory groups oversee at least the portfolio of research, if not the grant writing, data collection, and publication on specific projects.

In 1994, the Epidemiology Program Office (EPO) at CDC issued a program announcement to solicit cooperative agreement applications for "urban centers for applied research in public health" that would give greater emphasis to the participatory research mandate (Centers for Disease Control and Prevention, 1994). Three centers were funded in 1995 as extensions of the PRC program with a mandate to establish community partnerships governing the selection and execution of research projects and to participate in all phases of the research, from design to dissemination of results. Indeed, only one of the three centers is based primarily in a university. These three centers have leveraged federal core funds from CDC (EPO and Office of Extramural Prevention Research) of $705,000 to $1.6 million per year, to draw additional grants of $26 million from other centers and agencies of the federal government and from philanthropic foundations. The W. K. Kellogg Foundation has placed the national coordinating office for its Community Health Scholars postdoctoral program in one of these centers to foster the training of public health participatory research scholars.

The most generous CBPR initiative at CDC is the program announced in March 2002 for $13 million in investigator-initiated, peer-reviewed grants of up to $450,000 per year for three years for community based participatory prevention research. This grant program "seeks to support multi-disciplinary, multi-level, participatory research that will enhance the capacity of communities and population groups to address health promotion and the prevention of disease, disability and injury" (Centers for Disease Control and Prevention, 2002). "Multi-level" in this announcement signals an interest in applying participatory research not only with individual community residents and lay interest groups but also at the level of practitioners and policymakers whose participation can improve practice and resource allocation at the program, institution, and policy levels (Green & Mercer, 2001). Grantees will be expected to address or study their issues or interventions on at least two of these levels.

As of this writing, 560 letters of intent had been received in response to this call for proposals. This number greatly exceeds the response to most program announcements at CDC or requests for applications at NIH. It suggests a growing interest and perhaps a pent-up demand for opportunities to pursue this kind of research in public health and for the U.S. federal government to support it.

SOME FEDERAL QUANDARIES IN FURTHERING PARTICIPATORY RESEARCH

The first and most paradoxical of the issues confronting federal agencies in trying to support community based participatory research is the apparent contradiction of a centralized agency of government controlling the funds and selection of applicants for grants to support local initiative, autonomy, self-determination, and self-sufficiency. Federal agencies struggle to find the right posture to strike between restraining their own hegemony and that of research scientists in their collaboration with non-science-trained health professionals, policymakers, or local lay residents or citizens.

A related problem is that most of the federal funds for research are tied up in congressionally restricted vertical silos of categorical disease earmarks or line items in agency budgets. This makes the principle of local autonomy in selecting local needs to define research priorities seem somewhat hollow if the research funds can only be used in relation to specific diseases, age groups, risk factors, or other categories. This quandary is avoided in the latest CDC funding from the EPO and the Extramural Prevention Research Program of the Public Health Practice Program Office.

A third issue on which federal agencies and many participatory research scholars and practitioners disagree is how much involvement of the non-science-trained collaborators is needed in which phases and types of research. One widely adopted set of principles defines (or at least describes the purpose of) participatory research as seeking "to involve researchers and community participants as full partners in every phase of the research process." This expectation is adopted uncritically, even as many of the problems identified by those doing participatory research suggest that varying degrees of involvement of the two parties in different phases might avoid some of the strains. Clearly, involvement maximally of both parties in the first and last stages—the specification of the research questions and the interpretation and application of findings—is key to the purposes of ensuring that community interests are being represented in the research and its use. Involvement equally of the parties in these two phases would also achieve the intent of striking a better power balance between academic and community stakes in the research. Of equal concern in suggesting a more critical consideration of this expectation is the danger that community partners are usually volunteers contributing their time to the research partnership, so their devotion of time and effort to the technical phases of design and data collection could become itself an exploitive relationship. Add to this the more blatant imbalance of expertise at these technical phases, and the potential for exploitation grows. Some consideration of this variation in the necessity, trade-offs, and disadvantages of involvement in various stages requires further study and debate among all parties.

Finally, the logic and apparent advantages to a better fit for research with local or practitioner needs makes a strong but not compelling case for participatory research. Pressure will grow for more definitive evidence that these apparent advantages lead to better health outcomes where participatory approaches were applied. This will require research on participatory research and the continuing development of methodologies that suit participatory approaches without sacrificing too much internal and external validity.

References

Centers for Disease Control and Prevention, Epidemiology Program Office. (1994). *Cooperative agreement program for urban center(s) for applied research in public health.* Atlanta: Author.

Centers for Disease Control and Prevention, Public Health Practice Program Office, Office of Extramural Prevention Research. (2002). *Community-based participatory prevention research.* Atlanta: Author.

Dugan, M. A. (1996). Participatory and empowerment evaluation: Lessons learned in training and technical assistance. In D. M. Fetterman, S. J. Kaftarian, & A. Wandersman (Eds.), *Empowerment evaluation: Knowledge and tools for self-assessment and accountability* (pp. 277–303). Thousand Oaks, CA: Sage.

Fetterman, D. M. (1994). Empowerment evaluation. *Evaluation Practice, 15,* 1–15.

Green, L. W. (1986). The theory of participation: A qualitative analysis of its expression in national and international health policies. In W. B. Ward (Ed.), *Advances in health education and promotion* (Vol. 1, Part A, pp. 211–236). Greenwich, CT: JAI Press.

Green, L. W., George, M. A., Daniel, M., Frankish, C. J., Herbert, C. P., Bowie, W. R., & O'Neill, M. (1995). *Study of participatory research in health promotion: Review and recommendations for the development of participatory research in health promotion in Canada.* Vancouver, British Columbia: Royal Society of Canada.

Green, L. W., & Mercer, S. L. (2001). Participatory research: Can public health researchers and agencies reconcile the push from funding bodies and the pull from communities? *American Journal of Public Health, 91,* 1926–1929.

Moffett, T. (1971). *The participation put-on: Reflections of a disenchanted Washington youth expert.* New York: Dell.

Moynihan, D. P. (1969). *Maximum feasible misunderstanding: Community action in the War on Poverty.* New York: Free Press.

Mustard, H. S. (1948). *Government and public health.* New York: Commonwealth Fund.

National Institute of Environmental Health Sciences. (2002). Division of Extramural Research and Training [http://www.niehs.nih.gov/dert/programs/translat/cbpr/cbpr.htm].

Nix, H. L. (1970). *Identification of leaders and their involvement in the planning process.* Washington, DC: U.S. Department of Health, Education, and Welfare, Public Health Service, Bureau of Community Environmental Management.

Nutting, P. A. (Ed.). (1987). *Community-oriented primary care: From principle to practice.* Washington, DC: U.S. Department of Health and Human Services, Health Resources and Services Administration.

O'Fallon, L. R., Tyson, F. L., & Dearry, A. (Eds.). (2000). *Successful models of community-based participatory research: Final report.* Research Triangle Park, NC: National Institute for Environmental Health Science. [http://www.niehs.nih.gov/dert/programs/translat/cbr-final.pdf].

Park, P., Brydon-Miller, M., Hall, B. L., & Jackson, T. (Eds.). (1993). *Voices of change: Participatory research in the United States and Canada.* Westport, CT: Bergin & Garvey.

Stoto, M. A., Green, L. W., & Bailey, L. A. (Eds.). (1997). *Linking research and public health practice: A review of CDC's program of centers for research and demonstration of health promotion and disease prevention.* Washington, DC: National Academy Press.

Winslow, C.-E. A. (1920). The untilled fields of public health. *Science, 51,* 23.

Winslow, C.-E. A. (1984). *The evolution and significance of the modern public health movement.* New Haven, CT: Yale University Press. (Original work published 1923)

World Health Organization. (1986). *Ottawa charter for health promotion.* Copenhagen, Denmark: Author.

Yin, R. K., Kaftarian, S. J., & Jacobs, N. F. (1996). Empowerment evaluation at federal and local levels: Dealing with quality. In D. M. Fetterman, S. J. Kaftarian, & A. Wandersman (Eds.), *Empowerment evaluation: Knowledge and tools for self-assessment and accountability* (pp. 188–207). Thousand Oaks, CA: Sage.

Guidelines for Participatory Research in Health Promotion

Lawrence W. Green
M. Anne George
Mark Daniel
C. James Frankish
Carol P. Herbert
William R. Bowie
Michel O'Neill

In this appendix we present guidelines intended for use by grant application reviewers to appraise whether proposals for funding as participatory research meet participatory research criteria. These guidelines can also be used as a checklist by academic and community researchers in planning their projects.

As presented, the instrument employs what may be considered a generic set of guidelines that define participatory research. These guidelines represent a systematic attempt to make explicit and thus observable and possibly measurable the principles and defining characteristics of participatory research, from the perspective of health promotion. By objectifying these principles and characteristics, the guidelines will not find uniform favor with all who advocate a more unstructured form of participatory research. Nevertheless, if participatory research is to be funded as *research,* it is necessary (for reasons discussed throughout this book) to make the essential components of the process as explicit as possible.

In attempting to ascribe specificity and concreteness to participatory research practice, the guidelines risk denying a role for local adaptation. We therefore avoid attaching a single summative scoring procedure to the guidelines, and we caution the user that some of the classification categories do not follow

---

Note: Adapted with permission from the December 1994 report of the Royal Society of Canada titled *Study of Participatory Research in Health Promotion.*

a simple hierarchy from weak to strong participatory research. For example, guideline 1f suggests that "community participants should be able to contribute their physical and/or intellectual resources to the research process." The categories range from "no enabling of contribution from participants (researchers do it all)" to "full enabling of participants' resources (researchers act only as facilitators)." The latter category is not necessarily better than some of the middle categories, depending on the relationship called for or negotiated by the parties involved, including community members, researchers, and funding sponsors (Labonté, 1993). Another example of the need to decide on the appropriate weight to be given categories within guidelines is question 6a: "Do community participants benefit from the research outcomes?" At one end of the categories is "research benefits researchers or external bodies only." At the other is "research benefits community only." A preferable arrangement to the latter might be one of the middle categories in which both benefit.

This leaves open the choice of classification procedures and weights to the funding agency or project collaborators according to the relative importance they would attach to the various dimensions and to the categories within each criterion or guideline.

GUIDELINES AND CATEGORIES FOR CLASSIFYING PARTICIPATORY RESEARCH PROJECTS IN HEALTH PROMOTION

Definition

Participatory research is defined as systematic inquiry, with the collaboration of those affected by the issue being studied, for purposes of education and taking action or effecting change.

Instructions

The following guidelines can serve to appraise the extent to which research projects align with principles of participatory research.

For each guideline, check only one box. Some of the guidelines may not be applicable to the research project, in which case no boxes should be checked, or boxes labeled "Not Applicable" should be added to all the guidelines for users to check when appropriate. The categories identified by boxes for most guidelines increase in appropriateness to participatory research from top to bottom, but the most appropriate level for some projects on some guidelines might be more toward the middle or even to the bottom of the set of boxes.

Guidelines

1. Participants and the nature of their involvement:

(a) Is the community[1] of interest clearly described or defined?
   - ❑ no description
   - ❑ inexplicit/general description
   - ❑ general description but explicit
   - ❑ general/detailed description
   - ❑ detailed description

(b) Do members of the defined community participating in the research have concern or experience with the issue?
   - ❑ no concern or experience with the issue
   - ❑ little concern or experience with the issue
   - ❑ moderate concern or experience with the issue
   - ❑ much concern or experience with the issue
   - ❑ high concern or experience with the issue

(c) Are interested members of the defined community provided opportunities to participate in the research process?
   - ❑ no opportunity to participate
   - ❑ little opportunity to participate
   - ❑ more than one opportunity to participate
   - ❑ several opportunities to participate
   - ❑ many opportunities to participate

(d) Is attention given to barriers to participation, with consideration of those who have been underrepresented in the past?
   - ❑ no attention to offsetting barriers
   - ❑ low degree of attention to offsetting barriers
   - ❑ moderate degree of attention to offsetting barriers
   - ❑ moderate/high degree of attention to offsetting barriers
   - ❑ high degree of attention to offsetting barriers

(e) Has attention been given to establishing within the community an understanding of the researchers'[2] commitment to the issue?
   - ❑ no attention to the researchers' commitment
   - ❑ low attention to the researchers' commitment
   - ❑ moderate attention to the researchers' commitment
   - ❑ high attention to the researchers' commitment
   - ❑ explicit agreement on the researchers' commitment

(f) Are community participants enabled to contribute their physical and/or intellectual resources to the research process?
   - ❑ no enabling of contribution from participants (researchers do it all)

❏ mostly researcher effort; some support for contribution from participants
❏ about equal contributions from participants and researchers
❏ mostly resources and efforts of participants; researchers have some direct input
❏ full enabling of participants' resources (researchers act only as facilitators)

2. Origin of the research question:
   (a) Did the impetus for the research come from the defined community?
   ❏ issue posed by researchers or other external bodies
   ❏ impetus originated mainly from researchers; some input from community
   ❏ impetus shared about equally between researchers and community
   ❏ impetus originated mainly from community; some impetus from researchers
   ❏ issue posed by the community

   (b) Is an effort to research the issue supported by members of the defined community?
   ❏ support for research from very few, if any, community members
   ❏ less than half of the community supports research on the issue
   ❏ community is roughly divided on whether the issue should be researched
   ❏ more than half of the community supports research on the issue
   ❏ support for research from virtually all community members

3. Purpose of the research:
   (a) Can the research facilitate learning among community participants about individual and collective resources for self-determination?
   ❏ no provision for learning process
   ❏ low provision for learning process
   ❏ moderate provision for learning process
   ❏ moderate/high provision for learning process
   ❏ high provision for learning process

   (b) Can the research facilitate collaboration between community participants and resources external to the community?
   ❏ no potential for collaboration
   ❏ low potential for collaboration
   ❏ moderate potential for collaboration
   ❏ moderate/high potential for collaboration
   ❏ high potential for collaboration

(c) Is the purpose of the research to empower the community to address determinants of health?
- ❑ purpose devoid of empowerment objective
- ❑ low priority empowerment objective
- ❑ moderate priority empowerment objective
- ❑ moderate/high priority empowerment objective
- ❑ high priority empowerment objective

(d) Does the scope of the research encompass some combination of political, social, and economic determinants of health?
- ❑ no consideration of political, social, or economic determinants
- ❑ only one or two determinants are considered
- ❑ limited consideration of combined determinants of health
- ❑ moderate consideration of combined determinants of health
- ❑ comprehensive consideration of combined determinants

4. Process and context—methodological implications:

(a) Does the research process apply the knowledge of community participants in the phases of planning, implementation, and evaluation?
- ❑ no use of community knowledge in any phase
- ❑ use of community knowledge in one or two phases only
- ❑ limited use of community knowledge in all three phases
- ❑ moderate use of community knowledge in all three phases
- ❑ comprehensive use of community knowledge in all three phases

(b) For community participants, does the process allow for learning about research methods?
- ❑ no opportunity for learning about research
- ❑ low opportunity for learning about research
- ❑ moderate opportunity for learning about research
- ❑ moderate/high opportunity for learning about research
- ❑ high opportunity for learning about research

(c) For researchers, does the process allow for learning about the community health issue?
- ❑ no opportunity for learning about the community issue
- ❑ low opportunity for learning about the community issue
- ❑ moderate opportunity for learning about the community issue
- ❑ moderate/high opportunity for learning about the issue
- ❑ high opportunity for learning about the community issue

(d) Does the process allow for flexibility or change in research methods and focus, as necessary?
- ❑ methods and focus are predetermined; no potential for flexibility

     ❑ mostly predetermined methods and focus; limited flexibility
     ❑ about equal blend of predetermined methods and focus with flexibility
     ❑ high flexibility; some predetermined methods and focus
     ❑ complete flexibility; methods and focus not predetermined

(e) Are procedures in place for appraising experiences during implementation of the research?
     ❑ no procedures for appraising experiences
     ❑ few procedures for appraising experiences
     ❑ some procedures for appraising experiences
     ❑ many procedures for appraising experiences
     ❑ comprehensive procedures for appraising experiences

(f) Are community participants involved in analytic issues: interpretation, synthesis, and the verification of conclusions?
     ❑ no involvement of participants in any analytic issue
     ❑ involvement in one or two analytic issues only
     ❑ limited involvement of participants in all three analytic issues
     ❑ moderate involvement of participants in all three analytic issues
     ❑ comprehensive involvement all three analytic issues

5. Opportunities to address the issue of interest:

(a) Is the potential of the defined community for individual and collective learning reflected by the research process?
     ❑ research process not aligned with potential for learning
     ❑ limited alignment of research process with potential for learning
     ❑ moderate alignment of research process with potential for learning
     ❑ moderate/high alignment of research process with potential for learning
     ❑ comprehensive alignment of research process with potential for learning

(b) Is the potential of the defined community for action reflected by the research process?
     ❑ research process not aligned with potential for action
     ❑ limited alignment of research process with potential for action
     ❑ moderate alignment of research process with potential for action
     ❑ moderate/high alignment of research process with potential for action
     ❑ comprehensive alignment of research process with potential for action

(c) Does the process reflect a commitment by researchers and community participants to social, individual, or cultural actions consequent to the learning acquired through research?

❑ no commitment to action beyond data collection and analysis and writing report for funding agencies

❑ low commitment to social actions based on learning through research

❑ moderate commitment to social actions based on learning through research

❑ moderate/high commitment to social actions based on learning through research

❑ comprehensive commitment to social actions based on learning through research

6. Nature of the research outcomes:

(a) Do community participants benefit from the research outcomes?

❑ research benefits researchers or external bodies only

❑ research benefits researchers/external bodies primarily; community benefit is secondary

❑ about equal benefit of research for both researchers/external bodies, and community

❑ research benefits community primarily; benefit is secondary for researchers/external bodies

❑ explicit agreement on how the research will benefit the community

(b) Is there attention given to or an explicit agreement for acknowledging and resolving in a fair and open way any differences between researchers and community participants in the interpretation of the results?

❑ no attention to or any agreement regarding interpretation issues

❑ low attention to interpretation issues

❑ moderate consideration of interpretation issues

❑ high attention to interpretation issues; no explicit agreement

❑ explicit agreement on interpretation issues

(c) Is there attention given to or an explicit agreement between researchers and community participants with respect to ownership of the research data?

❑ no attention to or any agreement regarding ownership issues

❑ low attention to ownership issues

❑ moderate consideration of ownership issues

❑ high attention to ownership issues; no explicit agreement

❑ explicit agreement on ownership issues

(d) Is there attention given to or an explicit agreement between researchers and community participants with respect to the dissemination of the research results?
   ❑ no attention to or any agreement regarding dissemination issues
   ❑ low attention to dissemination issues
   ❑ moderate consideration of dissemination issues
   ❑ high attention to dissemination issues; no explicit agreement
   ❑ explicit agreement on dissemination issues

USING THE GUIDELINES FOR ASSESSING PARTICIPATORY RESEARCH PROJECTS

A project or funding proposal should be appraised in terms of each guideline, with only one box to be checked for each guideline. Classifications of "not applicable" should be added to the instrument throughout, as these may be as informative as other classifications. The purpose of the classifications is to create a profile of a project or funding proposal. This is not to imply that all projects or proposals need necessarily incorporate all guidelines. The specificity of the context of participatory research projects will decide not only which guidelines will apply but also the degree to which specific guidelines apply. Certain guidelines might not apply in a given context, and some might be emphasized to a greater degree than others. Variability between project profiles may reflect differences in alignment with principles of participatory research, but such differences may not necessarily reflect differences in the appropriate application of participatory research principles.

As categorical data, rather than ordinal data, the classifications can be counted as frequencies within individual categories. An overall score or a summation classification was not considered to be useful. It would be completely contrary to the intended purpose of the guidelines to attempt to infer from a single, total summary score or classification the degree to which a funding proposal followed principles of participatory research. Differing degrees and applications of participatory research are appropriate for different situations. Further, the use of a total score would complicate interpretation. The variable numbers of guidelines in different domains would present the paradox of a de facto weighting of domains (if guidelines were to be weighted equally) or an explicit differential weighting of guidelines (if domains were to be weighted equally). Some tendency toward weighting equally or differentially will occur whether a total summary score or classification is used or not, but the unexamined consequences of forcing a single weighting system a priori are lessened if one applies other methods to interpret the results as appropriate to the grant proposals in hand.

Given the manner by which the domains and their associated guidelines were extracted from the literature, a reasonable solution is to allow the guidelines each to be equally weighted. This choice accepts an implicit weighting of *domains.* It acknowledges the proportional contributions to the instrument of the more prevalent components of the participatory research literature, reflected by the number of guidelines included in the instrument for the particular domain to which they pertain. Interpretation could be based, therefore, on the frequency of classifications in each category. As each classification for each guideline is made by the user indicating where between bipolar extremes he or she feels a given proposal is best represented, these could be weighted according to the importance placed by the funding agency's own priorities on the various domains, guidelines, and classifications within guidelines.

Given the foregoing, projects or grant applications could be contrasted in terms of the distribution of classifications or ratings. Moving down the list, if the five categories are arbitrarily numbered from 1 to 5, a greater frequency of classifications in numerically lower categories over all guidelines would indicate a lesser alignment with the principles of participatory research. This approach avoids the limited perspective afforded by an overall arithmetic score or numerical classification, as it allows an appraisal of trends in the distribution of classifications. By category, overall frequencies could be expressed as counts or as percentages. Based on the emphasis of particular project goals or funding competitions, projects could be appraised and contrasted on the proportion of responses in, above, or below a certain category. Such decisions could be made at the discretion of project planners or funding agencies and would not be constrained by the format of the guidelines as presented here.

CONTENT VALIDITY: APPRAISAL BY EXTERNAL EXPERTS

The working definition and guidelines were presented for debate to two independent expert committees, both external to the project, over the course of two eight-hour workshops spaced six months apart. Each expert committee constituted, in effect, a convenience sample derived from our systematic networking strategy.

Questionnaires were mailed to a convenience sample composed of forty-one individuals who agreed to be surveyed about the representativeness of the guidelines. Each of these people had been identified as involved in participatory research projects in Canada; each represented an independent project. Of the twenty-nine people who returned completed survey instruments, some were associated with more than one project. Details of the methodology used in the survey to validate content are given in Appendix C of Green et al. (1995).

The results of this survey generated further revisions to the guidelines and hence further iterative revisions to the instrument. These revisions have been incorporated into the version of the instrument presented here (see Green et al., 1995, pp. 35–43). Improvements in the readability of the instrument were made in addition to content changes. We believe these results and improvements establish the feasibility of using the guidelines. It is also reasonable to assert that the content validity of the instrument has been established, but an ongoing appraisal of various forms of validity will continue to guide the evolution of the instrument. Validation studies are under way in the Office of Extramural Prevention Research, Public Health Practice Program Office, Centers for Disease Control and Prevention, U.S. Department of Health and Human Services.

Notes

1. The term *community* is defined in this context as any group of individuals sharing a given interest; this definition includes cultural, social, political, health, and economic issues that may link together individuals who may or may not share a particular geographic association. This definition also includes the traditional concept of community as a geographically distinct entity.

2. Though the general term *researcher* can refer to both the community participants involved and external persons with specialized training, this usage of *researcher* refers to external persons with specialized training in research methods. In a theoretical sense, the collaboration of people in participatory research makes the distinction of specialized researchers artificial.

References

Green, L. W., George, M. A., Daniel, M., Frankish, C. J., Herbert, C. P., Bowie, W. R., & O'Neill, M. (1995). *Study of participatory research in health promotion: Review and recommendations for the development of participatory research in health promotion in Canada.* Vancouver, British Columbia: Royal Society of Canada. [Available at http://www.ihpr.ubc.ca/guidelines.html].

Labonté, R. (1993). Community development and partnerships. *Canadian Journal of Public Health, 84,* 237–240.

Documenting and Assessing Community Based Scholarship
Resources for Faculty

Sarena D. Seifer

Our experience suggests that even those faculty with the belief that a participatory community based approach to research is appropriate and relevant to their work may find the process daunting, given the pressures of academic institutions on faculty to publish and obtain grant money.
—Israel, Schulz, Parker, & Becker (1998)

The most frequently cited barrier to faculty conducting community based participatory research (CBPR) is the risk associated with trying to achieve promotion and tenure (Israel, Schulz, Parker, & Becker, 1998, 2000; Maurana, Wolff, Beck, & Simpson, 2000). This appendix is intended primarily to serve as a resource for

- Faculty members who are engaged in CBPR and concerned about successfully preparing for and navigating their institution's review, promotion, and tenure process

- Faculty reviewers who are charged with assessing their colleagues' community based scholarship for the purpose of review, promotion, and tenure decisions

- Faculty members at health professional schools that are revising or plan to revise their review, promotion, and tenure policies

"The scholarship of engagement means connecting the rich resources of the university to our most pressing social, civic and ethical problems, to our children, to our schools, to our teachers and to our cities. . . . I have this growing conviction that what's also needed is not just more programs, but a larger purpose, a sense of mission, a larger clarity of direction in the nation's life as we move toward century twenty-one" (Boyer, 1996, p. 14).

Faculty members who are engaged in CBPR should be familiar with two landmark reports on scholarship in higher education: the Boyer report (Boyer, 1990) and the Glassick report (Glassick, Huber, & Maeroff, 1997). In 1987, the Carnegie Foundation for the Advancement of Teaching commissioned a report to examine the meaning of scholarship. *Scholarship Reconsidered,* by the late Ernest Boyer (1990), challenged higher education to embrace the full scope of academic work, moving beyond an exclusive focus on traditional and narrowly defined research as the only legitimate avenue to further knowledge. He proposed four interrelated dimensions of scholarship. The *scholarship of discovery* refers to the pursuit of inquiry and investigation in search of new knowledge. The *scholarship of integration* consists of making connections across disciplines and advancing knowledge through synthesis. The *scholarship of application* asks how knowledge can be applied to the social issues of the times in a dynamic process that generates and tests new theory and knowledge. The *scholarship of teaching* includes not only transmitting knowledge but also transforming and extending it. Subsequently, Boyer (1996) expanded his definition to include the *scholarship of engagement,* which regards service as scholarship when it requires the use of knowledge that results from one's role as a faculty member.

In an effort to move beyond basic research and peer-reviewed journal publication as the primary criteria for academic reward and promotion, Charles Glassick and his colleagues (Glassick, Huber, & Maeroff, 1997) built on Boyer's work to develop standards to assess the work of scholars: clear goals, adequate preparation, appropriate methods, significant results, effective presentation, and reflective critique.

Efforts are under way to apply the Boyer model and the Glassick standards in public health, medicine, nursing, and higher education as a whole:

- *Public Health:* The 1999 report of the Association of Schools of Public Health, *Demonstrating Excellence in Academic Public Health Practice* (Council of Practice Coordinators, 1999), encourages schools of public health to reconsider the definition and scope of what constitutes scholarship and how this relates to their mission, as reflected in their strategic objectives and reward structures.

- *Medicine:* An issue of the Association of American Medical Colleges' journal, *Academic Medicine,* was recently devoted to the theme of "expanding the view of scholarship," including the scholarship of application (Shapiro & Coleman, 2000).

- *Nursing:* The American Association of Colleges of Nursing (1999) issued a position statement on the definition of scholarship in nursing that supports Boyer's model and provides examples of the types of documentation needed for each dimension of scholarship in nursing.

- *Higher Education:* The American Association of Higher Education's Forum on Faculty Roles and Rewards sponsors an annual national conference and publishes resource materials (Driscoll & Lynton, 1999; Lynton, 1995). For more information, visit http://www.aahe.org/FFRR.

An increasing number of institutions of higher education are rewriting their review, promotion, and tenure policies to reflect the Boyer model. Readers may wish to consult the following Web sites to learn from several of these exemplary models:

Portland State University—http://www.oaa.pdx.edu/oaadoc/ptguide

University of North Carolina-Chapel Hill School of Public Health— http://www.sph.unc.edu/faculty/appointments

University of Wisconsin—http://www1.uwex.edu/secretary/$WPM79FB

STANDARDS OF DOCUMENTATION AND ASSESSMENT OF COMMUNITY BASED SCHOLARSHIP

"Applied scholarly research, teaching and service need clearly articulated scholarship criteria. More appropriate and inclusive forms of documentation and peer review standards should be established. Sustained recognition and support for the applied interdisciplinary scholarship of academic public health practice should be institutionalized both within each school and the university" (Council of Practice Coordinators, 1999, p. 12).

All forms of scholarship apply to CBPR, but the principles, processes, outcomes, and products may differ in a community setting. Community based participatory research requires the scholar to be engaged with the community in a mutually beneficial partnership. The role of expert is shared, and the relationship with the community must be reciprocal and dynamic. Community-defined needs direct the scholarly activities (see Chapters One, Three, and Six).

As with any form of scholarship, Glassick's six standards of assessment apply to CBPR. The challenge for faculty engaged in CBPR is to describe clearly how accepted standards of scholarship are implemented in the context of community. Cheryl Maurana and her colleagues (2000) elaborated on Glassick's work to articulate standards for the assessment of community based scholarship. These are summarized in Exhibit D.1. Complementing in many ways the guidelines presented by Green and his colleagues in Appendix 3, these questions can be used to guide the documentation needed for a faculty portfolio or dossier for review, promotion and tenure decisions. They can also be used by faculty review committees as a tool to assess community based scholarship.

Exhibit D.1. Standards for Assessment of Community Based Scholarship.

Clear Goals

1. Are the goals clearly stated, and jointly defined by community and academics?

2. Has the partnership developed its goals and objectives based upon community needs?

3. How do we identify the community issues? Are these needs and issues truly recognized by the scholar and institution?

4. Do both community and academia think the issue is significant and/or important?

5. Have the partners developed a definition of what the "common good" is?

6. Have the partners worked toward an agreed upon "common good"?

7. Is there a vision for the future of the partnership?

Adequate Preparation

1. Does the scholar have the knowledge and skills to conduct the assessment and implement the program?

2. Has the scholar laid the groundwork for the program based on most recent work in the field?

3. Were the needs and strengths of the community identified and assessed using appropriate method?

4. Have individual needs taken a back seat to group goals and needs?

5. Do the scholar and the community consider all the important economic, social, cultural and political factors that affect the issue?

6. Does the scholar recognize and respect community expertise?

7. Have the community-academic partners become a community of scholars?

8. Does the scholar recognize that the community can "teach," and that the community has expertise?

9. Does the scholar stay current in the field?

Appropriate Methods

1. Have all partners been actively involved at all levels of the partnership process—assessment, planning, implementation, evaluation?

2. Has the development of the partnership's work followed a planned process that has been tested in multiple environments, and proven to be effective?

3. Have partnerships been developed according to a nationally acceptable framework for building partnerships?

Approach

1. Are the methods used appropriately matched to the need?

2. Do the methods build in community involvement and sustainability?

3. What outcomes have occurred in program development and implementation?

4. Do the scholar and community select, adapt and modify the method with attention to local circumstances and continuous feedback from the community?

5. Do programs reflect the culture of the community?

6. Does the scholar use innovative and original approaches?

7. Does the approach emphasize sustainability?

Significant Results

1. Has the program resulted in positive health outcomes in the community?

2. Has the partnership effected positive change in the community and the academic institution?

3. Have models been developed that can be used by others?

4. What has been the impact on the community?

5. What has been the impact on the academic institution?

6. Have external resources (e.g., grant and fund raising) been affected by the program?

7. Are the results effective as judged by both the community and academia?

8. Do the scholar and community commit to a long-term partnership?

Effective Presentation

1. Has the work (outcomes and process) of the partnership been reviewed and disseminated in the community and academic institutions?

2. Have there been presentations/publications on community based efforts at both the community and academic levels?

3. Are the results disseminated in a wide variety of formats to the appropriate community and academic audiences?

Ongoing Reflective Critique

1. What evaluation has occurred?

2. Does the scholar constantly think and reflect about the activity?

3. Would the community work with the scholar again?

4. Would the scholar work with the community again?

Source: Reprinted with permission from C. Maurana, M. Wolff, B. J. Beck, & D. E. Simpson (2000). *Working with Our Communities: Moving from Service to Scholarship in the Health Professions.* San Francisco: Community-Campus Partnerships for Health.

PREPARING FOR THE REVIEW PROCESS

"A university's values are most clearly described by its promotion and tenure pol-icy and by the criteria used to evaluate faculty members" (Weiser, 1996, p. 1). High-quality community based scholarship that meets the Glassick standards of assessment does not guarantee a faculty member's success in the review, promo-tion, and tenure process. Tenured professors Sherril Gelmon and Susan Agre-Kippenhan (2002) have developed a set of guidelines for faculty on how to prepare for and navigate this complex process. Framing your work and dossier around the mission of your department, division, college, or university and creating linkages between your own work and more traditional scholarship in your discipline are among the recommendations they set forth, and the reader is encouraged to review their document for a fuller discussion of these and other guidelines.

"Publication in peer-reviewed journals is the typical end point in the mind of many researchers. For a results-oriented philanthropy, this is not enough" (Knickman & Schroeder, 2000, p. 781). For faculty who are concerned with goals such as social justice and eliminating health disparities, going beyond research for its own sake to work with communities on addressing the issues and con-cerns they identify should be embraced by health professional schools as central to the academic mission. As funding agencies and national professional orga-nizations increasingly seek to translate research into practice and to address the social determinants of health, the future appears bright for CBPR practitioners in the academy.

References

An extensive bibliography of relevant resources and Web links is available on the Community-Campus Partnerships for Health CBPR Web site at http://futurehealth.ucsf.edu/ccph/commbas.html.

American Association of Colleges of Nursing, Task Force on Defining Standards for the Scholarship of Nursing. (1999). *Position statement on defining scholarship for the discipline of nursing.* Washington, DC: Author.

Boyer, E. L. (1990). *Scholarship reconsidered: Priorities of the professorate.* Princeton, NJ: Carnegie Foundation for the Advancement of Teaching.

Boyer, E. L. (1996). The scholarship of engagement. *Journal of Public Services and Outreach, 1*(1), 11–20.

Council of Practice Coordinators. (1999). *Demonstrating excellence in academic public health practice.* Washington, DC: Association of Schools of Public Health.

Driscoll, A., & Lynton, E. A. (1999). *Making outreach visible: A guide to documenting professional service and outreach.* Washington, DC: American Association for Higher Education.

Gelmon, S., & Agre-Kippenhan, S. (2002, January). Promotion, tenure, and the engaged scholar: Keeping the scholarship of engagement in the review process. *AAHE Bulletin,* pp. 7–11.

Glassick, C. E., Huber, M. T., & Maeroff, G. I. (1997). *Scholarship assessed: Evaluation of the professorate.* San Francisco: Jossey-Bass.

Israel, B. A., Schulz, A. J., Parker, E. A., & Becker, A. B. (1998). Review of community-based research: Assessing partnership approaches to improve public health. *Annual Review of Public Health, 19,* 173–202.

Israel, B. A., Schulz, A. J., Parker, E. A., & Becker, A. B. (2000). *Community-based participatory research: Engaging communities as partners in health research.* San Francisco: Community-Campus Partnerships for Health.

Knickman, J. R., & Schroeder, S. A. (2000). Update from funders: The Robert Wood Johnson Foundation. *Medical Care, 38,* 781–784.

Lynton, E. A. (1995). *Making the case for professional service.* Washington, DC: American Association for Higher Education.

Maurana, C., Wolff, M., Beck, B. J., & Simpson, D. E. (2000). *Working with our communities: Moving from service to scholarship in the health professions.* San Francisco: Community-Campus Partnerships for Health.

Shapiro, E. D., & Coleman, D. L. (2000). The scholarship of application. *Academic Medicine, 75,* 895–898.

Weiser, C. J. (1996). *The value system of a university: Rethinking scholarship.* Corvallis: Oregon State University.

Thirteen Policy Principles for Advancing Collaborative Activity Among and Between Tribal Communities and Surrounding Jurisdictions

Turning Point/
National Association of County and City Health Officials

1. Don't plan for us without us.
2. Tribal consultation shall be the overarching principle.
3. No policies will be made for Tribes without the direct involvement of Tribes.
4. Tribal systems, traditional and governmental, shall be respected and followed by others working with Tribes.
5. Trust responsibilities between states and Tribes will be respected and honored, with emphasis on building a policy bridge, not a policy wall.
6. Policies shall not bypass Tribal government review and approval prior to implementation.
7. Tribally specific data shall not be used or published without prior consultation with the Tribe.
8. Policies shall respect Tribal belief in matrilineal and patrilineal ways of life, reverence for elders, and respect for children.

Note: This list was generated by Turning Point: Collaboration for a New Century of Public Health at its Spring Forum 2001 in Washington, D.C. Turning Point is an initiative of the National Association of County and City Health Officials (http://www.naccho.org) and is supported by the W. K. Kellogg Foundation and the Robert Wood Johnson Foundation. Reprinted with permission of the National Association of County and City Health Officials.

9. Policies shall respect humanitarian principles and values.

10. Policies shall be honored by actions.

11. Training policies shall include developing knowledge of American Indian and Alaska Native sovereignty.

12. Blanket policies shall be very broad, consider economic, social, regional, and cultural differences, and advance integration of public health and environmental health action.

13. Sovereignty includes an inherent right to be in search of life, liberty, and happiness as human beings.

Sample Community Health Indicators on the Neighborhood Level

Georg F. Bauer

Table F.1 presents a set of preliminary community health indicators (CHIs) developed for the Fruitvale/San Antonio District of Oakland, California, though a partnership coordinated by the author. The working group that developed these indicators included community residents and representatives of the Alameda County Health Department and the University of California, Berkeley, School of Public Health, collaborating through Oakland's Community Health Academy (see Chapter Seven). The list consists of ten categories and fifty-two components of community health. For most components, several indicators were suggested. For each indicator, the table shows the data source and the theoretical framework that guided its selection. Although not shown here, data were also collected on the percentages of survey respondents who subsequently reported that the indicator represented a topic with a high level of importance, as well as the percentage suggesting a high level of interest in taking action on a particular item.

Legend for Table

Frameworks guiding indicator selection
C = Issues identified by community
T = Theory of change of CCBI/Community Health Team
M = Empirical backup in literature: ecological model of community organizing
P = Public health mandates/objectives
Legend
CS — Community survey
CHT — Community Health Team
OS — Observational study
KII — Key informant interviews
ACPHD — Alameda County Public Health Department
— Number
(number in parentheses) — Identification number of indicators
% High importance — Percentage of survey respondents indicating a high level of importance of the particular issue on a 4-point scale
% High interest in action — Percentage of survey respondents indicating a high level of interest in action for the particular issue on a 5-point scale

Categories Components	Indicator	Source	Framework C T M P
1. Community Capacity Building/Empowerment			
Community involvement	% Membership/participation in community organization/ volunteer group (1)	CS		•	•	
	# Parents in PTA (2)	Schools				
Community involvement in policy making	% Registered to vote (3)	City	•	•		
Community organizing	% High importance	CS		•		
	% High interest in action (4)					
	# Grassroots groups × membership (5)	CHT/KII				
Shared community agenda	Mean % high importance of top 5 community issues	CS		•		
	Mean % high interest in action for top 5 community issues (6)					
Collaboration	# Grassroots groups in formal partnerships (7)	CHT/KII		•		
2. Community Relations			
Sense of community	% Valuing sense of community as very important (8)	CS		•	•	
	% Feeling good sense of community (9)					
Social support	% Having person in neighborhood to turn to for social support (10)	CS		•	•	
Neighborhood relations	% Neighborhood relations with at least a few people (11)	CS		•	•	
	% Comfortable borrowing a tool from at least a few people (12)					

Table F.1. Community Health Indicators.

			Framework			
Table F.1. (*Continued*)						
Categories *Components*	*Indicator*	*Source*	*C*	*T*	*M*	*P*
Neighborhood get-togethers	% High importance % High interest in action (13)	CS	•	•		
	# Neighborhood get-together/ year (14)	CHT/KII				
3. Community Attraction						
Neighborhood satisfaction	% Very/somewhat satisfied (15)	CS		•	•	
Stability	% Persons living in neighborhood = 5 years (16)	CS			•	
Intention to stay	% Intending to stay in neighborhood for next 5 years (17)	CS			•	
Main assets of neighborhood	% 5 top things to be maintained (18)	CS		•		
4. Cultural Affirmation						
Ethnic diversity	# Ethnic groups above 5% of population (19)	CS	•	•		
	% Members of these ethnic groups (20)					
Cultural awareness	# Ethnic events (21)	CHT/KII		•		
Cultural exchange	# Interethnic community groups × membership (22)	CHT/KII		•		
5. Youth Development						
Community meetings/ forums for youth	% High importance % High interest in action (23)	CS	•	•		
	# Community meetings × # participants (24)	CHT/KII				
Leadership training for youth	% High importance % High interest in action (25)	CS	•	•		
	# Youth through leadership training (26)	CHT				

(*Continued*)

Table F.1. Community Health Indicators. (*Continued*)						
Categories				*Framework*		
Components	*Indicator*	*Source*	*C*	*T*	*M*	*P*
Recreational/educational activities after school	% High importance % High interest in action (27) #Youth involved in organized activities (28)	CS CHT/KII	•			
Job training/vocational opportunities for youth	% High importance % High interest in action (29) # Youth through job/vocational training (30)	CS CHT/KII	•			
School education	% Completing high school (31) Public school budget/ student (32) Ratio of ethnic proportion of teachers versus students (33)	Schools	•			
Affordable child care	# Spots accessible for low-income families (34)	Social services				
6. Community Health and Safety						
Domestic violence	% High importance % High interest in action (35) # Reported domestic violence (36)	CS Police	•			
Street violence	% High importance % High interest in action (37) # Reported street violence (38)	CS Police	•			
Drug abuse	% High importance % High interest in action (39) # Reported/arrested drug users (40)	CS Police	•			
Drug dealing	% High importance % High interest in action (41) # Arrests drug dealers (42)	CS Police	•			

Table F.1. (*Continued*)						
Categories *Components*	*Indicator*	*Source*	*Framework* C T M P			
Crime prevention	% Area covered by community policing (43)	Police	•			
	% Area covered by neighborhood watch (44)	Police				
Traffic safety	% High importance % High interest in action (45)	CS	•			
	# Traffic accidents (46)	Police				
	Morbidity/mortality rate traffic injuries (47)	City				
	# Streets with speed barriers (48)					
7. Physical Environment						
Clean streets	% High importance % High interest in action (49)	CS	•		•	
Renovation of abandoned buildings	% High importance % High interest in action (50)	CS	•		•	
	# Abandoned buildings (51)	City				
Park/public space/ recreational facilities development	% High importance	CS	•			
	% High interest in action (52) Sq. ft. park/public space per resident (53)	City				
Gardening	% Houses with garden activity (54)	OS/survey			•	
Public transportation	# Bus lines serving the neighborhood (55)	AC transit	•			
Affordable housing	% of income spent on housing (56)	Census	•			
8. Economic Development						
Job development	Ratio seeking employment/ employed (57)	CS	•			

(*Continued*)

Table F.1. Community Health Indicators. (*Continued*)						
Categories			*Framework*			
Components	*Indicator*	*Source*	*C*	*T*	*M*	*P*
Local business development	# Small/medium licensed business (58)	City				
	# Liquor stores (59)	City				
Support of local economy	% Preferring small local stores (60)	CS				
	# Small stores and its tax revenue (61)	City				
Resources for basic needs	% Population above poverty (62)	Census				
Income equality	% Total income earned by households below median income (63)	Census				
9. Ecological Sustainability						
Population growth	# People in area (64)	Census				
	Birthrate (65)	ACPHD				
	Mortality rate (66)	ACPHD				
Residential and commercial water consumption	Gallons/day per capita (67)	EBMUD				
Residential and commercial energy consumption	BTUs gas and electricity/day per capita (68)	PGE				
Solid waste production	Pounds/day disposed per capita (69)	City				
	Pounds/day recycled per capita (70)					
Environmental hazards	# Registered toxic sites (71)	County				
Greening	# Trees on street (72)	OS				

Table F.1. (Continued)						

Categories Components	Indicator	Source	Framework C T M P			
10. Population Health						
Excess mortality	Years potential life lost for main causes of death (73)	ACPHD				•
Chronic disease mortality	CVD mortality rate (74) Cancer mortality rate (75)	ACPHD				•
Infectious disease morbidity	Incidence AIDS cases (76) Incidence tuberculosis cases (77)	ACPHD				•
Children and youth	Infant mortality rate (78) % Low-birthweight births <2500 gram (79) Birthrate teenagers <age 17 (80) Incidence vaccine preventable childhood disease (81)	ACPHD				•
Intentional injuries	Morbidity rate (82) Mortality rate (83)	ACPHD	•			•
Unintentional injuries (including traffic injuries)	Morbidity rate (84) Mortality rate (85)	ACPHD	•			•
Risk factors	Prevalence cigarette smokers (86) Prevalence alcohol consumption (87) # Tobacco/alcohol advertisement billboards (88)	ACPHD/ survey OS				•
Access to medical care	% Hospital patients with medical insurance (89) Asthma morbidity rate for hospital discharge (90) Diabetes morbidity rate for hospital discharge (91)	ACPHD				•

Risk Mapping as a Tool for Community Based Participatory Research and Organizing

Marianne P. Brown

The community members, all from the same neighborhood, gather around a large sheet of paper taped to the wall. One of them is creating a map of the neighborhood and marking where certain heath and safety hazards are. The others are giving guidance—"Don't forget the diesel exhaust from the idling trucks outside the frozen food plant." "Remember the broken concrete on the sidewalk in front of the corner store." "There's noise from the freeway that goes right by the elementary school."

This is what happens when people get together to develop a Risk Map—a visual representation of areas where there are hazards that could result in injury, illness, or even death. This appendix summarizes the Risk Map Method, an approach to action-oriented research and organizing that is increasingly being used to improve health and safety conditions in communities and workplaces around the United States.

WHY MAKE RISK MAPS?

The Risk Map Method lends itself to CBPR for several reasons:

- It draws on people's knowledge and insights about their community.

Note: Reprinted with permission from Alice Hamilton College, Inc./*New Solutions,* from "Worker Risk Mapping: An Education-for-Action Approach," by M. P. Brown, 1995, *New Solutions,* 5(2), pp. 22–30. Adapted by permission of the author.

- It helps people become active investigators.
- It incorporates experiential learning principles and offers a new method for involvement of study subjects.
- It is effective in a variety of settings.

Community Knowledge and Insight

In the United States, the people who assess community environmental hazards, recommend control measures, and see that they are implemented are typically health professionals—safety engineers, industrial hygienists, epidemiologists, physicians, nurses. These professionals use terms and concepts not commonly understood by laypersons, such as *dose-response, parts per million, ambient air levels, relative risk, particulates,* and *microns.* Consequently, their inspection reports, studies, and presentations are often written in a scientific jargon that is unclear to many who could benefit from the information provided. The Risk Map Method breaks from this traditional approach by acknowledging the vital contributions that people who might potentially be exposed to environmental hazards can make and by drawing on their knowledge when they develop risk maps based on their everyday experiences.

Health professionals use a "scientific approach" when they look at environmental hazards, relying heavily on quantitative measures to establish possible risks to humans. For example, industrial hygienists measure the levels of formaldehyde vapor in the air and then compare the results with what are considered acceptable levels previously established by a governmental agency through a process that is both scientific and political. Although such quantitative approaches are important, they need to be supplemented by the perceptions of community groups who can share vital information concerning when they experience irritation, smell odors, see dust. In this way, the worst exposure periods can be pinpointed. By more systematically combining the knowledge of community members with the expertise of outside professionals, a more complete picture of the hazards can be visualized.

Becoming Active Investigators

In the Risk Map Method, people are both the investigators and the subjects of their investigation. The standard approach used in a work setting is described by Jorge Mujica (1992, p. 767): "The participatory method draws on the established organization of workers in the workplace. For management purposes, workers are classified by the duties they perform, such as maintenance workers in a plant, assembly workers on an assembly line, and word processors in an office. By virtue of their shared work, these employees also share work hazards. This participatory method utilizes these existing groupings by bringing together these subgroups to both actively assess specific hazards and take action to correct them."

Experiential Learning and Involvement of Study Subjects

The Risk Map Method is very visual. People are asked to picture their neighborhood and then fill out a questionnaire or report on the hazards they know about. They are then asked to draw the hazards so that their neighbors can also see them. The method can be a very effective tool for those who have limited literacy or English reading or speaking skills.

The Risk Map Method can also help people learn to function effectively in a task based group. This in turn builds their confidence and shows them they can directly control aspects of their lives—and that environmental conditions in their community that could affect their health are not solely the purview of health and safety professionals. Such realizations can create a sense of ownership over such problems while also helping people see the collective, rather than individual, nature of the problems. Finally, in the process of prioritizing which problems to work on, participants gain perspective so that the small concerns of a few do not dominate.

Effectiveness in a Variety of Settings

The Risk Map Method evolved out of the experiences of workers in an auto plant in Italy in the early 1960s who identified workplace hazards by drawing on a blueprint of the factory circles of different colors and sizes indicating where the hazards were located. A group of scientists then verified the practical evidence. Since that time, versions of this approach have been used in a variety of settings around the world. In the United States, these have included state health departments, companies, labor unions, university labor centers, and community based organizations (see Chapter Seven).

LESSONS FOR ORGANIZERS OR RESEARCHERS ENGAGED IN COMMUNITY BASED PARTICIPATORY RESEARCH

Researchers who have used this method as part of a CBPR project or with community organizing efforts have found it effective for a variety of reasons. First and foremost, it is an approach people immediately respond to in a positive way. Risk mapping can be a confidence-building exercise and can also function as an immediate needs assessment tool. The outside researcher in a CBPR effort can see what the community members perceive the hazards to be and can use this information in subsequent work with the community to determine the specific health issue or issues to be studied. The Risk Map Method also provides

HOW TO MAKE A RISK MAP

Risk mapping is a technique to obtain information about hazards in the community or workplace. It can be useful in identifying hazards and developing priority issues and long-range goals. Risk mapping can be used as a way to visually portray the results of a previously conducted survey, or it can be engaged in at a group meeting by those present.

To make a risk map, follow these steps:

1. On a very large piece of paper, draw a picture of your neighborhood or community. Be sure to draw everything—streets and alleys; buildings such as homes, businesses, schools, and factories; parks; and all the other features of your neighborhood. For the workplace, draw a picture of the area where you spend most of your time. Be sure to draw everything—furniture, machinery, equipment and tools.

2. Label everything on your drawing.

3. With other community members or workers, draw any vehicular activity in your neighborhood or other mobile sources of hazards; draw stick figures where people live, work, go to school, or play. If it's a workplace, draw the flow of production and put stick figures where people work.

4. Mark where the hazards are using colored circles:

    Use *green* for physical safety hazards such as noise, heat or cold, leaks, slippery floors, unguarded equipment, radiation, electrical hazards.

    Use *red* for chemical hazards such as dusts, vapors, fumes, gases, and mists.

    Use *blue* for hazards related to physical exertion or bad ergonomics, which can cause musculoskeletal injuries.

    Use *purple* for hazards associated with work-related stress, such as lack of training, inadequate supervision, or too much overtime.

5. List hazards that would be simple to correct.

6. List items that require more information and investigation.

7. List priorities for research or change.

participants with a good way to learn about a neighborhood without asking a lot of questions.

On the down side, however, risk mapping takes a considerable amount of time. It takes about fifteen minutes for the map to be drawn and about twenty minutes for each individual or small group to explain its map. The outside researcher or organizer describes the exercise, provides the writing materials, and most important, asks probing questions about the maps. These questions can assist the outside researcher or group in then working with the community to further identify hazards and prioritize problems to form the basis of further action-oriented research.

Finally, and consistent with CBPR's emphasis on balancing research and action (Hall, 1981; Israel, Schulz, Parker, & Becker, 1998), there must be a commitment to follow through on the risk mapping effort. As noted, in CBPR this follow-up typically consists of a collaborative effort to identify specific problem areas for further study, conduct the research, and use the results as the basis of determining and implementing concrete action strategies to bring about change. For both organizers and partners in a CBPR project, the risk map serves as a powerful and evolving record of the hazards on which the group wants to work. When subsequent research and action take place and improvements in living or working conditions result, the risk map can further stand as a visual testimony of the participants' success.

References

Hall, B. L. (1981). Participatory research, popular knowledge, and power: A personal reflection. *Convergence, 14,* 6–19.

Israel, B. A., Schulz, A. J., Parker, E. A., & Becker, A. B. (1998). Review of community-based research: Assessing partnership approaches to improve public health. *Annual Review of Public Health, 19,* 173–202.

Mujica, J. (1992). Coloring the hazards: Risk maps, research, and education to fight health hazards. *American Journal of Industrial Medicine, 22,* 767–770.

Selected Centers and Other Resources for Participatory Research in North America

The last few years have seen an explosion of networks and centers engaged in, or supporting those who engage in, community based participatory research (CBPR). What follows is a partial list of local, regional, national, and international resources in the United States and Canada. Many other excellent centers and networks exist, and the reader is encouraged to use these as a "jumping-off point" for a fuller exploration.

NATIONAL AND INTERNATIONAL CENTERS AND NETWORKS HEADQUARTERED IN THE UNITED STATES AND CANADA

Campus Community Partnerships for Health
University of Washington School of Public Health and Community Medicine
UW Box 354809
Seattle, WA 98195
Phone: (206) 616-4305
Fax: (206) 616-6747
E-mail: sarena@u.washington.edu
Web: http://futurehealth.ucsf.edu/ccph.html
Contact: Sarena Seifer

Catalyst Centre
720 Bathurst Street
Toronto, Ontario M5S 2R4
Phone: (416) 516-9546
Fax: (416) 588-5725
E-mail: catalystcentre@web.ca
Web: http://www.catalystcentre.ca
Contact: Matt Adams

Community-Based Public Health Caucus
American Public Health Association
c/o School of Public Health
University of Michigan
M-4152, SPH-II
109 South Observatory
Ann Arbor, MI 48109
Phone: (734) 936-0936
Fax: (734) 936-0927
E-mail: tcitrin@umich.edu
Web: http://www.sph.umich.edu/cbph/caucus/index.html
Contact: Toby Citrin

Community Health Scholars Program
National Program Office
University of Michigan School of Public Health
109 Observatory, M3065
Ann Arbor, MI 48109
Phone: (734) 647-3065
Fax: (734) 936-0927
E-mail: chsp@umich.edu
Web: http://www.sph.umich.edu/chsp
Contact: Saundra Bailey

Community Research Project
The Bonner Foundation
10 Mercer Street
Princeton, NJ 08540
Phone: (609) 924-6663
Fax: (609) 983-4626
E-mail: rhackett@bonner.org
Web: www.bonner.org/campus/crp/objectives.htm
Contact: Bobby Hackett

Highlander Research and Education Center
1959 Highlander Way
New Market, TN 37820
Phone: (865) 933-3443
Fax: (865) 933-3424
Contact: Suzanne Pharr

International Council on Adult Education (ICAE)
720 Bathurst Street, Suite 500
Toronto, Ontario M5S 2R4
Phone: (416) 588-1211
Fax: (416) 588-5725
E-mail: acae@icae.ca *or* eva@icae.ca
Contact: Eva Kupidura

Institute for People's Education and Action (IPEA)
140 Pine Street, Room 10
Florence, MA 01062
Phone: (413) 585-8755
E-mail: ipea@peopleseducation.org
Web: http://www.peopleseducation.org
Contact: Chris Spicer
(publishes *Conversations* newsletter)

Loka Institute
P.O. Box 355
Amherst, MA 01004
Phone: (413) 559-5860
Fax: (413) 559-5811
E-mail: loka@loka.org
Web: http://www.loka.org
Mailing list: crn-list-subscribe@igc.topica.com
Contact: Rahi Kahn

National Network for Aboriginal Mental Health Researchers
Institute of Community and Family Psychiatry
Sir Mortimer B Davis–Jewish General Hospital
4333 Cote Ste Catherine Road
Montreal, Quebec H3T 1E4
Phone: (514) 340-8210
E-mail: laurence.kirmayer@mcgill.ca
Contact: Lawrence Kirmayer

National Network on Environments and Women's Health
c/o Centre for Health Studies, York University
4700 Keele Street, 214 York Lanes
Toronto, Ontario M3J 1P3
Phone: (416) 736-5941
Fax: (416) 736-5986
Web: http://www.yorku.ca/nnewh

Participatory Development Forum
1404 Scott Street
P.O. Box 3000, Station C
Ottawa, Ontario K1Y 4MB
Phone: (613) 792-1006
Fax: (613) 792-1206
E-mail: pdforum@pdforum.org
Web: http://www.pdforum.org

Society for Community Research and Action
1800 Canyon Park Circle, Bldg. 4 Suite 403
Edmond, OK 73013
Phone: (405) 341-4960
E-mail: SCRA@telepath.com
Web: apa.org/divisions/div27/
Contact: Janet Singer

U.S. LOCAL AND REGIONAL CENTERS

Allied Research Center
3781 Broadway
Oakland, CA 94611
Phone: (510) 653-3415
Fax: (510) 653-3427
E-mail: arc@arc.org
Web: http://www.arc.org
Contact: Sonia Peña

Center on AIDS, Drugs and Community Health
Hunter College, City University of New York
425 East 25th Street
New York, NY 10010

Phone: (212) 481-5111
E-mail: nfreunden@hunter.cuny.edu
Contact: Nicholas Freundenberg

Center for AIDS Prevention Studies (CAPS)
University of California, San Francisco
74 New Montgomery Street, Room 600
San Francisco, CA 94105
Phone: (415) 597-9159
Fax: (415) 597-9213
E-mail: skegeles@psg.ucsf.edu
Web: http://www.caps.ucsf.edu
Contact: Susan Kegeles

Center for Community Education and Action
901 North Washington Street, Suite 201
Wilmington, DE 19801
Phone: (302) 777-7479
Fax: (302) 762-5370
E-mail: ppark@fielding.edu
Contact: Peter Park

Center for Community Partnerships
University of Pennsylvania
133 South 36th Street, Room 519
Philadelphia PA 19104
Phone: (215) 898-5351
E-mail: weeks@pobox.upenn.edu/ccp *or* harkavy@pobox.upenn.edu
Web: http://www.upenn.edu/ccp
Contact: Ian Harkavy

Center for Community Research
Institute on Sexuality, Health and Inequality
San Francisco State University
3004 16th Street, Suite 301
San Francisco, CA 94103
Phone: (415) 522-5879
Fax: (415) 522-5899
E-mail: ccr@sfsu.edu
Web: http://www.ccr.sfsu.edu
Contact: Rafael Diaz

Center for Health, Environment and Justice
P.O. Box 6806
Falls Church, VA 22040
Phone: (703) 237-2249
E-mail: chej@chej.org
Web: http://www.chej.org
Contact: Barbara Sullivan

Center for Popular Education and Participatory Research (CPEPR)
University of California, Berkeley
4501 Tolman Hall, Room 1670
Berkeley, CA. 94720
Phone: (510) 642-2856
E-mail: cpepr@uclink.berkeley.edu
Contact: John Hurst

Center for Research on Women
University of Memphis
Memphis, TN 38512
Phone: (901) 678-2770
Fax: (901) 678-3652
E-mail: pbetts@memphis.edu
Web: http://cas.memphis.edu/isc/crow
Contact: Phyllis Betts

Center for Urban Research and Learning
Loyola University Chicago
820 North Michigan Avenue, 10th floor
Chicago, IL 60611
Phone: (312) 915-7760
Fax: (312) 915-7770
E-mail: pnyden@luc.edu
Web: http://www.luc.edu.curl
Contact: Philip Nyden

College of Public and Community Service
University of Massachusetts, Boston
100 Morissey Blvd.
Boston, MA 02124
Phone: (617) 287-7262 *or* (617) 287-7100
E-mail: marie.kennedy@umb.edu
Contact: Marie Kennedy

Community Research, Education and Practice Consortium
School of Hygiene and Public Health
Johns Hopkins University
624 North Broadway, Fifth Floor
Baltimore, MD 21205
Phone: (410) 502-8671
Fax: (410) 614-2797
E-mail: sdefranc@jhsph.edu
Contact: Susan De Francesco

Community Resource and Research Center
6930 Carroll Avenue, Suite 600
Takoma Park, MD 20912
Phone: (301) 891-0570
Fax: (301) 891-0571
E-mail: crrc@earthlink.net
Web: http://www.crrcenter.org
Contact: Bristow Hardin

Datacenter
1904 Franklin Street, Suite 900
Oakland, CA 94612
Phone: (510) 835-4692, ext. 312
Fax: (510) 835-3017
E-mail: datacenter@datacenter.org
Web: http://www.datacenter.org
Contact: Leon Sompolinsky

Detroit Community-Academic Urban Research Center
School of Public Health and Medical Sciences
University of Michigan
1420 Washington Heights
Ann Arbor, MI 48109
Phone: (734) 764-5171
Fax: (734) 763-7379
E-mail: rojomcg@umich.edu
Web: http://www.sph.umich.edu/urc/
Contact: Robert J. McGranagham

Harlem Health Promotion Center
Mailman School of Public Health
Columbia University

600 West 168th Street
New York, NY 10032
Phone: (212) 342-2303
Fax: (212) 342-2320
E-mail: men11@columbia.edu
Web: http://www.harlemhealth.org
Contact: Mary Northridge (c/o Cynthia Dunbar)

Healthy Neighborhoods Project
Contra Costa County Department of Public Health
597 Center Street, Suite 325
Martinez, CA 94553
Phone: (925) 313-6810
Fax: (925) 313-6864
E-mail: rcarill@hsd.co.contra-costa.ca.us
Contact: Roxanne Carillo

Institute for Community Research
2 Hartford Square West
Hartford, CT 06106
Phone: (860) 278-2044
Fax: (860) 278-2141
E-mail: info@incommunityresearch.org
Web: http://www.incommunityresearch.org
Contact: Jean J. Schensul

Neighborhood Planning for Community Revitalization
330 Humphrey Center
301 19th Avenue South
Minneapolis, MN 55455
Phone: (612) 625-5584
Fax: (612) 626-0273
E-mail: npcr@freenet.msp.mn.us
Web: http://www.npcr.org
Contact: Kris S. Nelson

New York Urban Research Center
Center for Urban Epidemiological Studies
New York Academy of Medicine
1216 Fifth Avenue

New York, NY 10029
Phone: (212) 822-7382
E-mail: dvlahov@nyam.org
Web site: http://www.nyam.org
Contact: Dr. David Vlahov, Director

Partnership for the Public's Health
505 Fourteenth Street, Suite 810
Oakland,CA 94612
Phone: (510) 451-8600
Fax: (510) 451-8606
Web: http://www.PartnershipPH.org
Contact: Maria Campbell Casey

Poverty and Race Research Action Council
3000 Connecticut Avenue N.W., Suite 200
Washington, DC 20008
Phone: (202) 387-9887
E-mail: chartman@prrac.org
Web: http://www.prrac.org/
Contact: Chester Hartman

Project South
Institute for the Elimination of Poverty and Genocide
9 Gammon Avenue S.W.
Atlanta, GA 30315
Phone: (404) 622-0602
Fax: (404) 622-6618
Web: http://www.projectsouth.org
Contact: Duane Edwards, Research Director

Seattle Partners for Healthy Communities
First Interstate Building
999 Third Avenue, Suite 1200
Seattle, WA 98104
Phone: (206) 296-6817
Fax: (206) 205-5314
E-mail: james.krieger@metrokc.gov *or* sandra.ciske@metrokc.gov
Web: http://depts.washington.edu/hprc/seattlepartners
Contact: Jim Krieger *or* Sandy Ciske

Southern Regional Council
133 Carnegie Way N.W., Suite 900
Atlanta, GA 30303
Phone: (404) 522-8764, ext. 21
Fax: (404) 522-8791
E-mail: wjohnson@southerncouncil.org
Web: http://www.southerncouncil.org
Contact: Wendy Johnson

Sustainable Urban Neighborhoods
Urban Studies Institute
University of Louisville
426 West Bloom Street
Louisville, KY 40208
Phone:(502) 852-8543
Fax: (502) 852-4580
Web: http://www.louisville.edu/org/sun
Contact: John Gilderbloom

CANADIAN LOCAL AND REGIONAL CENTERS

Atlantic Centre of Excellence for Women's Health
5940 South Street, P.O. Box 3070
Halifax, Nova Scotia B3J 3G9
Phone: (902) 470-6725
Fax: (902) 470-6752
Web: http://www.medicine.dal.ca/mcewh

Atlantic Health Promotion Research Centre
Dalhousie University
Dentistry Building
5981 University Avenue, Room 5200
Halifax, Nova Scotia B3H 3J5
Phone: (902) 494-2240
Fax: (902) 494-3594
Web: http://www.medicine.dal.ca/ahprc
Contact: Renee Lyons

BC Centre of Excellence for Women's Health
E311-4500 Oak Street
Vancouver, British Columbia V6H 3N1
Phone: (604) 875-2633
Fax: (604) 875-3716
Web: http://www.bccewh.bc.ca
Contact: Dr. Lorraine Greaves

Centre for Health Promotion
University of Toronto
100 College Street, Suite 207
Toronto, Ontario M5G 1L5
Phone: (416) 978-1100
Web: http://www.utoronto.ca/chp
Contact: Suzanne Jackson

Centre for Health Promotion Studies
5–10 University Extension Centre
8303 112th Street
Edmonton, Alberta T6G 2T4
Phone: (780) 492-4039
Fax: (780) 492-9579
Web: http://www.chps.ualberta.ca
Contact: Kim Raine

Centre for Human Settlements
University of British Columbia
2206 East Mall
Vancouver, British Columbia V6T 1Z3
Phone: (604) 822-5254
Fax: (604) 822-6164
E-mail: chs@interchange.ubc.ca
Contact: Peter Boothroyd *or* Leonora Angeles

Community Health Promotion Coalition
University of Victoria
University House 2, Room 107
P.O.Box 3060, Stn CSC
Victoria, British Columbia V8W 3R4
Phone: (250) 472-4102

Fax: (250) 472-4836
Web: http://web.uvic.ca/ ~ chpc
Contact: Marcia Hills *or* Budd Hall

Équipe de recherche en promotion de la santé
GRIS, Université de Montréal
P.O. Box 6128, Station Centre-Ville
Montréal, Québec H3C 3J7
Phone: (514) 343-6185
Fax: (514) 343-2207
Principal Investigator: Lucie Richard
Contact: Louise Potvin

Groupe de recherche et d'intervention en promotion de la santé de l'Université
Laval (GRIPSUL)
École des sciences infirmières
Université Laval
Pavillion Comtios Y108-5
Québec, Québec G1K 7P4
Phone: (418) 656-2131
Fax: (418) 656-7747
Web: http://www.ulaval.ca/fsi/gripsul.html
Contact: Michel O'Neill

Health Promotion Research Group
University of Calgary, Community Health Sciences
3330 Hospital Drive N.W.
Calgary, Alberta T2N 4N1
Phone: (403) 220-8242
Contact: Dr. Penny Hawe

Institute of Health Promotion Research
University of British Columbia
2206 East Mall, Room 324
Vancouver, British Columbia V6T 1Z4
Phone: (604) 822-2258
Web: http://www.ihpr.ubc.ca
Contact: C. James Frankish

Kahnawake Schools Diabetes Prevention Project
Kahnawake Education Center
P.O. Box 100

Kahnawake Territory, Mohawk Nation
Via Quebec J0L 1B0
Phone: (450) 635-4374
Fax: (450) 635-7279
E-mail: info@ksdpp.org
Web: http://www.ksdpp.org
Contact: Ann Macaulay

Prairie Region Health Promotion Research Centre
University of Saskatchewan
Health Sciences Building
107 Wiggins Road
Saskatoon, Saskatchewan S7N 5E5
Phone: (306) 966-7939
Fax: (306) 966-7920
Web: http://www.usask.ca/healthsci/che/prhprc
Contact: Joan Feather
Prairie Women's Health Centre of Excellence
56 The Promenade
Winnipeg, Manitoba R3B 3H9
Phone: (204) 982-6630
Fax: (204) 982-6637
E-mail: pwhce@uwinnipeg.ca
Web: http://www.pwhce.ca
Contact: Margaret Haworth-Brockman

Rural Development Institute
Brandon University
270 18th Street
Brandon, Manitoba R7A 6A9
Phone: (204) 571-8518
Web: http://www.brandonu.ca/rdi
Contact: Robert Annis

Aboriginal Capacity and Developmental Research Environments (ACADRES)

Community Information and Epidemiological Technologies (CIET) Canada
478 Rideau Street, Suite 3
Ottawa, Ontario K1N 5Z4
Phone: (613) 241-2081
E-mail: CIETinter@compuserve.com
Contact: Neil Andersen

Saskatchewan Indian Federated College
President's Office
CW Building, Room 227
3737 Wascana Parkway
Regina, Saskatchewan S4S 0A2
Phone: (306) 779-6211
E-mail:eber@sifc.edu
Contact: Eber Hampton

173 Heritage Medical Research Centre
University of Alberta
Edmonton, Alberta T6G 3S2
Phone: (780) 492-6703
E-mail: malcolm.king@ualberta.ca
Contact: Malcolm King

Centre for Aboriginal Health Research
Department of Community Health Sciences
Faculty of Medicine
University of Manitoba
750 Bannatyne Avenue
Winnipeg, Manitoba R3T 2N2
Phone: (204) 789-3677
E-mail: oneilj@ms.umanitoba.ca
Contact: John O'Neil

Dialogue Questions

National Coalition for Healthier Cities and Communities
National Civic League

These seven questions may form the "backbone" of your dialogue. This ensures that the perspectives of your group can be included in the Healthy Communities Agenda process. Several subquestions are offered as prompts to assist you in deepening the dialogue. You decide which questions to spend more time on. It is not necessary to get consensus, but do seek focus. Ideas for further conversation can be found by accessing www.healthycommunities.org.

Community

1. What do you believe are the two or three most important characteristics of a healthy community?

   • When you picture a healthy community, what stands out?

2. What makes you most proud of our community?

What's Working?

3. Give some specific examples of people or groups working together to improve the health and quality of life of our community. (Listen for and record compelling statements and stories.)

   • How did these come about? Who was involved? How did they access needed resources? What was accomplished?

Note: Permission to reprint granted by the National Coalition for Healthier Cities and Communities and the National Civic League.

- How do you think some of these efforts could be expanded?
- What are the most important lessons you have learned from both successful and unsuccessful community efforts?

Issues

4. What do you believe are the two or three most important issues that must be addressed to improve the health and quality of life in our community?

- If you could improve one thing in our community right now, what would it be?
- What are the two or three most important challenges we face in the next five to ten years?

Causes and Barriers

5. What do you believe is keeping our community from doing what needs to be done to improve health and quality of life? (Refer to issues identified in question 4.)

- What do you believe are the underlying causes or reasons for these barriers?
- What is our community currently doing to address these issues?
- What makes leadership difficult on these issues?

Policy and Practice

6. What action, policy, or funding priorities would you support to build a healthier community?

- Would you support the priorities if they meant an increase in taxes? (At what level—federal, state, local?)
- What changes in how our community spends its time and resources would make our community better? (Think of work, school, worship, recreation, civic life, other areas.)
- What is the responsibility of community members in building a healthy community?

Community Action

7. What would excite you enough to become involved (or more involved) in improving our community?

- What is the best way to engage other community members?

- What is the best way to get youth, parents, organizations, businesses, the faith community, schools, media, and other groups involved?

- How can we build on the assets and strengths of our community?

- How could learning from this conversation apply to your current activities?

- Are there any obvious next steps?

NAME INDEX

Flax, J., 27
Forget, G., 278
Foucault, M., 38, 78, 83, 86
Fox, R., 106
Francis, P., 35
Francisco, V. T., 155, 156, 158, 159, 170, 366
Franczak, M., 384
Franken, H. P., 265
Freeman, H., 375
Freire, P., 6, 9, 15, 18, 30, 36, 41–44, 56, 88, 91, 103, 132, 147, 157, 181, 272
Freudenberg, N., 294, 371, 374, 378, 379
Fricke, J. G., 266
Friedland, R., 37
Fuerstein, M. T., 265, 271
Fulbright-Anderson, K., 272
Fullerton-Gleason, L., 33
Fullilove, M. T., 375
Fullilove, R. E., 375
Furnell, R., 275
Furuseth, O., 223

G

Gaiter, J., 378
Galea, S., 371, 375, 376
Gardner, J., 161
Garrett, L., 83
Gatenby, B., 269
Gaventa, J., 4, 10, 13, 31, 32, 35, 37, 44, 54, 58, 86, 99, 101, 106, 182, 210, 222, 251, 259, 277, 349, 367
Gayle, H., 53
Gedicks, A., 100
Genat, W., 6, 10
George, M. A., 3, 14, 34, 157, 251
Geronimus, A. T., 294, 371, 384
Gershman, J., 83
Gibson, R. P., 83
Giddens, A., 212
Giddings, P., 300
Gilkes, C., 294, 296, 300, 302
Gill, R., 266
Gillette, A., 10, 28
Gilmartin, C., 40
Gitlin, T., 34
Goetchius, C., 390
Goette, C., 18, 259
Goldberger, N., 208
Goldenberg, K., 113
Goldfader, R., 184
Gooden, S., 365
Goodman, R. M., 14, 32, 34, 167, 235, 243, 270, 350, 361, 371
Goodwin, B. C., 204

Gottemoeller, M., 147
Gottlieb, N. H., 57
Graham, B. G., 224
Grant, G., 135, 224, 225
Greany, M. L., 137, 182
Green, L. W., 3, 4, 12, 14, 34, 54, 55, 56, 57, 58, 156, 157, 159, 163, 182, 233, 251, 268, 271, 279, 281, 289, 294, 295, 309, 341, 342, 384, 391, 395
Green, M., 135, 224
Greene, J. C., 264, 278
Greenwood, D. J., 6, 30, 32, 208, 213, 269, 274
Guiterrez, L., 92
Gustafson, D. H., 143
Gustavsen, B., 205, 209, 268
Gutierrez, L. M., 78, 128, 256, 294, 301
Guzman, J. R., 53, 58, 59, 127, 294, 296

H

Habermas, J., 9, 32, 36, 205, 270
Hagey, R. S., 4, 251, 391, 392, 395, 398
Hall, B. L., 4, 6–7, 10, 14, 28, 30, 35, 54, 56, 58, 137, 211, 242, 245, 295, 304, 310, 333, 339, 349
Hall, J., 188
Halpern, R., 384
Ham, C., 278
Hammett, T. M., 378
Hancock, T., 16, 57, 131, 135, 140, 143, 144, 145, 146, 147
Hargraves, M. A., 83
Harkavy, I., 30, 269, 274
Harper, G. W., 18, 316
Harrison, J., 371
Harrison, L., 273
Hart, D., 267
Hatch, J., 28, 53, 54, 55, 56, 85, 90, 294, 295, 297
Hazen, M. A., 268, 270
Heaney, K., 182
Heaney, T. W., 99, 100
Heath, G. W., 53
Henderson, D., 28
Henkel, M., 263, 270
Herman, A. A., 8, 53, 83, 371
Herman, D. B., 188
Heron, J., 28, 207, 212, 214
Hesse-Biber, S., 40
Hewell, H., 270, 277
Higgins, D. L., 374, 383
Hills, M., 28
Hill, Y. R., 293
Hoffman, D. L, 172
Hoffman, S., 113

SUBJECT INDEX

Society for Participatory Research in Asia, 14

South Carolina Fair Share, 367

Southeast Halifax Environmental Reawakening, 225. *See also* CHER (Community Health and Environmental Reawakening) partnership [North Carolina]

Southern Organizing Committee, 366

Southern tradition: described, 28–29; origins of, 30–31

STDs (sexually transmitted diseases), 325

Structured dialogue, 42

Studies/moratoriums, 358

Substance abuse issues: CAB (Community Action Board) of CUES work on, 374–375; CUES CAB study on Harlem, 375–379; NCY jail discharge policies and impact on, 379–382

Sun Microsystems, 168

Sustainable Communities Network Web site, 162

SWOT (strengths, weaknesses, opportunities, threats) analysis, 364

T

"Teacher learners" dialogic method, 320–321

Teaching to Transgress (hooks), 43

"Terminal hardening of the categories" malady, 136

Theater of the Oppressed, 42

Third World countries, 364

"Town criers" on AIDS (San Francisco), 181

Transgender community: CAB (community advisory board) made up from, 335–342; described, 333–334; project interviews with, 335. *See also* Vulnerable populations

Transgender Community Health Project: co-learning process during, 337–338; collaboration between San Francisco Health Department and, 340; empowering process during, 338–339; initiation and organization of, 335–337; participatory and cooperative nature of, 335–337; research and action balance during, 339–342; system development during, 338

Tuskegee study, 321

"Two languages of race," 90–91

Tyranny of decision making, 35

Tyranny of the group, 35

Tyranny of methods, 35

U

UNC Department of Epidemiology, 228

UNC News Service, 226

Unconscious racism, 91

UNC (University of North Carolina), 224. *See also* CHER (Community Health and Environmental Reawakening) partnership [North Carolina]

United Kingdom participatory health initiatives, 271–272

University of Kansas, 156

University of North Carolina's School of Public Health, 135

University of South Carolina, 367

University of Toledo Urban Affairs Center, 98

Urban Quality Indicators Newsletter Web site, 162

URC (Detroit Community-Academic Urban Research Center) partnership: Community Action Against Asthma, 61, 64, 66–67, 69, 70; East Side Village Health Worker Partnership, 61, 65, 66, 67; establishing the "community" in partnership, 60–61; establishing set of CBPR principles, 59; establishment of, 71n.1, 373–374; ongoing evaluation of CBPR principles implementation by, 70–71; procedures for CBPR principles by, 68; strategies to create collaborative/equitable, 62–63

U.S. Administration on Aging Web site, 163

U.S. Centers for Disease Control and Prevention's Evaluation Working Group, 162, 373

U.S. Department of Agriculture, 229

U.S. Department of Health and Human Services, 11, 163, 357

U.S. Environmental Protection Agency Web site, 163

U.S. Health Resources and Services Administration (HRSA) Web site, 162

V

Vacco v. Quill, 244

VHW (Village Health Worker): building mutual support, 304–306; differing agendas/priorities of, 307–309; discussion of findings on, 309–311; health concerns of, 302–303; limited resources/influence of, 303–304; mistrust of research by, 306–307; process of becoming, 299–301; time/multiple commitments of, 301–302. *See also* East Side Village Health Worker Partnership (ESVHWP)

Virginia Polytechnic University, 365

Virginia Tech, 357

Visioning processes, 146–147

Voluntary agreements, 356–357